Oxygen Transport:
Principles and Practice

Oxygen Transport: Principles and Practice

edited by

J.D. Edwards
Consultant Physician, Director,
Intensive Care Unit,
University Hospital of South Manchester, UK.

W.C. Shoemaker
Professor of Surgery,
Vice Chairman of Academic Affairs,
Martin Luther King Jr/Charles R. Drew Medical Center,
Los Angeles, USA.

J.-L. Vincent
Professor and Clinical Director,
Department of Intensive Care,
Hôpital Universitaire Erasme,
Brussels, Belgium.

W.B. Saunders Company Ltd
London · Philadelphia · Toronto
Sydney · Tokyo

W.B. Saunders 24–28 Oval Road
Company Ltd London NW1 7DX, UK
Baillière Tindall
The Curtis Center
Independence Square West
Philadelphia, PA 19106–3399, USA

55 Horner Avenue
Toronto, Ontario M8Z 4X6, Canada

Harcourt Brace & Company, Australia
(Australia) Pty Ltd
30–52 Smidmore Street
Marrickville, NSW 2204, Australia

Harcourt Brace & Company, Japan
Ichibancho Central Building,
22–1 Ichibancho
Chiyoda-ku, Tokyo 102, Japan

© 1993 W.B. Saunders Company Ltd

First published 1993
Second printing 1995

A catalogue record for this book is available from the
British Library

ISBN 0–7020–1576–8

This book is printed on acid-free paper

Typeset by Phoenix Photosetting, Chatham, Kent
Printed and bound in Great Britain at the
University Press, Cambridge

Contents

List of Contributors

E. Abraham
UCLA School of Medicine, Division of Pulmonary and Critical Care Medicine, 37–131 CHS, 10833 Le Conte Avenue, Los Angeles, California 90024–1690, USA

G.I.J.M. Beerthuizen
Martini-Hospital, Van Swietenlaan 4, Groningen, The Netherlands

J.E. Calvin
Department of Medicine, Section of Cardiology, RUSH-Presbyterian St, Luke's Medical Center, Room 1021 Jelke, 1653 West Congress Parkway, Chicago, Illinois 60612, USA

Aurel C. Cernaianu
University of Medicine and Dentistry of New Jersey, Robert Wood Johnson Medical School at Camden, 3 Cooper Plaza, Suite 411, Camden, New Jersey 08103, USA

Kevin M. Chan
UCLA School of Medicine, Division of Pulmonary and Critical Care Medicine, 37–131 CHS, 10833 Le Conte Avenue, Los Angeles, California 90024 1690, USA

Pierre-Georges Durand
Hôpital Cardiolgique L Pradel, BP Lyon-Montchat, 69394 Lyon Cedex 03, France

J. Denis Edwards
Intensive Care Unit, University Hospital of South Manchester, Nell Lane, Withington, Manchester M20 8LR, UK

R.J.A. Goris
Department of General Surgery, University Hospital Nijmegen, PO Box 9101, 6500 HB Nijmegen, The Netherlands

Guillermo Gutierrez
Pulmonary and Critical Care Medicine Division, University of Texas Health
Science Center, 6431 Fannin, Suite 1274, Houston, Texas 77030, USA

K.B. Hankeln
Department of Anesthesiology and Intensive Care Medicine, Zentralkran-
kenhaus Bremen Nord 2820, Bremen 70, Germany

M.T. Haupt
Medical Intensive Care Unit, Detroit Receiving Hospital, RM 55–10, School
of Medicine, 4201 St Antoine, Detroit, Michigan 48202, USA

U. Kreimeier
Institute for Anaesthesiology, Ludwig-Maximilian University Munich,
Klinikum Grosshadern, Marchioninistrasse 15, D-8000 Munich 70,
Germany

Iain McA. Ledingham
Department of Emergency and Critical Care Medicine, Faculty of Medicine
& Health Sciences, UAE University, Al Ain, United Arab Emirates

Jean-Jacques Lehot
Hôpital Cardiologique L Pradel, BP Lyon-Montchat, 69394 Lyon Cedex 03,
France

R.A. Little
North Western Injury Research Centre, University of Manchester, Stopford
Building, Oxford Road, Manchester M13 0PT, UK

K. Messmer
Institute for Surgical Research, Klinikum Grosshadern, University of
Munich, Marchioninistr 15, 8000 Munich 70, Germany

Mohamed Naguib
Department of Emergency and Critical Care Medicine, Faculty of Medicine
& Health Sciences, UAE University, Al Ain, United Arab Emirates

Loren D. Nelson
Vanderbilt University, 218 Medical Center, South Nashville, Tennessee
37232, USA

P. Nightingale
Department of Intensive Care, University Hospital of South Manchester,
Nell Lane, Withington, Manchester M20 8LR, UK

Luis Ortiz
Pulmonary and Critical Care Medicine Division, University of Texas Health
Science Center, 6431 Fannin, Suite 1274, Houston, Texas 77030, USA

Richard W. Samsel
Department of Medicine MC6026, 5841 South Maryland Avenue, Chicago,
Illinois 60637, USA

Paul T. Schumacker
Department of Medicine MC6026, 5841 South Maryland Avenue, Chicago,
Illinois 60637, USA

William C. Shoemaker
Department of Emergency Medicine and Surgery, King-Drew Medical
Center and UCLA School of Medicine, 12021 South Wilmington Avenue,
Los Angeles, California 90059, USA

R.J. Snell
Department of Medicine, Section of Cardiology, RUSH-Presbyterian St
Luke's Medical Center, Room 1021 Jelke, 1653 West Congress Parkway,
Chicago, Illinois 60612, USA

Jean-Louis Teboul
Intensive Care Unit, Hôpital de Bicêtre, 78 Rue de Général Leclerc, 94275 Le
Kremlin Bicêtre, Cedex, France

P. van der Linden
Service d'Anesthesiologie, Hôpital Universitaire Erasme, Route de Lennik
808, B-1070 Brussels, Belgium

Jean-Louis Vincent
Department of Intensive Care, Hôpital Universitaire Erasme, Route de
Lennik 808, B-1070 Brussels, Belgium

Preface

Shortly after oxygen was discovered by Priestley in 1774, Lavoisier demonstrated that it was essential for life in both plants and animals. Subsequently, the importance of the combustion of oxygen as the essential component of metabolic processes was recognized. Over the past century, measurement of the rate of oxygen consumption ($\dot{V}O_2$ has become an accepted standard to evaluate body metabolism. Oxygen is the most important substrate carried by the circulation and, compared to its rate of utilization, it has the lowest stores.

Having developed quite independently from biochemistry, circulatory physiology initially focused on pressure, flow and other haemodynamic parameters. After the invention of the sphygmomanometer by Roca Riva, blood pressure measurements dominated circulatory monitoring.

Circulatory physiology came of age after two major contributions, one theoretical and the other demonstrably practical. Barcroft in 1920 defined shock as three types of anoxia: stagnant (low cardiac output), anoxic (arterial hypoxaemia) and anaemic (reduced haemoglobin concentration). Shortly after their demonstration of cardiac catheterization, the Nobel laureates, Cournand, Richards and associates applied this technique to the investigation of traumatic shock. They calculated cardiac output by the direct Fick method by measuring oxygen contents of arterial and mixed venous blood concomitantly with $\dot{V}O_2$ from expired gas collected in Douglas bags. In this classical study of severely traumatized shock patients, they demonstrated low flow and hypovolaemia.

Despite the intellectually compelling nature of these early studies, it was not until Swan and his colleagues developed the balloon-tipped, flow-directed pulmonary artery (PA) catheter and the thermodilution method for cardiac output measurements that these concepts were routinely applied to critically ill patients. In essence, the major contribution by Swan and colleagues was that they moved the cardiac catheterization laboratory to the bedside of the critically ill patient. These cardiologists applied their method for cardiac output measurements to the classic Starling and Sarnoff myocardial performance curves. Based on cardiac index greater or less than $2.5 \, l min.m^2$ and pulmonary wedge pressures greater or less than 20 mmHg, tour clinical subsets were defined and appropriate therapy proposed.

This approach has since become accepted as the standard of care for patients following acute myocardial infarction. This therapeutic paradigm has not been tested for non-cardiac conditions. However, circulatory function cannot be confined only to cardiac contractility. The circulation is comprised of three major components: cardiac function, pulmonary function, and tissue perfusion. Cardiac performance can be measured precisely by, for instance, multiple-gated acquisition (MUGA) scans, echocardiography, myocardial performance curves and dP/dt measurements in addition to routine electrocardiographs, radiography, and cardiac enzymes. Similarly pulmonary function may be evaluated by technetium scanning, carbon monoxide diffusion, and nitrogen washout curves in addition to the standard arterial blood gases with estimates of extent of pulmonary venous admixture by such indices as PaO_2/FiO_2, PAO_2/PaO_2, $P(A-a)O_2$ and respiratory index. Sampling of mixed venous blood allows calculation of the shunt fraction. By contrast, tissue perfusion and tissue oxygenation has conventionally and routinely been evaluated by unreliable signs such as cold clammy skin, weak thready pulse, altered mental status, and other so-called vital signs. Now, however, global tissue oxygenation, may be evaluated objectively by the calculation of delivery of oxygen (DO_2) to the tissues and assessment of its adequacy by measurement of mixed venous oxyhaemoglobin saturation $S\bar{v}O_2$, blood lactate and calculation of oxygen extraction ratio (OER).

A fresh look at critical illness clearly reveals four aspects of the underlying circulatory impairment: First, that the major function of the circulation is to transport the necessary supply of oxygen and oxidative substrates, including glucose, amino acids, and fatty acids that are needed to support body metabolism. Second, oxygen delivery may be rate-limiting for body metabolism and vital organ function. Third, multiple organ failure, which is the most common cause of death in ICU patients, has an underlying antecedent circulatory impairment that can be described by DO_2 and VO_2 relationships. Finally the $\dot{D}O_2$, $\dot{V}O_2$ relationships provide the means to objectively evaluate the tissue perfusion component of circulatory function. The importance of this can not be over-emphasised since decreased tissue perfusion and tissue oxygenation characterised by inadequate $\dot{D}O_2$ are the major initiating events that set in motion the subsequent pathophysiologic complications of haemorrhagic, traumatic, postoperative, and septic shock. By contrast, normal tissue perfusion documented by an adequate $\dot{D}O_2$ and lower blood lactate levels was shown to be associated with improved survival.

These studies opened the way to more detailed investigations in other forms of cardiorespiratory failure, as determinants of outcome and logical goals of therapy, in various clinical circumstances. Because this approach is novel, controversial, and contrary to conventional wisdom (assuming the latter is not a contradiction in terms), the present monograph had aimed to bring together recent contributions by leaders in the field for the purpose of summarizing more rational and effective methods of therapy for critically ill patients.

J. Denis Edwards
William C. Shoemaker
Jean-Louis Vincent

Part One

Principles

1 Overview: Evolution of the Concept from Fick to the Present Day

Iain McA. Ledingham and Mohamed Naguib

'Let not my heart be taken from me, let it not be wounded, and may neither swords nor gashes be dealt upon me because it hath been taken from me.'
Anonymous author of the *Book of the Dead*

The concept of oxygen transport is one of central importance both to the physiologist and to the clinician. A firm grasp of the basic principles and current measurement techniques is of particular significance to those working in the field of emergency and critical care medicine. This overview will address the evolution of the concept from its early development more than a century ago to its present increasingly sophisticated role in the management of the critically ill patient.

One of the fascinating aspects of this story is the continually changing, dynamic interplay between theory and practice with, on the one hand, the emergence of a physiological principle often many years before appropriate technology (and therefore practical application), whilst on the other, technological advance facilitating understanding of pathophysiological mechanisms. Interwoven throughout this patchwork are the often disconnected threads of therapeutic empiricism.

Primary Concepts and Related Developments

In 1870, the German physiologist, Adolph Fick, demonstrated that by adding a substance to a column of biological flowing fluid, the rate of flow could be calculated. From this emerged one of the most celebrated principles in biology: *'During any interval of time, the amount of a substance entering a given compartment in the inflowing blood must be equal to the quantity of the substance being removed from the blood by the compartment plus the quantity of the substance leaving in the outflowing blood.'*

At about the same time a fellow countryman, Pflüger (1872) wrote: *'Arterial oxygen content, arterial pressures, velocity of blood stream, mode of cardiac work, mode of respiration are all incidental and subordinate; they all combine their actions only in service to the cells.'*

The main ingredients of oxygen transport and exchange in the body were thus identified at an early stage although it was many years before physiologists were able to capitalize on these observations in a practical sense and considerably longer before there was any apparent impact in the management of the acutely ill patient.

The Fick Principle

The Fick principle is really a statement of the conservation of matter and is valid whether the compartment involved is accumulating, metabolizing or excreting the marker substance from the bloodstream.

Consider the system illustrated in Fig. 1.1. H is the compartment supplied by an inflow of blood $\dot{V}$in containing the substance at a concentration of Cin,t. The outflow of blood is $\dot{V}$out with a concentration Cout,t. For simplicity, we shall assume that the system is removing the substance from the bloodstream.

Since by simple mathematical computation quantity equals volume multiplied by concentration, the quantity of the substance entering the compartment (H) in the inflowing blood is equal to $\dot{V}$ entering H multiplied by the concentration of the substance of the inflowing blood:

$$dQin/dt = \dot{Q}in = \dot{V}Cin,t \qquad (1.1)$$

Similarly, the quantity of the substance leaving H in the outflowing blood is:

$$dQout/dt = \dot{Q}out = \dot{V}Cout,t \qquad (1.2)$$

The quantity of the substance removed during passage through the compartment (H) is:

$$dQremoved/dt = \dot{Q}removed = V_H (dC_H/dt) \qquad (1.3)$$

Now the Fick principle states that during any interval of time

$$\dot{Q}in = \dot{Q}removed + \dot{Q}out \qquad (1.4)$$

Substituting in Eqn (1.4) the values given by Eqns (1.1)–(1.3)

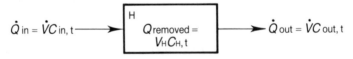

$$\dot{Q}in = \dot{V}Cin,t \longrightarrow \boxed{\begin{array}{c} H \\ Qremoved = \\ V_HC_H,t \end{array}} \longrightarrow \dot{Q}out = \dot{V}Cout,t$$

Figure 1.1   The meaning of the symbols depicted in this figure are as follows: $\dot{V}$ = volume per unit time; $\dot{Q}$ = quantity per unit time; Q = quantity, which equals volume (V) multiplied by concentration (C), i.e. $V \times C$. The subscript, t = at particular time, and is used to indicate the time-dependent variables. The compartment (H) is being washed by a column of fluid passing through it. Assume that the volume of the compartment (H) and the flows ($\dot{V}$) are constant, then the Fick principle requires that during any time interval (t) the quantity of the substance ($\dot{Q}$in) entering the compartment (H) be equal to the quantity of the substance leaving the compartment ($\dot{Q}$out) plus the quantity of the substance removed during passage through the compartment ($\dot{Q}$removed).

$$\dot{V}Cin,t = \dot{V}Cout,t + V_H(dC_H/dt) \tag{1.5}$$

rearrange

$$V_H (dC_H/dt) = \dot{V}(Cin,t - Cout,t) \tag{1.6}$$

It can be seen from Eqn (1.6) that pulmonary oxygen uptake (or expired carbon dioxide) could be related to cardiac output and arterial and mixed venous gas concentrations.

In the case of oxygen uptake, let the compartment be the entire body, let the substance be oxygen; the blood flow is assumed to be equal to cardiac output. The Fick principle becomes:

$$\dot{V}O_2 = \dot{Q} (CaO_2 - C\bar{v}O_2) \tag{1.7}$$

or

$$\dot{Q} = \dot{V}O_2/(CaO_2 - C\bar{v}O_2) \tag{1.8}$$

where $\dot{V}O_2$ is the total body oxygen consumption in millilitres O_2 per minute, $\dot{Q}$ is cardiac output in litres per minute and CaO_2 and $C\bar{v}O_2$ are, respectively, the arterial and mixed venous oxygen contents in millilitres of oxygen per 100 ml blood. Normally

$$\dot{Q} = 250 \text{ ml min}^{-1}/(200 - 150) \text{ ml min}^{-1} = 5.0 \text{ litres min}^{-1}$$

A similar formula applies to carbon dioxide production.

The 'Direct Fick Method'

Determination of cardiac output by this method required a measurement of oxygen uptake and arterial and mixed venous blood oxygen content. $\dot{V}O_2$ was determined by collecting the expired gas in a large bag (Douglas, 1911) or spirometer (Tissot, 1904) and measuring its oxygen concentration. Mixed venous blood was taken via a catheter in the pulmonary artery, and arterial blood by puncture of any peripheral artery (e.g. radial, femoral or brachial artery). The application of the Fick principle was therefore limited to steady-state cardiac output estimation.

Accurate and reliable techniques for measurement of oxygen in respiratory gases and blood were developed in the 1920s and remain the gold standards of accuracy (Haldane, 1920; Van Slyke & Neill, 1924) in healthy volunteers. Visscher and Johnson (1953) discussed the limiting factors of the Fick technique and pointed out the technical difficulties of maintaining a steady state in relation to measurements of oxygen and carbon dioxide production. In 1959, Guyton described a continuous cardiac output recorder employing the Fick principle for use in animals. This system was able to record dynamic changes in flow.

In the clinical setting, especially in critically ill patients, a non-steady-state condition exists. With the recent introduction of mass spectrometry and oximetry to clinical practice, continuous cardiac output in non-steady-state conditions can be determined using the Fick principle (Neuhof & Wolf, 1978; Davies *et al.*, 1987).

The 'Indirect Fick Method'

The Fick principle may also be used indirectly to measure blood flow. In methods based on the absorption of a foreign gas, e.g. krypton and xenon, during its passage through the lungs, if the solubility of the gas in the blood is known and its uptake is measured, blood flow can be calculated. A variation of the Fick approach is employed in indicator dilution methods using such markers as hypertonic saline, brilliant red and methylene blue.

After the problem of recirculation of the indicator had been resolved, the first measurement of cardiac output in man was reported by Hamilton and co-workers in 1932. A good correlation was shown to exist between the Fick and the dye dilution methods (Hamilton *et al.*, 1948). The indicator dilution method using indocyanine green dye has now been largely replaced by the thermodilution technique using a flow-directed pulmonary artery catheter which is positioned in the proximal branch of the pulmonary artery (Ganz *et al.*, 1971; Forrester *et al.*, 1972). Comparison of the Fick and thermodilution methods shows good correlation, although the Fick values are usually lower (Davies *et al.*, 1986).

New, non-invasive methods to measure cardiac output include aortic pulse-wave contour analysis (English *et al.*, 1980), thoracic electrical bio-impedance (Bernstein, 1986), laser Doppler velocimetry (Eyer *et al.*, 1987), and the transtracheal Doppler technique (Abrams *et al.*, 1989). However, large variabilities are observed in these methods, as compared with the thermodilution technique.

Use of the Fick Principle to Determine Oxygen Consumption

Equation (1.7) states that oxygen consumption is equal to cardiac output times the difference between arterial and mixed venous oxygen contents. From Eqn (1.8) it can be seen that, when $\dot{V}O_2$ is constant, the arterial–mixed venous oxygen content difference is reciprocally related to cardiac output. It follows that if $\dot{V}O_2$ is constant, extraction of oxygen from the blood must be increased at lower cardiac outputs. If we rearrange the Fick equation

$$C\bar{v}O_2 = CaO_2 - (\dot{V}O_2/\dot{Q}) \tag{1.9}$$

it can be seen that alteration of mixed venous oxygen content will follow any imbalance between oxygen supply and demand. Oxygen delivery ($\dot{D}O_2$) equals the arterial oxygen content (CaO_2) times cardiac output $\dot{Q}$):

$$\dot{D}O_2 = (CaO_2)\,(\dot{Q}) \tag{1.10}$$

The content of oxygen (CO_2) is expressed in millilitres of oxygen per decilitre of blood and is the sum of the oxygen bound to haemoglobin and that dissolved in plasma. The latter amount is very small since the solubility of oxygen in blood is only 0.003 ml O_2 per dl of blood per mm Hg PO_2. The amount of oxygen bound to haemoglobin is determined by the amount of haemoglobin present, the binding capacity of oxygen to haemoglobin and the partial pressure of oxygen (PO_2).

$$CO_2 = (Hb \times 1.38 \times SO_2) + (PO_2 \times 0.003) \tag{1.11}$$

where CO_2 = oxygen content (ml dl^{-1} blood); Hb = haemoglobin content (g dl^{-1} blood); SO_2 = oxygen saturation (%); and PO_2 = partial pressure of oxygen (mm Hg).

Normally, arterial oxygen content

$$CaO_2 = (15 \times 1.38 \times 1.00) + (100 \times 0.003)$$

$$= \quad 20.7 \quad + \quad 0.3 \quad = 21 \text{ ml } dl^{-1} \text{ blood}$$

If we ignore the dissolved oxygen content in Eqn (1.11), which is usually insignificant, and substitute for the oxygen contents of arterial and mixed venous blood in Eqn (1.9), then

$$S\bar{v}O_2 \times Hb \times 1.38 = (Hb \times 1.38 \times SaO_2) - (\dot{V}O_2/\dot{Q}) \tag{1.12}$$

This gives us

$$S\bar{v}O_2 = SaO_2 - (\dot{V}O_2/\dot{Q} \times Hb \times 1.38) \tag{1.13}$$

where $S\bar{v}O_2$ = mixed venous oxygen saturation and SaO_2 = arterial oxygen saturation.

Equation (1.13) indicates that $S\bar{v}O_2$ varies directly with $\dot{Q}$, Hb and SaO_2 and inversely with $\dot{V}O_2$ if both variables do not change. Mixed venous oxygen saturation ($S\bar{v}O_2$) can be measured continuously using oximeters incorporated into pulmonary artery catheters. The normal $S\bar{v}O_2$ is 75% ($P\bar{v}O_2 = 40$ mm Hg (5.3 kPa), which indicates that normal metabolic needs are met by extraction of 25% of delivered oxygen.

Reduction in Oxygen Delivery

Around the time the original techniques were being developed for measurement of respiratory and blood gas contents, Barcroft (1920) published his hypothesis on the classification of the 'anoxaemias'. His description of deficits in oxygen transport as hypoxic (reduced PaO_2), anaemic (reduced Hb) and stagnant (reduced blood flow or cardiac output) was based on reduced haemoglobin oxygen saturation, haemoglobin concentration and blood flow respectively. Following this, histotoxic hypoxia was perceived to reflect an inability of haemoglobin to unload oxygen to the tissues (Peters & Van Slyke, 1931).

The integral components of oxygen transport from the lung to the mitochondria are described with reference to the conventional oxygen cascade (Fig. 1.2). Clinical and laboratory experience has revealed that the body can tolerate a reduction of 50% in any of the three components of oxygen transport – oxygen saturation, haemoglobin concentration and blood flow (Crowell *et al.*, 1959); Gaston *et al.*, 1973). The general rule is that the reduction of a single component is followed by compensatory changes in the others to restore the normality and maintain adequate tissue oxygenation. If all three components decrease simultaneously, as may occur in critical illness, reductions of as little as 30% of each component may prove intolerable unless rapidly corrected (Freeman & Nunn, 1963).

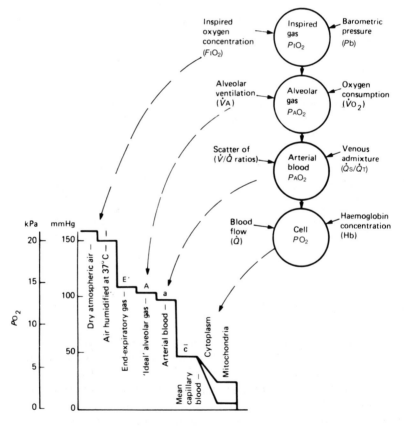

Figure 1.2 Oxygen cascade. (With permission from Nunn, 1989.)

Hypoxaemia

Hypoxaemia is defined as a relative deficiency of oxygen tension in arterial blood, a PaO_2 of less than 80 mm Hg (10.6 kPa). Although a PaO_2 between 80 and 95 mm Hg (10.7–12.6 kPa) cannot be considered 'normal' (other than in relation to the ageing process or high altitudes), it may not represent a direct threat to tissues (Shapiro, 1979). Arterial oxygen tensions between 60 and 80 mm Hg (8–10.7 kPa) have been described as 'mild hypoxaemia' and between 40 and 60 mm Hg (5.3–8 kPa) as 'moderate hypoxaemia'. Values less than 40 mm Hg (5.3 kPa) represent 'severe hypoxaemia'. At the latter values the oxygen pressure gradient between capillaries and mitochondria is diminished. A fall in $P\bar{v}O_2$ below 30 mm Hg (4 kPa) usually signifies tissue hypoxia. The stepwise deterioration in cerebral function in relation to progressive hypoxaemia is indicated in Table 1.1. One of the cardinal features of hypoxia is the cessation of oxidative phosphorylation when mitochondrial PO_2 falls below a critical level (less than 1 mm Hg (0.1 kPa)).

Adaptive responses mediated by the chemoreceptors may favour survival of the organism by diverting oxygen to organs such as the heart and brain at the expense of splanchnic organs and skeletal muscles.

Anaemia

Acute reduction in haemoglobin without reduction in blood volume may be associated with remarkably little change in oxygen transport because of the accompanying increase in cardiac output (Gruber *et al.*, 1976). Studies by Messmer and his colleagues (1973) confirmed that tissue oxygenation in a number of organs, including the liver, remains essentially unchanged with a reduction in haematocrit to 20%. On the other hand, chronic anaemia is not associated with a rise in cardiac output until the haemoglobin falls below 7 g dl^{-1}. More moderate degrees of anaemia are associated with elevation of 2,3-diphosphoglycerate and decrease in oxyhaemoglobin oxygen affinity.

Hypoperfusion – Low or Inadequate Cardiac Output

The Second World War proved a major stimulus to investigation of the pathophysiological disturbances of shock. From the many laboratory studies performed during the 1940s and 1950s (Wiggers, 1942; Frank & Fine, 1943) reduced or inadequate circulating blood volume emerged as a common feature of most types of shock. In the case of a haemorrhagic shock a reduction in total body oxygen consumption was observed and an apparent relationship established between the magnitude of oxygen debt, first enunciated by Hill in 1931, and irreversibility of the shock process (Crowell & Smith, 1964). The concept of target organs to account for irreversibility became popular and the heart (Guyton & Crowell, 1961) and adrenal

Table 1.1 Effects of hypoxic cerebral hypoxia

Arterial PO_2	Biochemical change in brain	Physiological change
50 mm Hg (6.7 kPa)	Glycolysis starts with production of lactate Phosphocreatine and ATP still normal Serotonin, noradrenaline, dopamine and acetylcholine levels fall	Cerebral blood flow increases Minor changes in the EEG Memory impairment on testing
35 mm Hg (4.7 kPa)	Glycolysis pronounced Phosphocreatine levels fall but ATP still normal	EEG clearly abnormal Judgement and behaviour impaired
20 mm Hg (2.7 kPa)	ATP levels fall Brain lipid metabolism impaired	EEG slowing (1–2 Hz) or absence of activity Coma (response only to pain)
< 5 mm Hg (0.7 kPa)	Mitochondria cease function, cell damage (cerebellum, cerebral cortex and hippocampus)	Death from cardiovascular failure

With permission from Davidson *et al.*, 1988.

gland were considered frontrunners for this role. While the target organ concept was constantly challenged a marked difference in the vulnerability of the organs of the body to low flow states was undeniable. Later it was possible to attribute some of the observed changes to reflex neurogenic mechanisms, to the release into the circulation of a range of vasoactive substances and to the phenomenon of autoregulation.

Much of this important basic experimental work had no apparent immediate clinical impact. Apart from insufficient awareness of the published evidence and uncertainty about the applicability of the laboratory data to the shocked patient there was, of course, the problem of lack of appropriate convenient technology. As a result of the latter a series of indirect measurements including the so-called 'vital signs', peripheral skin temperature, urine output, and occasionally blood volume and arterial lactate were used to gauge the severity of the shock state. This combination of factors led to a preoccupation in the clinical situation with hypotension rather than hypoperfusion and to the development of therapeutic regimens to restore arterial blood pressure and the other vital signs to within the normal range. Vasopressor agents were widely used to elevate arterial diastolic pressure with the aim of improving coronary perfusion (Weil, 1955).

The next major step in an understanding of the pathophysiology of shock was human cardiac catheterization, and an annotation in the *British Medical Journal* of 1944 attests to the major contribution made by the pioneers in this field:

> the techniques of study developed by Cournand and his colleagues (1943) show the way in which these problems (viz, the treatment of shock) may be approached; their bold, brilliant and apparently safe technique of intra-cardiac catheterization seems to open a new era in the research study of human cardio-dynamics.

The basis of the modern approach to treatment of shock can be traced to the introduction of the bedside technique of flow-directed pulmonary artery catheterization (Ganz et al., 1971; Swan & Ganz, 1975) which transformed the management of the shocked patient and transplanted much of the laboratory expertise into the emergency and operating rooms and the intensive care unit.

The concept of oxygen availability and the importance of its relationship to tissue oxygen consumption gathered practical momentum in the early 1960s when investigators such as Fine and Gelin defined shock as '*a poly-etiologic syndrome characterized by a decrease in tissular blood flow below a certain critical level necessary for the normal display of the obligate metabolic processes*' (see Suteu et al., 1977).

Thus the concept of oxygen transport and availability of oxygen is by no means new. The novel concept is that it can, with motivation, be applied at the bedside in critically ill patients and be applied to the management of their shock.

Increase in Oxygen Availability

Increased oxygen transport may be achieved by augmenting any of its three components – oxygen concentration, haemoglobin concentration and blood flow (or any combination of the three). Since the ultimate object of the exercise is to restore normal cellular oxygenation, the optimum method of increasing oxygen transport depends on the underlying pathophysiological disturbance.

Oxygen therapy has been used for more than a century (Haldane, 1917) and the classical indications for increasing inspired oxygen concentration include ventilatory failure and pulmonary shunting. The range of concentrations vary as indicated from 30 to 100%, the precise value influenced in part by factors other than optimization of tissue oxygenation, e.g. avoidance of hypercapnia. Alveolar oxygen stores can be substantially increased by oxygen administration and the period of safe respiratory arrest may thereby be increased fourfold. The role of oxygen therapy in anaemia and ischaemia is much less clear, the clinical benefits appearing to be marginal. Attempts to improve the situation using hyperbaric oxygen in the treatment of hypoperfusion and to prolong the period of safe circulatory arrest have met with only limited success (Ledingham *et al.*, 1971). Even in the presence of tissue hypoxia the vasoconstrictive effect of hyperoxia is manifest, thus counteracting the raised transmural PO_2 gradient. The vasoconstrictive action can be overcome by pharmacological means (Schraibman & Ledingham, 1969), the spectre of oxygen toxicity looms large. Experimental and clinical evidence indicates a well-marked threshold for sensitivity to oxygen around 450 mm Hg (60 kPa) and the more prolonged the exposure the greater the risk.

The concept of 'optimum haematocrit' has been debated for many years. Laboratory studies demonstrated that capillary red cell flow is optimized at an haematocrit of around 30% (Klitzman & Dulin, 1979). In a recent clinical investigation, volume-repleted critically ill patients given packed red cells to raise haemoglobin to 10.5 g dl^{-1} showed no improvement in haemodynamic, metabolic or biochemical markers of tissue hypoxia (Dietrich *et al.*, 1990). While this effect may be modified by the degree of dysfunction of tissue oxygen exchange, current evidence would suggest that volume-resuscitated patients with haemoglobin concentrations of less than 7 g dl^{-1} should be transfused. Transfusion above that level should be considered on individual merit based upon the patient's cardiopulmonary reserve and tissue oxygen consumption (Cane, 1990).

Over the years, alternative methods of increasing oxygen carriage, bypassing the haemoglobin mechanism, have been explored. Perfluorochemical (PFC) emulsions are chemically and pharmacologically inert liquids that dissolve oxygen in very large quantities. They also dissolve carbon dioxide in quantities approximately four times those of oxygen. Since neither gas is attracted to fluorocarbons *per se*, it is assumed that the gas molecules are lodged in the spaces between the fluorocarbon molecules (Clark, 1985). On addition of PFC emulsions to whole blood, oxygen is therefore carried by three mechanisms, namely haemoglobin, PFC and plasma. Rosen *et al.* (1985) reported that the oxygen contact curve of Fluosol-DA (20%) – a PFC emulsion – obeyed Henry's law and that the extrapolated increase in oxygen content at a PO_2 of 760 mm Hg (101 kPa) and at 37°C was 5.6 ml dl^{-1}.

Increase in cardiac output is usually considered in conjunction with the other components of oxygen transport. Optimization of total oxygen delivery (Fig. 1.3) is normally achieved using a combination of intravenous fluids and increased oxygen concentration. Further sophistication of this process involves improving microvascular flow, pulmonary ventilation/perfusion ratios and individual organ perfusion. Finally, judicious control of factors leading to increased oxygen consumption (e.g. pain and fever) is important.

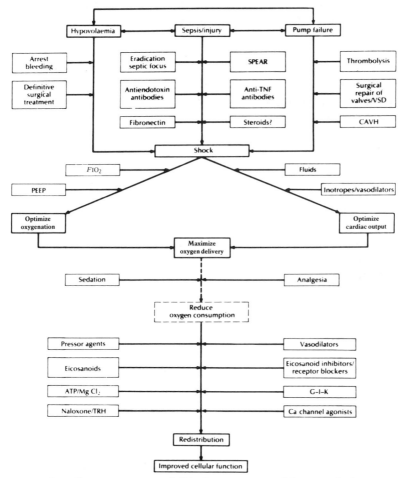

Figure 1.3 Specific treatment modelitis in treatment of hypoperfusion states of various aetiology. (With permission from Ledingham & Wright, 1990.)

Cardiac output is increased in the first instance by adjusting intravascular volume such that end-diastolic volume (i.e. preload) is optimal; the use of inotropic and/or vasodilator drugs may be indicated in the event of a poor response to the use of fluids alone. Many shocked patients manifest hypoxaemia of varying degree and multifactorial aetiology. Rapid correction of disturbed pulmonary gas exchange is an important component of primary care, normally involving the use of mechanical ventilation and augmented inspired oxygen. Judicious use of positive end-expiratory pressure may improve gas exchange by increasing alveolar volume but possible adverse effects include hepatorenal dysfunction and pulmonary barotrauma. Recent attention has been directed to improving regional blood flow using a variety of pharmacological agents but this development is still in its infancy and its effectiveness remains to be established (Ledingham & Wright, 1990). Even more embryonic are those therapies aimed at protecting or improving cellular function (Chernow & Roth, 1986).

The standard approach to the treatment of hypoperfusion outlined above is undoubtedly logical, but restoration of normal haemodynamic and respiratory values does not consistently lead to clinical recovery (Shoemaker et al., 1973). In traumatic and septic shock, for example, improved oxygen consumption and survival appear to be associated with a hyperdynamic circulatory response to resuscitation (Shoemaker et al., 1983), an observation in keeping with the delivery-dependent oxygen consumption phenomenon. Clinical trials involving the achievement of supranormal physiological values have been associated with improved clinical outcome (Shoemaker et al., 1988; Tuchschmidt et al., 1991).

While the first priority in the treatment of hypoperfusion is augmentation of oxygen delivery, interventions that decrease oxygen demand are occasionally appropriate. Analgesic and sedative drugs are not only relevant for the relief of pain and distress but may well beneficially reduce total body oxygen consumption (Wallace et al., 1988). Likewise, mechanical ventilation is used primarily to improve pulmonary gas exchange but additional benefit may accrue from reducing the oxygen demands of the increased work of breathing commonly seen in, for example, septic patients. Finally, while decreased body temperature is associated with a lowered metabolic rate (if shivering is prevented), induced hypothermia has not been shown to be of value in the clinical setting. Nevertheless avoidance of sustained extreme elevations of core temperature (more than 40°C) is rational.

Future Developments

The monitoring devices of the future should enable us to assess accurately, in a non-invasive fashion, the dynamic changes in physiological and biochemical functions of the cell. Several new techniques and methods have considerable potential for future developments for clinical application in the critically ill patient. Nuclear magnetic resonance (NMR) spectroscopy and especially ^{31}P-NMR spectroscopy has been used to evaluate myocardial energy metabolism under different conditions both *in vitro* (Lewandowski *et al.*, 1987) and *in vivo* (Bottomley, 1985). This technique permits the non-invasive measurements of free cytosolic phosphorus-containing compounds such as ATP, inorganic phosphate (P_i) and phosphocreatine (PCr), as well as intracellular pH. During hypoxia the ATP and PCr levels are decreased with a parallel increase in P_i (Bailey *et al.*, 1981). In addition *in situ* enzyme function, glycogen metabolism and changes in intracellular sodium content can be assessed by different NMR spectroscopy techniques.

The use of positron-emitting isotopes of carbon, oxygen, nitrogen and fluorine permit quantification of changes in cellular metabolism during hypoxia in individual organs (Phelps & Mazziotta, 1985). Recently, it has been possible to look at the state of reduction of cytochrome-a,a_3 through the skin by using near-infrared (NIR) radiation. This non-invasive technique has the potential for measuring changes in tissue oxygenation (Wharton & Tzagoloff, 1964). NIR optical spectroscopy has been employed in patients for continuous monitoring of regional cerebral oxygen saturation and intermittent monitoring of regional cerebral transit time (McCormick *et al.*, 1991). Simultaneous use of NMR and NIR spectroscopy in animal models of cerebral hypoxia demonstrates the ability of the latter technique to detect hypoxia earlier than NMR spectroscopy (Tamaura *et al.*, 1988).

These examples of advanced technology, recently introduced into the clinical setting, raise the hope that the present gulf between global haemodynamic and respiratory measurements and organ cellular function will in due course be bridged. The probable payoff is that early detection and correction of regional oxygen exchange disturbances will lead to a reduction both in early mortality and in the frequency of multiple organ failure (Cerra, 1991). Amongst the several potentially exciting possibilities in goal-directed optimization of cellular function are more selective opiate antagonists and thyrotropin-releasing hormone, ATP/MgCl$_2$ and calcium antagonists which bypass the adrenergic receptor (Chernow & Roth, 1986). Complementary manoeuvres aimed at improving microcirculatory function include the use of drugs with intravascular effects, e.g. pentoxifylline (Waxman, 1990) haemodilution techniques and small-volume resuscitation by means of hypertonic saline-dextran infusions (Holcroft *et al.*, 1987; Kreimeier *et al.*, 1991).

Clinical experience indicates that oxygen transport disturbances are usually part of a multifactorial homeostatic insult, with trauma and sepsis being frequent concomitant phenomena. Hypoxia itself may set the scene for additional injury, e.g. gut mucosal disruption leading to bacterial translocation and endotoxaemia, thereby initiating the cascade of mediator and cytokine release. Furthermore, the presence of pre-existing organ dysfunction may render the patient selectively vulnerable. New therapeutic strategy is being developed to address these problems.

However, even when hypoxia has been relieved, all may not be well. Post-hypoxic cellular injury is now an acknowledged complication of resuscitation attributable to the production of large quantities of superoxide radical and hydrogen peroxide and leading to histologically demonstrable cell damage (Granger *et al.*, 1986).

The therapeutic implications of these observations remain to be determined but optimization of oxygen transport, whilst attractive in the light of present laboratory and clinical evidence, will clearly require constant review as further information on possible adverse cellular effects comes to hand. Of particular interest is the recent finding that acidosis and lactate appear to have a protective effect on post-hypoxic cellular injury (Kowalski *et al.*, 1990).

Summary

The past 100 years have witnessed a stepwise progressive improvement in understanding of the pathophysiological disturbances that can occur in the process of oxygen transport. Intermittent spectacular technological achievements have accelerated the rate of progress. Therapeutic advances have been particularly impressive during recent decades. Nevertheless, the loop remains to be closed in terms of demonstrable optimization of tissue oxygen delivery. Once achieved, the essential validity of the pronouncements of the several distinguished physiologists, including Adolph Fick, who wrote the early chapters of this story more than 100 years ago, will have been confirmed.

This brief introductory overview does scant justice to a very broad and rapidly expanding area of medical knowledge. The following chapters will help to provide more substance to the topics covered in the chapter as well as dealing with a number of additional issues of interest to both the medical scientist and the clinician.

References

Abrams JH, Weber RE & Holmen KD (1989) Transtracheal Doppler: a new method of continuous cardiac output measurement. *Anaesthesiology* **70:** 134–8.
Annotation (1944) Heat in the treatment of shock. *Br. Med. J.* **1:** 49–50.
Bailey IA, Seymour A-M & Radda GK (1981) A ^{31}P nuclear magnetic resonance study of the effects of reflow on the ischemic rat heart. *Biochim. Biophys. Acta* **637:** 1–7.

Barcroft J (1920) On anoxaemia. *Lancet* **ii:** 485–9.

Bernstein DP (1986) Continuous non-invasive real-time monitoring of stroke volume and cardiac output by thoracic electrical bioimpedance. *Crit. Care Med.* **14:** 898–901.

Bihari DJ (1987) Mismatch of the oxygen supply and demand in septic shock. In Vincent JL & Thijs LG (eds) *Update in Intensive Care and Emergency Medicine*, pp 148–60. Berlin: Springer-Verlag.

Bottomley PA (1985) Noninvasive study of high energy phosphate metabolism in human heart by depth resolved 31-P NMR spectroscopy. *Science* **229:** 769–72.

Cane RD (1990) Hemoglobin: How much is enough? *Crit. Care Med.* **18:** 1046.

Cerra FB (1991) Multiple organ failure: Is it only hypoxia? In Gutierrez G & Vincent JL (eds), *Update in Intensive Care and Emergency Medicine (12) Tissue Oxygen Utilization*, pp. 242–51. Berlin: Springer-Verlag.

Chernow B & Roth BL (1986) Pharmacologic manipulation of the peripheral vasculative in shock, clinical and experimental approaches. *Circ. Shock* **18:** 141–55.

Clark Jr LC (1985) Introduction to fluorocarbon. *Int. Anesth. Clin.* **23:** 1–9.

Cournand A, Riley RL, Bradley SE *et al.* (1943) Studies of circulation in clinical shock. *Surgery* **13:** 964–95.

Crowell JW & Smith EE (1964) Oxygen deficiency and irreversible hemorrhagic shock. *Am. J. Physiol. Rev.* **206:** 313.

Crowell JW, Ford RG & Lewis VM (1959) Oxygen transport in hemorrhagic shock as a function of the hematocrit ratio. *Am J. Physiol.* **196:** 1033.

Davidson JF, Douglas AS & Erskine JG (1988) Central nervous system. In Ledingham IMcA & Mackay C (eds), *Jamieson & Kay's Textbook of Surgical Physiology*, pp. 219–35. London: Churchill-Livingstone.

Davies G, Jebson P & Hess D (1986) Continuous Fick cardiac output compared to thermodilution. *Crit. Care Med.* **14:** 881–5.

Davies G, Hess D & Jebson P (1987) Continuous Fick cardiac output compared to continuous pulmonary artery electromagnetic flow measurement in pigs. *Anesthesiology* **66:** 805–9.

Dietrich KA, Conrad SA, Hebert CA *et al.* (1990) Cardiovascular and metabolic response to red blood cell transfusion in critically ill volume-resuscitated nonsurgical patients. *Crit. Care Med.* **18:** 940–4.

Douglas CG (1911) A method of determining the total respiratory exchange. *J. Physiol.* **42:** 17.

English JB, Hodges MR, Sentker C *et al.* (1980) Comparison of aortic pulse-wave contour analysis and thermodilution methods of measuring cardiac output during anesthesia in the dog. *Anesthesiology* **52:** 56–61.

Eyer S, Borgos J & Strate RG (1987) Laser Doppler flowmetry and cardiac output in critically ill surgical patients. *Crit. Care Med.* **15:** 778–9.

Fick A (1870) Uber die Messung des Blutquantums in den Herzventriklen. Reprinted and translated in Hoff HE & Scott HJ (1948) Physiology. *New Engl. J. Med.* **239:** 120–6.

Forrester JS, Ganz W, Diamond G *et al.* (1972) Thermodilution cardiac output determination with a single flow directed catheter. *Am. Heart J.* **83:** 306–11.

Frank HA & Fine J (1943) Traumatic shock: A study of the effect of oxygen on hemorrhagic shock. *J. Clin. Invest.* **22:** 205.

Freeman J & Nunn JF (1963) Ventilation-perfusion relationships after haemorrhage. *Clin. Sci.* **24:** 135–47.

Ganz W, Donoso R, Marcus HS *et al.* (1971) A new technique for measurement of cardiac output by thermodilution in man. *Am. J. Cardiol.* **27:** 392–6.

Gaston C, Rodriquez JA, Dzindzio B *et al.* (1973) Effect of acute isovolemic anemia on cardial output and estimated hepatic blood flow in the conscious dog. *Circ. Res.* **32:** 530.

Granger DN, Hollwarth ME & Park DA (1986) Ischaemia-reperfusion injury: Role of oxygen-derived free radicals. *Acta Physiol. Scand.* (Suppl.) **548:** 47–63.

Gruber UF, Sturm V & Messmer K (1976) Fluid replacement in shock. In Ledingham IMcA (ed.), *Monographs in Anaesthesiology*, Vol. 4, p. 231. Amsterdam: Excerpta Medica America, Elsevier.

Guierrez G & Pohil RJ (1986) Oxygenation consumption is linearly related to oxygen supply in critically ill patients. *J. Crit. Care* **1:** 45.

Guyton AC (1959) A continuous cardiac output recorder employing the Fick principle. *Circ. Res.* **7:** 661.

Guyton AC & Crowell JM (1961) Dynamics of the heart in shock. *Fedn. Proc.* **20**(Suppl. 9): 51–60.

Haldane JS (1917) The therapeutic administration of oxygen. *Br. Med. J.* **1:** 181–3.

Haldane JS (1920) *Methods of Air Analysis* (3rd edition). London: Griffin.

Hamilton WF, Moore JW, Kinsman JM *et al.* (1932) Studies on the circulation. IV. Further analysis of the injection method, and changes in hemodynamics under physiological and pathological condition. *Am. J. Physiol.* **99:** 534.

Hamilton WF, Riley RL, Attyah AM *et al.* (1948) Comparison of the Fick and dye injection methods of measuring the cardiac output in man. *Am. J. Physiol.* **153:** 309–21.

Hill AV (1931) *Adventures in Biophysics*. Pennsylvania: University of Pennsylvania Press.

Holcroft JW, Vassar MJ, Turner JE *et al.* (1987) 3% NaCl and 7.5% NaCl/ dextran 70 in the resuscitation of severely injured patients. *Ann. Surg.* **206:** 279–88.

Klitzman BM & Dulin BR (1979) Microvascular hematocrit and red cell flow in resting and contracting striated muscle. *Am. J. Physiol.* **237:** H481.

Kowalski DP, Aw TY & Jones DP (1990) Lactate protects against oxidative injury in post-anoxic hepatocytes. *Fed. Am. Soc. Exp. Biol. J* **4:** A898.

Kreimeier E, Frey L, Dentz J *et al.* (1991) Hypertonic saline dextran resuscitation during the initial phase of acute endotoxemia: Effect on regional blood flow. *Crit. Care Med.* **19:** 801–9.

Ledingham IMcA & Wright I (1990) Shock. In Cohen RD, Lewis B, Alberti KGMM & Denham AM (eds), *The Metabolic and Molecular Basis of Acquired Disease*, pp. 718–41. London: Ballière Tindall.

Ledingham IMcA, Parratt JR, Smith G *et al.* (1971) Haemodynamic and myocardial effects of hyperbaric oxygen in dogs subjected to haemorrhage. *Cardiovasc. Res.* **5**: 277–85.

Lewandowski ED, Devous MD & Nunnally RL (1987) High energy phosphates and function in isolated working rabbit hearts. *Am. J. Physiol.* **253**: H1215–23.

McCormick PW, Stewart M, Goetting *et al.* (1991) Noninvasive cerebral optical spectroscopy for monitoring cerebral oxygen delivery and hemodynamics. *Crit. Care Med.* **19**: 89–97.

Messmer K, Sunder-Plassmann L, Jesch F *et al.* (1973) Oxygen supply to the tissues during limited normovolemic hemodilution. *Res. Exp. Med.* **159**: 152–66.

Neuhoff H & Wolf H (1978) Method for continuously measured oxygen consumption and cardiac output for use in critically ill patients. *Crit. Care Med.* **6**: 155–61.

Nunn JF (1989) Effects of anaesthesia on respiration. In Nunn JF, Utting JE & Brown Jr (eds), *General Anaesthesia*, pp. 185–209. London: Butterworths.

Peters JP & Van Slyke DD (1931) *Quantitative Clinical Chemistry*, p. 579. Baltimore: Williams & Wilkins Co.

Pflüger E (1872) Uber die Diffusion des Sauerstoffs, den Ord und die grenze der Oxydationsprozesse im thierischen organismus. *Pflüger's Arch. Gesamte Physiologie Menschen Thiere* **6**: 43–64.

Phelps ME & Mazziotta JC (1985) Positron emisson tomography: Human brain function and biochemistry. *Science* **228**: 799–809.

Reinhart K (1989) Oxygen transport and tissue oxygenation in sepsis and septic shock. In Reinhart K & Eyrick K (eds), *Sepsis – An Interdisciplinary Challenge*, pp. 125–39. Berlin: Springer.

Rosen AL, Sehgal LR, Gould S *et al.* (1985). Transport of oxygen by perfluorochemical emulsion. *Int. Anesth. Clin.* **23**: 95–103.

Schraibman IG & Ledingham IMcA (1969) Hyperbaric oxygen and regional vasodilation in pedal ischemia. *Surg. Gynecol. Obstet.* **129**: 761–7.

Shapiro BA (1979) Oxygenation; measurement and clinical assessment. *ASA Refresher Courses Anesth.* **7**: 189–202.

Shoemaker WC, Montgomery ES, Kaplan E *et al.* (1973) Physiologic patterns in surviving and non-surviving shock patients. *Arch. Surg.* **106**: 630–6.

Shoemaker WC, Appel P & Bland R (1983) Use of physiologic monitoring to predict outcome and to assist in clinical decisions in critical ill postoperative patients. *Am. J. Surg.* **146**: 43–50.

Shoemaker WC, Appel PL, Kram HB *et al.* (1988) Prospective trial of supranormal values of survivors as therapeutic goals in high-risk surgical patients. *Chest* **94**: 1176–86.

Suteu I, Bandila T, Cafrita A *et al.* (1977) *Shock: Pathology, Metabolism, Shock Cell, Treatment*, p. 17. Abacus: Tunbridge Wells.

Swan HJC & Ganz W (1975) Use of balloon flotation catheters in critically ill patients. *Surg. Clin. North Am.* **55**: 501–9.

Tamaura M, Hazeki O, Nioka S *et al.* (1988) The simultaneous measurements of tissue oxygen concentration and energy state by near infrared and nuclear magnetic resonance spectroscopy. *Adv. Exp. Med. Biol.* **222**: 359–63.

Tissot J (1904) Nouvelle methode de mesure et d'inscription du debit et des mouvements respiratoires de l'homme et des animaux. *J. Physiol.* **6:** 688.

Tuchschmidt J, Fried J, Astiz M *et al.* (1991) Supranormal oxygen delivery improves mortality in septic shock patients. *Crit. Care Med.* **19:** S66.

Van Slyke DD & Neill JM (1924) The determination of gases in blood and other solutions by vacuum extraction and manometric measurements. *J. Biol. Chem.* **61:** 523.

Visscher MB & Johnson JA (1953) The Fick principle: Analysis of potential errors in its conventional application. *J. Appl. Physiol.* **5:** 635–40.

Wallace PGM, Bion JF & Ledingham IMcA (1988), The changing face of sedative practice. In Ledingham IMcA (ed.), *Recent Advances in Critical Care Medicine*, No. 3, pp. 69–94. Edinburgh: Churchill Livingstone.

Waxman K (1990) Pentoxifylline in septic shock. *Crit. Care Med.* **18:** 243–4.

Weil MH (1955) Clinical studies on a vasopressor agent: metaraminol (aramine) II observations on its use in the management of shock. *Am. J. Med. Sci.* **230:** 357–69.

Wharton DC & Tzagoloff A (1964) Studies on the electron transfer system. LVII: The near infrared absorption band of cytochrome oxidase. *J. Biol. Chem.* **239:** 2036–41.

Wiggers CJ (1942) Present status of shock problem. *Physiol. Rev.* **22:** 74.

2 Applied Physiology

Roderick A. Little and J. Denis Edwards

Oxygen enables the energy contained in food to be converted into a form which can be used to maintain higher forms of life. Ingested carbohydrates, fats and proteins are oxidized and a proportion of the free energy released is then transformed, for controlled release, in adenosine triphosphate (ATP). As discussed below, one molecule of glucose yields on complete intracellular oxidation 38 molecules of ATP. The unique property of ATP resides in two 'high-energy' phosphate bonds which, on hydrolysis, release free energy. Such hydrolysis releases 12 kcal (1 kcal = 4.2 kJ) per mole of ATP; thus the oxidation of 1 mole of glucose will generate 456 kcal. This contrasts with the 686 kcal released by total combustion in oxygen and represents an efficiency of *in vivo* energy transfer of 66% (the 'lost' 34% is dissipated as heat).

As the ATP–ADP cycle is fundamental to the integrity of life, a more detailed discussion of ATP formation is warranted. Glucose, absorbed from the gut or derived within the liver from other carbohydrates, enters cells by a process of facilitated or carrier-mediated diffusion which, with the exception of liver and brain cells, is enhanced by insulin. Once in a cell the glucose is converted to glucose-6-phosphate and then can be used immediately for the release of energy or stored as glycogen. The release of energy (generation of ATP) is accomplished by the formation of pyruvic acid from the glucose (glycolysis) and its subsequent oxidation in the citric or tricarboxylic acid (TCA) cycle (Fig. 2.1). Glycolysis involves a sequence of ten reactions which occurs within the cytosol and ends in the formation of two molecules of pyruvate from one molecule of glucose with the net gain of two molecules of ATP. There is also a release of hydrogen atoms which combine with nicotinamide adenine dinucleotide (NAD^+) to form NADH and free hydrogen ions.

The next step in the generation of energy from glucose is the transport of pyruvate into the mitochondrial matrix and its combination with a co-enzyme A to form acetyl CoA, carbon dioxide and further hydrogen atoms. The acetyl CoA then condenses with oxaloacetate to form citric acid at the start of the TCA cycle. The nine stages in this cycle end with the regeneration of oxaloacetate and the production of two further molecules of ATP and 16 hydrogen atoms. Up to this point, only four molecules of ATP have been generated and it is the oxidation of the large amounts of hydrogen formed that will form the other 34 molecules of ATP. The oxidation of hydrogen is accomplished within the mitochondria by a complex process known as

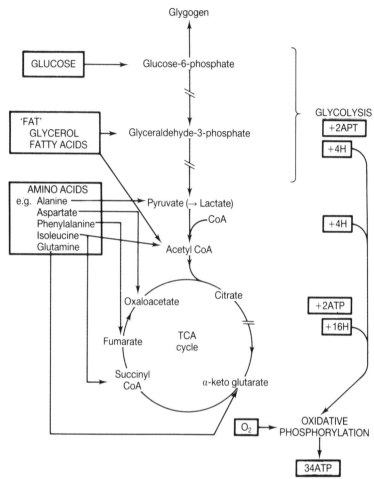

Figure 2.1 Schematic showing glycolytic pathway and tricarboxylic acid cycle by which substrates (carbohydrate, fat and protein) are converted into energy (ATP).

oxidative phosphorylation in which the electron transport chain situated on the inner mitochondrial membranes plays a key role. The final component in this chain is cytochrome oxidase which transfers electrons to oxygen to form water. It is the flux of electrons through the electron transport chain and the associated movements of protons across the inner mitochondrial membrane that drives ATP synthesis.

In the absence of oxygen there is no regeneration of NAD^+, with the result that the TCA cycle and oxidative phosphorylation stop and pyruvate is converted to lactate. A small amount of energy can, however, still be released by glycolysis but such anaerobic glycolysis is very wasteful as only two ATP molecules (24 kcal) are released per molecule of glucose (686 kcal), an efficiency of 3.5%. Thus very large amounts of glucose are needed to sustain energy production under anaerobic conditions and only those organs with substantial stores of glycogen (e.g. skeletal muscle) can do so. The brain, which has no such stores, is very susceptible to lack of oxygen and the subsequent production of lactate (for review see Nunn, 1987). The extent of anaerobic glycolysis can be quantified in terms of 'oxygen debt'. This is the extra O_2 consumption required to replenish O_2 stores (e.g. in myoglobin) and high-energy phosphate stores and dispose of the accumulated lactate once the imbalance between O_2 supply and demand has been corrected. The magnitude of this 'oxygen debt' has been directly related to the severity of shock and mortality in clinical and experimental studies (Crowell & Smith, 1964; Shoemaker et al., 1988).

The other energy substrates, fat and protein, are also oxidized through the TCA cycle. Fat or triacylglycerol is first oxidized to fatty acids and glycerol. The glycerol is converted to glyceraldehyde-3-phosphate which is an intermediate in the glycolytic pathway. The fatty acids are transported into the mitochondria where, by β-oxidation, they are degraded to acetyl CoA which enters the TCA cycle. If the supply of oxaloactetate is limited the acetyl CoA may condense to form ketone bodies (acetoacetate and β-hydroxybutyrate) which are themselves used as energy sources (e.g. by cardiac muscle). Amino acids can also be used as a source of energy. The degradation of amino acids by aminotransferases occurs mainly in liver and involves the removal of α-amino groups and the conversion of the remaining carbon skeleton into intermediates in the glycolytic chain or TCA cycle (Fig. 2.1).

It is clear that oxygen is vital for oxidative phosphorylation and the generation of ATP, but at what level does aerobic metabolism become compromised? The consensus is that the critical level of mitochondrial PO_2 is in the range 1–2 mm Hg (0.1–0.3 kPa), although the exact figure may vary between tissues (Nunn, 1987). Such values are only some 1% of the partial pressure of oxygen in the atmosphere and the maintenance and manipulation of this gradient from air to mitochondrion (the oxygen cascade) will now be discussed (Fig. 2.2).

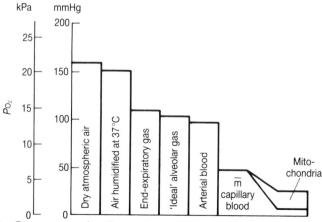

Figure 2.2 Oxygen cascade. (From Nunn, 1987.)

Inspired and Alveolar Gas

The fractional concentration of oxygen (FIO_2) in air is 0.2093 with a partial pressure (PO_2) in the dry gas phase of 158 mm Hg (21 kPa). However, air in the airways and alveoli is saturated with water vapour at 37°C and as total pressure remains unaltered the effective inspired partial pressure (PIO_2) exerted by oxygen will be reduced. Thus:

PIO_2 = FIO_2 − (barometric pressure − saturated water vapour pressure)
    = 149 mm Hg (19.9 kPa)

However by the time the humidified inspired air has reached the alveoli its composition and the partial pressure of oxygen will be further modified (Table 2.1). Alveolar oxygen tension (PAO_2) represents the balance between that delivered by alveolar ventilation ($\dot{V}A$) and that removed by the blood perfusing the alveoli, oxygen consumption ($\dot{V}O_2$). As $\dot{V}O_2$ can be considered relatively constant, the major determinant of PAO_2 is $\dot{V}A$. The relationship between PAO_2 and $\dot{V}A$ is described by a rectangular hyperbola with the horizontal asymptote being the partial pressure of oxygen (PO_2) in the inspired air (Fig. 2.3a). It is evident from this relationship that hyperventilation has little influence on PAO_2 whereas hypoventilation can have a very marked effect. This relationship can be modified by either exogenous factors such as changing the FIO_2 (and hence PO_2) (Fig. 2.3b) or endogenous factors such as an increase in oxygen consumption ($\dot{V}O_2$) (Fig. 2.3c). As discussed comprehensively by Nunn (1987), increasing the percentage of oxygen in inspired air from 20.9 to 30% is sufficient to correct falls in PAO_2 (and hence arterial oxygen tension) which are due to hypoventilation. However, the situation is very different when hypoxaemia is due to venous admixture (see below). An increase in $\dot{V}O_2$ which is a characteristic feature of the 'flow' or hypermetabolic response to critical illness (Wilmore, 1977) will also modify the relationship between PAO_2 and $\dot{V}A$. It becomes progressively more difficult as $\dot{V}O_2$ increases, to maintain PAO_2 by increasing $\dot{V}A$ and once again the problem can be ameliorated by increasing FIO_2.

Table 2.1 Normal values of fractional concentrations of gases under differing environments

	Dry atmospheric[a]	Humidified[b]	Alveolar[c]
Oxygen	21.1	19.9	13.9
Nitrogen	80.2	75.1	75.9
Carbon dioxide	<0.1	<0.1	5.2
Water	0	6.3	6.3
Total concentration	101.3	101.3	101.3

[a] Room air without additional humidification.
[b] Room air with a humidity of 6.3%.
[c] Alveolar concentration or predicted values for relative percentage of each gas present in the alveolar environment.

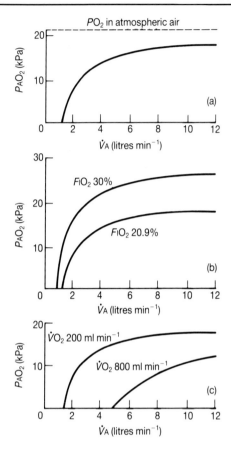

Figure 2.3 (a) The relationship between alveolar ventilation($\dot{V}_A$) and alveolar PO_2 in a subject breathing room air ($\dot{V}O_2 = 200\,ml\,min^{-1}$). (b) The effect of increasing F_IO_2 from 20.93 to 30% on the relationship between alveolar ventilation ($\dot{V}_A$) and alveolar PO_2 ($\dot{V}O_2 = 200\,ml\,min^{-1}$). (c) The effect of increasing $\dot{V}O_2$ from 200 to 800 ml min^{-1} on the relationship between alveolar ventilation ($\dot{V}_A$) and alveolar PO_2 in a subject breathing room air. (Modified from Nunn, 1987.)

Alveolar/Arterial PO_2 Difference

In healthy young adults the difference between alveolar and arterial PO_2 is small (less than 15 mm Hg (2 kPa)), but it increases in the elderly and may reach very high values in diseased states characterized by, for example, inequalities in ventilation/perfusion (see below). Oxygen moves by passive diffusion from the alveoli across the respiratory or pulmonary membrane into the capillaries. This membrane is very thin (approximately 0.6 μm) but is composed of a number of layers; a fluid or surfactant layer, alveolar epithelium, epithelial basement membrane, interstitial space, capillary basement membrane and capillary endothelium. The rate of diffusion of oxygen across this membrane is determined by the partial pressure difference across it, the solubility coefficient of oxygen and its thickness. Rapid diffusion is aided by the large surface area ($160\,m^2$) available for equilibration with the total pulmonary capillary blood volume of no more than 100 ml. The diameter of these capillaries is less than that of the blood cells which means that the cells traversing the capillaries are pressed against endothelial cells, further reducing the diffusion path for oxygen. The average time required for a red blood cell to traverse a pulmonary capillary is 0.75 s, which compares very favourably with the time of 0.25 s for equilibration of haemoglobin with alveolar gas. Thus, a delay in diffusion may not adversely effect oxygenation.

An important cause for an increase in the alveolar/arterial PO_2 difference is an increase in the degree of pulmonary venous admixture or 'intrapulmonary shunting', which is due to venous blood effectively by-passing the areas of gas exchange and then mixing with oxygenated blood leaving the pulmonary capillaries due to regional differences in the ventilation/perfusion ratio ($\dot{V}/\dot{Q}$) rather than anatomical right to left shunts. The magnitude of venous admixture is calculated as the amount of mixed venous blood which has to be added to reduce the P_AO_2 to the measured arterial PO_2 (PaO_2). Thus the lower the PaO_2 the greater the extent of venous admixture. The difference between the calculated venous admixture and the actual amount can be ascribed to the influence of arterial blood draining alveoli with a ventilation/perfusion ratio greater than 0 but less than normal. The effects of venous admixture on the relationship betwen F_IO_2 and PaO_2 are of greater clinical importance. Even a small degree (5%) of shunting can significantly reduce PaO_2 although because of the slope of the haemoglobin/oxygen dissociation curve (see below) the effects on oxygen content and saturation will be small. The relationship between F_IO_2 and PaO_2 at different levels of venous admixture have been described in the iso-shunt diagram by Nunn and his colleagues (Benatar et al., 1973; Nunn, 1987) (Fig. 2.4). It can be seen from this diagram (which, however, assumes an arterial–mixed venous oxygen content difference of $5\,ml\,dl^{-1}$) that with a shunt of 25% or more it is impossible to achieve a normal P_AO_2 even with an F_IO_2 of 1 (100% inspired O_2).

As mentioned above, alveolar ventilation $\dot{V}_A$ with air and perfusion ($\dot{Q}$) with blood are rarely closely matched in critically ill patients. Thus areas in which ventilation exceeds perfusion (as in the upper part of the lung in an upright subject) have a $\dot{V}/\dot{Q}$ ratio greater than 1 and when flow exceeds perfusion (as in the lower parts of the lung) $\dot{V}/\dot{Q}$ is less than 1. Thus in the extreme case of flow without ventilation (i.e. the anatomic shunt discussed above) $\dot{V}/\dot{Q}$ is zero. The influence of regional differences in $\dot{V}/\dot{Q}$ on the alveolar/arterial O_2 difference is complex; however, it does seem that the adverse influence of areas with a low ratio is not fully compensated by those

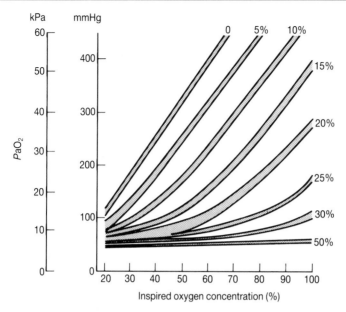

Figure 2.4   Iso-shunt diagram showing the iso-shunt bands (%) drawn to include values of Hb ($10–14\,g\,dl^{-1}$), $PaCO_2$, ($25–40\,mm\,Hg$) and an arterio-mixed venous oxygen content difference of $5\,ml\,dl^{-1}$. (From Nunn, 1987.)

with a high ratio. This is due to the greater amount of blood flowing through the under-ventilated areas and to the non-linearity of the dissociation curve which means that the fall in saturation from areas with a low $\dot{V}/\dot{Q}$ is greater than the increase in saturation from areas with a high $\dot{V}/\dot{Q}$.

Carriage of Oxygen in Arterial Blood

Oxygen is mainly carried in the blood bound to haemoglobin within the red blood cells and a small amount is dissolved in plasma. The latter component is normally a small part (1.5%) of the total but can be raised when FiO_2 and PaO_2 are increased (Bernstein, 1991).

$$
\begin{aligned}
\text{Dissolved oxygen } (\text{ml/dl}^{-1}) \text{ blood} &= \text{solubility coefficient } (0.003) \times PaO_2 \\
&\quad (\text{mm Hg}) \\
&= \text{solubility coefficient } (0.0225) \times \\
&\quad PaO_2 \text{ (kPa)}
\end{aligned}
$$

The majority is carried by haemoglobin (molecular weight 67 000) which is composed of four subunits (molecular weight 16 800), each consisting of a protein chain with a haem group attached to a histidine residue. One molecule of oxygen is bound loosely with one of the six coordinate valencies of each of the haem iron atoms, hence each molecule of haemoglobin is associated with four molecules of oxygen. The kinetics of the association are such that all the molecules of O_2 bind at the same rate (Staub, 1963). The amount of oxygen bound to haemoglobin (HbO_2) is calculated from the equation

$$HbO_2 = Hb \times SaO_2 \times 1.34$$

where Hb is the haemoglobin content ($g\,dl^{-1}$ blood), SaO_2 is the arterial saturation of haemoglobin with O_2, and 1.34 is the oxygen-carrying capacity of haemoglobin when fully saturated (ml $O_2\,g^{-1}$ haemoglobin).

Therefore, arterial oxygen content (CaO_2) can be calculated from:

$$CaO_2 = HbO_2 + \text{dissolved } O_2$$

Thus the amount of oxygen carried is influenced by changes in haemoglobin concentration and in the arterial saturation of haemoglobin with O_2. The relationship between PO_2 and the percentage saturation of haemoglobin with O_2 is described by the oxyhaemoglobin dissociation curve (Fig. 2.5). The position of this sigmoid curve is described most precisely by the P_{50}, the PO_2 at which haemoglobin is 50% saturated, which lies on the steep linear part of the curve. Under normal conditions the P_{50} is 26.3 mm Hg (3.5 kPa) (Nunn, 1987). It can be seen that arterial blood with a PaO_2 of approximately 95 mm Hg (12.5 kPa) will have an oxygen saturation in excess of 95%, whereas mixed venous blood with a PaO_2 of approximately 40 mm Hg (5.5 kPa) will have a saturation of 75%. As arterial blood is normally some 95–98% saturated with O_2 then raising the FiO_2 and hence PAO_2 or PaO_2 to supranormal levels can only have a small effect on the arterial oxygen content in a normal individual.

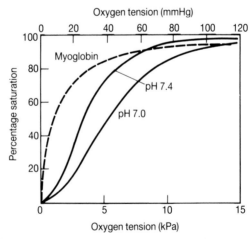

Figure 2.5   The relationship between oxygen tension (PO_2) and percentage saturation of myoglobin (----) and haemoglobin (——) with O_2. The effect of a fall in pH from 7.4 to 7.2 on the oxyhaemoglobin dissociation curve is also shown.

If the haemoglobin concentration is taken as $145\,g\,l^{-1}$ then it can be calculated that the amount of oxygen carried by haemoglobin in arterial blood is some $188\,ml\,l^{-1}$ blood ($145.0 \times 0.97 \times 1.34$). Similarly, the oxygen content of mixed venous blood is approximately $146\,ml\,l^{-1}$ blood ($145 \times 0.75 \times 1.34$) representing, in this example, an uptake by the tissues in excess of $40\,ml\,O_2\,dl^{-1}$ blood or an extraction of just over 20%.

The position of the dissociation curve is not fixed in critically ill patients. The P_{50} can increase, shifting the curve to the right, or decrease, shifting the curve to the left by a number of factors. Increases in hydrogen ion concentration (reduction in pH), PCO_2, temperature and haemoglobin concentration all move the curve to the right (the Bohr effect) (Fig. 2.5). One other factor which effects the position of the oxyhaemoglobin dissociation curve is 2,3-diphosphoglycerate (2,3-DPG) which is formed in a 'shunt' off the main glycolytic pathway (Fig. 2.1). One molecule of 2,3-DPG binds to the β-chain of deoxygenated (but not oxygenated haemoglobin), resulting in a conformational change which reduces oxygen affinity (i.e. moves the curve to the right). A reduction in 2,3-DPG concentration has been reported in a number of 'shock' states and also in stored blood, but although these changes will impair O_2 supply to tissues, they do not seem to be of great clinical significance. Oxygen also combines in muscle with myoglobin (molecular weight 16 800) which contains one atom of iron per molecule. The oxygen association curve of myoglobin is a rectangular hyperbola which lies very much to the left of the haemoglobin–oxygen dissociation curve (Fig. 2.5). Thus myoglobin takes up and releases oxygen much more readily at a low PO_2 than haemoglobin. For example, the P_{50} of myoglobin is as low as 5 mm Hg (0.7 kPa), a value which is not unrepresentative of tissue PO_2 (Fig. 2.2). The oxygen combined with myoglobin can be considered as a store (approximately 200 ml) for use when muscle blood is reduced, for example during contraction.

Delivery of Oxygen to the Tissues

Oxygen delivery ($\dot{D}O_2$) is the product of oxygen content of the blood and the volume of blood perfusing a tissue, organ, or the whole body ($\dot{Q}$), i.e.

$$\dot{D}O_2 = CaO_2 \times \dot{Q}\,ml\,min^{-1}$$

As the factors determining CaO_2 have been considered above, those influencing $\dot{Q}$ will now be discussed. It is customary in clinical practice to consider oxygen delivery in terms of the whole body and in this case $\dot{Q}$ is equal to cardiac output. Cardiac output (litres min^{-1}) is determined by the amount of blood ejected during each systolic contraction (stroke volume) and the heart rate; the stroke volume from each ventricle coupled in series (right to the lungs, left to the rest of the body) is the same (approximately 70–80 ml).

Variations in cardiac output can therefore be achieved by changes in heart rate and/or stroke volume. Heart rate reflects the balance between the chronotropic influences of the efferent sympathetic and parasympathetic (vagal) cardiac innervations. An increase in sympathetic activity leading to an increase in heart rate (tachycardia) and an increase in vagal activity reducing heart rate (brady-cardia). Most stress or shock states (e.g. the 'flow' phase responses to trauma or sepsis) are characterized by a global increase in efferent sympathetic activity and, not surprisingly, this is usually accompanied by a tachycardia. The increase in efferent cardiac sympathetic activity, augmented by the increase in circulating catecholamine levels, will also increase the strength of contraction by the ventricles (positive inotropic effect). Thus for a given degree of cardiac filling (atrial pressure or preload) the ventricular stroke work or output is increased by sympathetic stimulation. This effect can be, to some extent, offset by an increase in peripheral resistance (afterload).

The opposing sympathetic and vagal influences on heart rate can be quite complex, as illustrated by the acute response to haemorrhage (Kirkman & Little, 1988). Initially, a progressive blood loss reduces venous return to the heart which leads to a fall in cardiac output and hence in arterial blood pressure. This hypotension reduces the efferent input to the central nervous system from the aterial baro- or stretch receptors which normally exert an inhibitory influence on efferent sympathetic activity. A reduction in this inhibition therefore increases sympathetic outflow with all its cardiovascular and metabolic sequelae. Heart rate increases and there is a concomitant constriction of vascular smooth muscle, increasing peripheral resistance to blood flow and reducing the size of the venous (capicitance) side of the circulation. All of these homeostatic responses are an attempt to maintain cardiac output and blood pressure in the face of falling blood volume. The vasoconstriction is not, however, uniform: it tends to be more intense in vascular beds such as skeletal muscle and skin whilst sparing the cerebral and coronary beds (Chien, 1967). When the blood loss exceeds some 20% of blood volume there is a dramatic change in the pattern of response with the appearance of a marked bradycardia and vasodilatation in skeletal muscle (Barcroft et al., 1944). This bradycardia does not reflect the imminent demise of the heart but is a reflex triggered by 'distortion' receptors in the myo-cardium. The bradycardia which is mediated by the vagus can be interpreted as protective, reducing myocardial work at a time when coronary blood flow may be compromised, and may also serve to maintain output as cardiac filling is markedly reduced. These homeostatic responses can only serve to maintain blood flow to 'essential areas for a limited period and clearly the deficit in intravascular blood volume must be corrected as soon as possible especially if, as discussed elsewhere, increases in cardiac output and oxygen delivery are indicated in 'shock'. The increase in sympathetic activity also mediates the mobilization, and modulates the utilization, of energy substrates (carbo-hydrate and fat) which will fuel this hypermetabolism.

The distribution of blood flow within a tissue will be determined both by the number of open capillaries and the resistance to the flow. In the smallest arterial vessels the main influence on resistance is the diameter of the vessel (resistance is inversely proportional to the fourth power of the radius) whereas in the exchange vessels or capillaries the viscosity of blood may be more important. Viscosity or the inherent resistance to flow is dependent on a number of factors including velocity of flow, haematocrit, temperature, red cell deformability and the presence of microaggregates. Viscosity increases disproportionately as haematocrit rises and the effect is most marked at low velocities or shear rates (Messmer, 1975). However, the haematocrit in the capillaries may be as low as 10% and the major influence on capillary blood flow in, for example, shock are changes in red cell deformability and the formation of blood cell aggregates which can plug vessels.

A reduction in haematocrit induced by normovolaemic haemodilution reduces $\dot{D}O_2$ despite an increase in cardiac output (see Bernstein, 1991). The increase in cardiac output is thought to be mediated by an increase in venous return (preload). $\dot{D}O_2$ can, however, be maintained if intravascular volume is increased (hypervolaemia) and in this situation maximum values for $\dot{D}O_2$ are found at an haematocrit of 30%. In this situation $\dot{V}O_2$ is well-maintained until haematocrit falls below approximately 20%, although this may not be the case if a hypermetabolic stimulus such as sepsis or trauma is superimposed. As $\dot{D}O_2$ falls, $\dot{V}O_2$ can be maintained by an increase in the extraction of O_2 delivered to the tissues.

$$\text{Oxygen extraction ratio (OER)} = \frac{CaO_2 = C\overline{v}O_2}{CaO_2}$$

Those tissues which have a low resting OER will have most resistance whereas organs such as the heart which normally have a high OER will be most susceptible to an impairment in $\dot{D}O_2$. Thus the maintenance of an adequate myocardial O_2 delivery may determine total body resistance to a reduction in $\dot{D}O_2$.

The presence of arterio-venous anastomoses can reduce the effective delivery of oxygen to tissues by diverting blood flow from the capillaries. Thus, paradoxically, an increase in blood flow can be associated with a reduction in 'nutritive blood flow' or tissue oxygen delivery. The overall importance of such anastomoses is unclear although they clearly have a role in the skin where they are important in the control of the rate of heat loss.

Tissue PO_2

As oxygen is needed to maintain cellular aerobic metabolism it would seem that the most meaningful site for the measurement of PO_2 would be in the tissues (or ideally within the cells). Electrodes based on the polarographic principle described by Clark (1956) can be used in the form of a multiwire assembly placed on the surface of, for example, a muscle or as a needle inserted into tissue. A different approach is to implant a silastic tonometer within the tissue and measure the PO_2 of the fluid inside the tonometer after a suitable equilibration period (Niinikoski & Halkola, 1978). A recent innovation has been the use of such a tonometer implanted in the lumen of the intestine to measure the intracellular acid–base status of the mucosa, the integrity of which may be an important factor in determining outcome in a number of shock states (e.g. Deitch, 1990). The values obtained for tissue PO_2 in skeletal muscle show a wide distribution, reflecting the O_2 gradient within a tissue predicted from the Krogh model (Krogh, 1919), with a median of some 3.15 mm Hg (4.2 kPa) (Beerthuizen et al., 1989) (Fig. 2.6). A reduction in this median PO_2 value preceding a reduction in arterial blood pressure has been observed in a number of models of haemorrhagic and septic shock suggesting the tissue PO_2 may be a sensitive indicator of an early reduction in $\dot{D}O_2$. Reassuringly, significant correlations have been found in critically ill patients and experimental animals between skeletal muscle PO_2 (median) and SaO_2 (+), $S\bar{v}O_2$ (+), arterio-venous oxygen difference (−) and blood lactate concentration (−) (Beerthuizen et al., 1989).

Oxygen Consumption ($\dot{V}O_2$)

The rates at which the processes of aerobic metabolism take place can be assessed by measuring the rates of oxygen consumption ($\dot{V}O_2$) and carbon dioxide production ($\dot{V}CO_2$). Whole body $\dot{V}O_2$ is most conveniently measured in clinical practice by the application of the Fick principle or by indirect calorimetry.

The Fick principle states that the rate of which a substance (e.g. oxygen) is taken up by an organ or the whole body is equal to the arterio-venous difference in concentration of the substance multiplied by blood flow. Thus if cardiac output ($\dot{Q}$), CaO_2 and $C\bar{v}O_2$ (ideally measured in the pulmonary artery) are known, then the Fick equation can be rearranged to derive $\dot{V}O_2$:

$$\dot{V}O_2 = (CaO_2 - C\bar{v}O_2)\dot{Q}$$

The technique of indirect calorimetry involves the measurement of the oxygen and carbon dioxide concentrations of inspired (FI) and expired (FE) and the volumes of inspired ($\dot{V}I$) and expired ($\dot{V}E$) air. Thus $\dot{V}O_2$ = amount of O_2 inspired − amount of O_2 expired:

$$\dot{V}O_2 = (\dot{V}I \times FIO_2) - (\dot{V}E \times FEO_2)$$

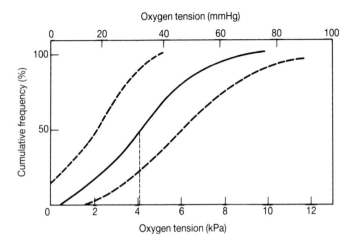

Figure 2.6 Cumulative distribution (±SD) of oxygen tension in human skeletal muscle, based on 100 measurements in each of 31 healthy subjects (median value = 31.5 mm Hg (4.2 kPa)). (From Beerthuizen, 1987.)

O_2 and CO_2 concentrations are usually measured with paramagnetic and infrared analysers and $\dot{V}E$ with a rotameter. $\dot{V}I$ is then calculated from $\dot{V}E$ (and the amount of nitrogen which does not participate in gas exchange) in inspired and expired gas:

$$\dot{V}I = \frac{\dot{V}E \times F_EN_2}{F_IN_2}$$

However, nitrogen concentrations are not usually measured directly but are calculated as the 'balance' after measurement of the other gases:

$$F_IN_2 = 1 - F_IO_2$$

and

$$F_EN_2 = 1 - \left(F_EO_2 + F_ECO_2 + \frac{P_{H_2O}}{\text{Barometric pressure}}\right)$$

In a similar manner $\dot{V}CO_2$ can be calculated:

$$\dot{V}CO_2 = (\dot{V}E \times F_ECO_2) - (\dot{V}I \times F_ICO_2)$$

In normal room air the F_ICO_2 is negligible and the calculation can be simplified:

$$\dot{V}CO_2 = \dot{V}E \times F_ECO_2$$

Table 2.2 Volumes of oxygen consumed, carbon dioxide produced, respiratory quotients (RQ) and energy equivalents involved in the oxidation of various energy sources

Energy in source	VO_2 (litres g^{-1})	VCO_2 (litres g^{-1})	RQ	Energy expenditure (kcal litre^{-1} O_2)
Glucose	0.746	0.746	1.00	5.01
Fat	2.03	1.43	0.70	4.70
Protein	0.966	0.782	0.81	4.60

Modified from Frayn (1983).

Metabolic rate (MR) is often calculated from $\dot{V}O_2$ and a figure for the energy equivalent (the amount of energy liberated per litre of O_2 consumed) of 4.82 kcal:

$$MR \text{ (kcal day}^{-1}) = \dot{V}O_2 \text{ (litres min}^{-1}) \times 4.82 \times 60 \times 24$$

More precise information about the substrate being oxidized can be obtained by using both $\dot{V}O_2$ and $\dot{V}CO_2$ to obtain the respiratory quotient (RQ) or respiratory exchange ratio (RER) (Table 2.2) (Frayn, 1983).

$$RQ = \dot{V}CO_2/\dot{V}O_2$$

From the data shown in Table 2.2 and assuming that the amount of protein oxidized can be estimated from urinary nitrogen excretion (n) it can be calculated that:

$$\dot{V}O_2 \text{ (litres min}^{-1}) = 0.746 \text{ carbohydrate (g min}^{-1}) + 2.03 \text{ fat (g min}^{-1})$$
$$+ 6.25 \times 0.966 \text{ protein (g min}^{-1})$$

and

$$\dot{V}CO_2 \text{ (litres min}^{-1}) = 0.746 \text{ carbohydrate (g min}^{-1}) + 1.43 \text{ fat (g min}^{-1})$$
$$+ 6.25 \times 0.782 \text{ protein (g min}^{-1})$$

Thus the rates of carbohydrate (c) and fat (f) oxidation can be derived:

$$c = 4.55\dot{V}CO_2 - 3.21\dot{V}O_2 - 2.87n$$
$$f = 1.67\dot{V}O_2 - 1.67\dot{V}CO_2 - 1.92n$$

The influence of other metabolic processes such as lipogenesis, gluconeogenesis, lactate and ketone body formation on these calculations of substrate oxidation are reviewed by Frayn (1983).

Clinical Relationship Between Oxygen Delivery and Oxygen Consumption

In clinical practice the units used for assessment and manipulation are different from those used in the physiology laboratory. First, $\dot{D}O_2$ and $\dot{V}O_2$ are indexed to some estimates of the patient's size. This may be indexed to weight – the results being expressed in millilitres per minute per kilogram – or to body surface area (BSA), the results then being expressed as millilitres per minute per square metre. The BSA is determined from standard nomograms based on measurements of the patient's height and weight. The height is easily determined with a tape measure. Weight is determined by use of a bedside weighing machine, which entails lifting the patient from the bed. This needs to be done with caution in a mechanically ventilated hypotensive patient. The cardiac output therefore become cardiac index (CI). All variables derived from the cardiac output such as stroke volume, left ventricular stroke work index are routinely indexed to BSA. Also CaO_2 and $C\bar{v}O_2$ are calculated in millilitres per decilitre by modern blood-gas analysers. In terms of oxygen transport the values that are most important in routine clinical use are the $\dot{D}O_2$ and the $\dot{V}O_2$ given by the equations:

$$\dot{D}O_2 = CI \times CaO_2 \times 10\,\text{ml}\,\text{min}^{-1}\,\text{m}^{-2}$$

$$\dot{V}O_2 = CI \times (CaO_2 - C\bar{v}O_2) \times 10\ \text{ml}\,\text{min}^{-1}\,\text{m}^{-2} \times 10$$

The relationship between $\dot{D}O_2$ and $\dot{V}O_2$ is indexed mathematically by the OER. In a normal resting individual OER is 25%. Thus with a Hb value of $15\,\text{g}\,\text{dl}^{-1}$ and 95% oxyhaemoglobin saturation, CaO_2 could be calculated to be

$$\text{Normal } CaO_2 = 15 \times 1.34 \times 0.95 = 19.1\,\text{ml}\,\text{dl}^{-1}$$

In this case the contribution of dissolved oxygen would be trivial and can therefore be discounted. With a cardiac output of 5.0 litres min^{-1} and a BSA of $1.8\,\text{m}^2$ we can calculate CI:

$$CI = \frac{5}{1.8} = 2.8 \text{ litres min}^{-1}\,\text{m}^{-2}$$

and $\dot{D}O_2$:

$$\dot{D}O_2 = 2.8 \times 19.1 \times 10 = 535\ \text{ml}\,\text{min}^{-1}\,\text{m}^{-2}$$

If the OER is 25% (normal requirement at rest) then if 25% of the oxyhaemoglobin is removed during circulation of the blood through the systemic capillary bed then the mixed venous saturation would be 75%, with the $C\bar{v}O_2$ being calculated as

$$C\bar{v}O_2 = Hb \times 1.34 = 0.75 = 15.1\,\text{ml}\,\text{min}^{-1}\,\text{m}^{-2}$$

The fall in saturation from 95 to 75% is dependent on the shape of the oxyhaemoglobin dissociation curve. As the PaO_2 approaches that in the capillaries, the tissue at the venous end of the capillary circulation, it becomes the mixed venous oxygen tension ($P\bar{v}O_2$) and the mixed venous saturation ($S\bar{v}O_2$).

Using the Fick principle the $\dot{V}O_2$ is the sum of the CI and the difference between CaO_2 and $C\bar{v}O_2$, therefore,

$$\dot{V}O_2 = 2.8 \times (19.1 - 15.1) \times 10 = 140\,\text{ml}\,\text{min}^{-1}\,\text{m}^{-2}$$

The values of $P\bar{v}O_2$ and $S\bar{v}O_2$ are such that they lie on the linear portion of the oxyhaemoglobin dissociation curve. These normal relationships are depicted in Figure 2.5.

The $\dot{D}O_2$ $\dot{V}O_2$ Relationship in Shock States

An Absolute Reduction in Oxygen Delivery

The easiest form of acute circulatory failure to understand in terms of oxygen transport is that of pure flow, i.e. low cardiac output without an increase or decrease in oxygen demand and, therefore, no major change in $\dot{V}O_2$. Let us take the example of a typical patient in cardiogenic shock following acute myocardial infarction.

The CI is 2.0 litres min^{-1} m^{-2}, Hb 14.0 g dl^{-1} and, after correction of hypoxaemia, SaO_2 is 95%. Thus we can calculate CaO_2

$$CaO_2 = 14.0 \times 1.34 \times 0.95 = 17.8\,\text{ml}\,\text{dl}^{-1}$$

and $\dot{D}O_2$

$$\dot{D}O_2 = 2.0 \times 17.8 \times 10 = 356\,\text{ml}\,\text{min}^{-1}\,\text{m}^{-2}$$

However, as this patient maintains a normal $\dot{V}O_2$ the OER rises dramatically and $S\bar{v}O_2$ falls. In this case to a value of 57% we can calculate $C\bar{v}O_2$ as

$$C\bar{v}O_2 = 14.0 \times 1.34 \times 0.57 = 10.7\,\text{ml}\,\text{min}^{-1}\,\text{m}^{-2}$$

We can now calculate $\dot{V}O_2$

$$\dot{V}O_2 = 2.0 \times (17.8 - 10.7) \times 10 = 142\,\text{ml}\,\text{min}^{-1}\,\text{m}^{-2}$$

Although $\dot{V}O_2$ has been maintained, it is at the expense of a critical reduction in $S\bar{v}O_2$ which may limit oxygenation to some tissues. This issue is discussed elsewhere in this text and will not be elaborated on here.

Take another example – that of a patient with sudden blood loss whose cardiac output was fixed. In this example the Hb falls to 6.0 g dl^{-1} and there is no hypoxaemia.

$$CaO_2 = 6.0 \times 1.34 \times 0.95 = 7.6\,ml\,dl^{-1}$$

CI is 3.0 litres $min^{-1}\,m^{-2}$. So we can calculate $\dot{D}O_2$:

$$\dot{D}O_2 = 3.0 \times 7.6 \times 10 = 228\,ml\,min^{-1}\,m^{-2}$$

$S\bar{v}O_2$ is measured as 45%, so we can calculate $C\bar{v}O_2$:

$$CO_2\,O_2 = 3.8\,ml\,dl^{-1}$$

and

$$\dot{V}O_2 = 3.0 \times (7.7 - 3.8) \times 10 = 114\,ml\,min^{-1}\,m^{-2}$$

In the first case

$$OER = \frac{CaO_2 - C\bar{v}O_2}{CaO_2} = \frac{7.1}{17.8} = 40\%$$

and in the second

$$OER = \frac{CaO_2 - C\bar{v}O_2}{CaO_2} = \frac{3.8}{7.8} = 49\%$$

Of course in clinical practice in the anaemic patient there may well be a compensatory increase in cardiac output.

The final common mechanism for reduction in $\dot{D}O_2$ is hypoxaemia. If we again consider a theoretical patient, this time with profound arterial desaturation (SaO_2 55%) and a fixed cardiac output (3.0 litres $min^{-1}\,m^{-2}$) and an Hb concentration of 15 $g\,dl^{-1}$:

$$CaO_2 = 15 \times 1.34 \times 0.55 = 11\,ml\,min^{-1}\,m^{-2}$$

and

$$\dot{D}O_2 = 3.0 \times 11 \times 10 = 330\,ml\,min^{-1}\,m^{-2}$$

If this patient was to maintain a $\dot{V}O_2$ of 140 $ml\,min^{-1}\,m^{-2}$ then we could calculate the level of $S\bar{v}O_2$ necessary to achieve this as:

$$\dot{V}O_2 = CI \times (CaO_2 - C\bar{v}O_2) \times 10\,ml\,min^{-1}\,m^{-2}$$

$$CaO_2 - C\bar{v}O_2 = \frac{\dot{V}O_2}{CI \times 10} = \frac{140}{30} = 4.6\,ml\,dl^{-1}$$

As

$$C\bar{v}O_2 = CaO_2 - (CaO_2 - C\bar{v}O_2)\,ml\,dl^{-1}$$

then in this patient

$$C\bar{v}O_2 = 11.00 - 4.6 = 6.4\,ml\,dl^{-1}$$

and as $C\bar{v}O_2 = Hb \times 1.34 \times S\bar{v}O_2$, then

$$S\bar{v}O_2 = \frac{C\bar{v}O_2}{Hb \times 1.34} = \frac{6.4}{15.0 \times 1.34} = 32\%$$

This would, of course, represent a severe level of reduced oxygen availability at the venous end of the capillary circulation. In fact, if there were no shift in the oxyhaemoglobin dissociation curve, the $P\bar{v}O_2$ would be of the order of 20 mm Hg (2.6 kPa). Of course, this is a theoretical situation. If the arterial desaturation was to occur acutely in a patient, the physiological response would be an increase in cardiac output. Patients with chronic cardiorespiratory disease adapt to such low values of $S\bar{v}O2$ and $P\bar{v}O_2$ as they develop very slowly. However, if in the acute situation cardiac output cannot increase, then this extreme mixed venous desaturation and hypoxia could be found in clinical practice.

We could take these considerations further. Consider a patient with cardiogenic shock and arterial desaturation – a not uncommon clinical situation. If we take a representative value of CI as 1.8 litres $min^{-1} m^{-2}$, an SaO_2 of 75% with a normal Hb, then

$$CaO_2 = 15.0 \times 1.34 \times 0.75 = 15.0 \text{ ml dl}^{-1}$$

and

$$\dot{D}O_2 = 2.0 \times 15.0 \times 10 = 300 \text{ ml min}^{-1} m^{-2}$$

If this patient was even modestly anaemic with an Hb of 10.00 g dl^{-1}, then

$$CaO_2 = 10.0 \times 1.34 \times 0.75 = 10.0 \text{ ml dl}^{-1}$$

and

$$\dot{D}O_2 = 2.0 \times 10 \times 10 = 200 \text{ ml min}^{-1} m^{-2}$$

In this situation even a low normal values of $\dot{V}O_2$ could only be achieved by large increases in OER and once again very low values of $S\bar{v}O_2$ and $P\bar{v}O_2$. For instance, if the patient's $\dot{V}O_2$ was to be maintained at 110 ml $min^{-1} m^{-2}$, which is generally considered to be the low end of the normal range, we could repeat the calculations used above as if

$$\dot{V}O_2 = 110 \text{ ml min}^{-1} m^{-2} \text{ and } \dot{V}O_2 = CI \times (CaO_2 - C\bar{v}O_2) \times 10 \text{ ml min}^{-1} m^{-2}$$

then $CaO_2 - C\bar{v}O_2$ must be 5.5 ml dl^{-1} and $C\bar{v}O_2$ must be 4.5 ml dl^{-1} and $S\bar{v}O_2$ must be 34% with $P\bar{v}O_2$ being less than 23 mm Hg (3 kPa), assuming no shift in the oxyhaemoglobin dissociation curve. OER under these circumstances is 55%.

In terms of management of this patient we could consider the effects of blood transfusion to increase Hb to $14 \cdot 0 \, g \, dl^{-1}$ and supplemental inspired oxygen to increase SaO_2 to 95% then

$$\dot{D}O_2 = 2.0 \times 17.8 \times 10 = 356 \, ml \, min^{-1} \, m^{-2}$$

At the same level of $\dot{V}O_2$ we could recalculate $C\bar{v}O_2$ and $S\bar{v}O_2$:

$$C\bar{v}O_2 = CaO_2 - (CaO_2 - C\bar{v}O_2) = 17.8 - 5.5 = 12.3 \, ml \, min^{-1} \, m^{-2}$$

and

$$S\bar{v}O_2 = \frac{C\bar{v}O_2}{Hb \times 1.34} = \frac{12.3}{14.0 \times 1.34} = 65\%$$

These two relatively simple manoeuvres have increased the arterial global level of $\dot{D}O_2$ and availability at the venous end of the capillary circulation, so if once again we assume there is no shift in the oxyhaemoglobin dissociation curve, the $P\bar{v}O_2$ would have risen to approximately 34 mm Hg (4.5 kPa).

In all these examples we have assumed that the ability of the tissues to extract oxygen has not been impaired either by alterations at a microcirculatory level or by the phenomenon of so-called flow dependency.

A Relative Reduction in Oxygen Delivery

This represents a completely different manifestation of the relationship between $\dot{D}O_2$ and $\dot{V}O_2$. In these general clinical circumstances the absolute value of $\dot{D}O_2$ may be within the normal range but the level of delivery is not adequate. This may be because the demand for oxygen is increased above normal levels (the reasons for this are discussed in other chapters of this book) or that the delivery which is supplied is not associated with the expected level of uptake of oxygen. This latter situation has been said to be seen classically in patients with severe sepsis or adult respiratory distress syndrome (ARDS).

References

Barcroft H, Edholm OG, McMichael J & Sharpey-Schafer EP (1944) Post haemorrhagic fainting. Study by cardiac output and forearm flow. *Lancet* i: 489–91.

Beerthuizen GIJM (1987) Skeletal muscle PO_2 assessment during imminent shock. Thesis, Catholic University of Nijmegen.

Beerthuizen GIJM, Goris RJA & Kreuzer FJA (1989) Skeletal PO_2 during imminent shock. *Arch. Emerg. Med.* **6**: 172–182.

Benatar SR, Hewlett AM & Nunn JF (1973) The use of iso-shunt lines for control of oxygen therapy. *Br. J. Anaesth.* **45:** 711–18.

Bernstein DP (1991) Oxygen transport and utilization in trauma. In Capan LM, Miller SM & Turndorf H (eds), *Trauma Anaesthesia and Intensive Care*, pp. 115–65. Philadelphia: J.B. Lippincott.

Chein S (1967) Role of the sympathetic nervous system in haemorrhage. *Physiol. Rev.* **47:** 214–28.

Clark LC (1956) Monitor and control of blood and tissue oxygen tensions. *Trans. Am. Soc. Artif. Intern. Organs* **2:** 41–8.

Crowell JW & Smith EE (1964) Oxygen deficit and irreversible hemorrhagic shock. *Am. J. Physiol.* **206:** 313–16.

Deitch EA (1990) Gut failure: its role in the multiple organ failure syndrome. In Deitch EA (ed.), *Multiple Organ Failure*, pp. 40–59. New York: Thieme.

Frayn KN (1983) Calculation of substrate oxidation rates in vivo from gaseous exchange. *J. Appl. Physiol.* **55:** 628–34.

Kirkman E & Little RA (1988) The pathophysiology of trauma and shock. In Kox W & Gamble J (eds), *Fluid Resuscitation. Baillière's Clinical Anaesthesiology*, pp. 467–82. London: Baillière Tindall.

Krogh A (1919) The member and distribution of capillaries in muscles with calculations of the oxygen pressure head necessary for supplying the tissue. *J. Physiol.* **52:** 409–15.

Messmer K (1975) Hemodilution. *Surg. Clin. North Am.* **55:** 659–78.

Niinikoski J & Halkola L (1978) Skeletal muscle PO_2: indicator of peripheral tissue perfusion in haemorrhagic shock. *Adv. Exp. Med. Biol.* **94:** 585–92.

Nunn JF (1987) *Applied Respiratory Physiology*. London: Butterworth.

Shoemaker WC, Appel PL & Kram HB (1988) Tissue oxygen debt as a determinant of lethal and non-lethal postoperative organ failure. *Crit. Care Med.* **16:** 1117–20.

Staub NC (1963) Alveolar–arterial oxygen tension gradient due to diffusion. *J. Appl. Physiol.* **18:** 673–80.

Wilmore DW (1977) *The Metabolic Management of the Critically Ill*. New York: Plenum.

3 Measurements, Technical Problems and Inaccuracies

Peter Nightingale

Introduction

The practical application of oxygen transport principles is only possible when repeated and accurate measurements of oxygen transport variables can be made at the bedside. The only method which is widely available is to measure cardiac output using the thermodilution technique, and the oxygen content of arterial and mixed venous blood using a blood-gas analyser linked to a cooximeter. This requires insertion of a pulmonary artery flotation catheter, the use of which has recently been reviewed by an expert panel (Bennett *et al.*, 1991). Systemic and pulmonary arterial pressures must also be measured, and derived haemodynamic values calculated, to guide resuscitation and therapy.

This chapter reviews the theory and practice of making these measurements, and highlights potential pitfalls in obtaining and interpreting them. Clinicians must have a clear understanding of these pitfalls to avoid making interventions based on erroneous data.

Pressure Measurements

An appreciation of the theory underlying arterial pressure monitoring is necessary to ensure high-fidelity recordings and to prevent errors in interpretation. Pressure monitoring systems consist of several interacting parts with their associated interfaces (Gardner, 1986).

CATHETER IN VESSEL

↓   Sampling stopcocks

CONNECTING TUBING

↓   Continuous flush device

PRESSURE TRANSDUCER

↓   Electronics

WAVEFORM DISPLAY

The Electro-Hydraulic System

This consists of a sterile system of tubing filled with heparinized saline connected to the pressure transducer. Specifications for amplifier systems have been described (Gardner, 1981). A band width of DC to 50 Hz is required to reproduce pressure waveforms accurately without distortion. Zero stability should be ± 1 mm Hg. Sensitivity and stability should be ± 1% over time and within the physiological temperature range.

The hydraulic system incorporates a continuous flush device to reduce clot formation at the end of the monitoring catheter and maintain patency. Normal saline with 1 iu ml^{-1} of heparin pressurized to 300 mm Hg is used, typically at 1–3 ml h^{-1}. A fast flush override is used to remove air bubbles and blood from the system during priming and after sampling. This may deliver fluid volumes that are significant in neonates, and prolonged activation can lead to retrograde flushing of the proximal arterial system and affect the cerebral circulation. The fast flush actuator should respond rapidly so that a square waveform is produced when assessing the dynamic characteristics of the system as described below (fast flush test).

The pressure transducer should be carefully applied to the membrane at the base of the disposal dome designed to separate the sterile-fluid-filled system from the reusable transducer. The use of a few drops of sterile saline is permissible to ensure a good seal, but air bubbles must be scrupulously avoided if the system is not to become excessively damped. Failure to obtain a good seal at this interface can lead to erroneously low pressures being displayed. Nosocomial infections have been traced to contaminated transducers and strict sterility is needed.

To reduce nosocomial infection the flushing system is changed regularly at 24–48 h intervals. Since infection usually occurs through stopcocks during blood sampling, these sites should be handled with scrupulous care using a set protocol to minimize contamination (remember that stopcocks do not stop cocci!).

Reusable transducers are being superseded by disposable transducers incorporated into the fast flush device. These systems are smaller and have a straight through design to minimize dead space and areas where small bubbles can collect. The electronic characteristics are also better with improved stability and accuracy.

Before use the transducer system should be zeroed and calibrated. Modern transducers are linear typically to 1% of stated accuracy, and for practical purposes need only be zeroed. It is useful, however, when first bringing a transducer into use, to calibrate against a mercury column. Readings are taken at 0, 50, 100, 150 and 300 mm Hg to check for accuracy and linearity of response at the extremes of range.

The mid-axillary line in the fourth intercostal space is the reference point used for zeroing vascular pressures. With the usual arrangement of placing transducers at the bedside, zeroing involves opening the stopcock above the transducer dome to air and using a spirit-level to adjust the air–fluid interface so as to be level with the reference point. It is good practice to re-zero frequently, especially if therapeutic interventions are being contemplated.

For optimum dynamic response the length of tubing connecting the arterial catheter to the transducer should be non-compliant and as short as possible. Although the transducer should ideally be mounted close to the patient, in practice it is not uncommon for 100 cm or more of tubing to lead to transducers mounted at the bedside. This may be clinically convenient, but haemodynamic responsiveness is degraded and the longer the tubing the more the signal will be distorted. Sampling sites with compliant membranes should not be in contact with the transduced column of saline.

Frequency Response

Understanding the concept of frequency response ensures optimum fidelity of pressure recordings and enables aberrant displayed waveforms and pressures to be interpreted.

If displacement takes place in a fluid-filled column, the fluid will oscillate for a short period before coming to a rest, similar to a spring with a weight attached. Damping of the oscillations depends on the elasticity of the system, and on the mass of fluid and friction generated. This can be expressed by a factor known as the damping coefficient. The elasticity of the system is determined by the degree of movement of the various parts including the transducer diaphragm, connecting tubing and sampling sites, and by the presence of air bubbles.

The dynamic response of a monitoring system is also influenced by its natural frequency. If energy is fed into the system at gradually increasing frequencies, then the amplitude of oscillations will increase up to a maximum – the resonant frequency. Ideally the resonant frequency should be above the range of frequencies measured in clinical practice to prevent distortion of the displayed waveform.

To reproduce the original waveform faithfully, the frequency response of a system should be flat up to a frequency that contains 10 harmonics of the original. For pressure waves in the arterial system at a rate of 120 beats min^{-1}, that is 2 Hz, a flat response to 20 Hz is needed (Gardner, 1986). In clinical practice, pressure monitoring systems are almost always underdamped, and the natural frequency is often barely high enough.

The equations for natural frequency and damping coefficient can be defined for a fluid-filled monitoring system:

$$\text{Natural frequency} = 1.4 \times 10^3 \times \frac{d}{\sqrt{Vd \times L}}$$

$$\text{Damping coefficient} = 1.36 \times 10^3 \, \frac{\sqrt{Vd \times L}}{d^3}$$

where d = catheter diameter; L = catheter length; Vd = volume displacement.

A damping coefficient < 1 indicates an underdamped system that will oscillate. A damping coefficient > 1 indicates that the system is overdamped and will not oscillate, but features such as the dicrotic notch will be lost from the waveform. These dynamic characteristics can be assessed at the bedside using the fast flush test (Gardner, 1981), and compared to a plot of damping coefficient against natural frequency.

The diagrams shown in Fig. 3.1a should be available on all intensive care units and defines the limits within which an adequate dynamic response is to be found. Systems falling outside these recommendations will produce waveforms distorted by under- or over-damping.

Fast Flush Test

The fast flush test should be taught to all staff and done regularly to confirm an adequate dynamic response. With a paper chart recorder running and recording the arterial waveform, actuate and release the fast flush device. A square wave pulse of 300 mm Hg is thus imposed on the printed arterial waveform. The paper recorder must be capable of responding to systems with natural frequencies at least up to 20 Hz. The test may need to be repeated in order to obtain a trace which has the down slope of the square wave in the diastolic region of the pressure waveform. A typical printout is shown in Fig. 3.1b.

To determine the natural frequency of the system, the distance between successive peaks is carefully measured and divided into the paper speed. In the example in Fig. 3.1b the paper speed is 25 mm s^{-1} and the peak-to-peak distance is 2 mm, the natural frequency is therefore 12.5 Hz.

To determine the damping coefficient, the amplitudes of two successive peaks are measured and the ratio of the second to the first calculated. The damping coefficient can be solved using this ratio but is more conveniently obtained from Fig. 3.1a. The amplitude ratio in the example is 22 ÷ 27 or 0.81, equivalent to a damping coefficient of 0.1. It can be seen that this system falls short of adequate. The system is underdamped and the displayed waveforms will be distorted, producing excessive systolic overshoot. Reference to Fig. 3.1a shows that it is possible to vary either the natural frequency or the damping coefficient in order to improve dynamic performance. However, if the natural frequency is below 7.5 Hz, no alteration in damping coefficient can produce an acceptable signal. Most systems produce an underdamped response, therefore it is important to have as high a natural frequency as possible (at least > 12.5 Hz). This is done by eliminating

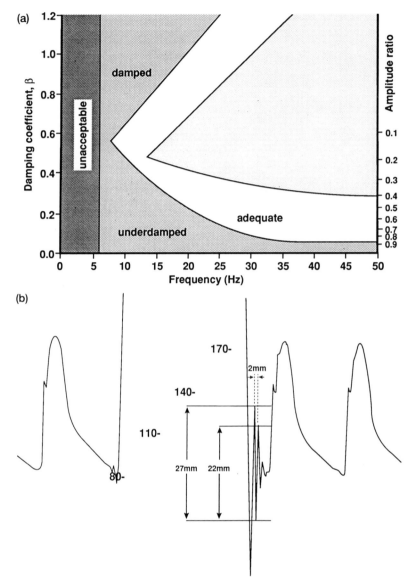

Figure 3.1 (a) Relationship between frequency response and damping coefficient. (b) Example of fastflush test. See text for explanation.

all air bubbles, using short wide catheters, short lengths of non-compliant tubing and ensuring all components have small volume displacements. Commercial devices such as the ROSE or Accudynamic try to compensate for underdamped systems by altering the damping coefficient without decreasing the natural frequency (Allan *et al.*, 1988). The effects of the Accudynamic, and the beneficial effects of using shorter lengths of tubing are shown in Fig. 3.2.

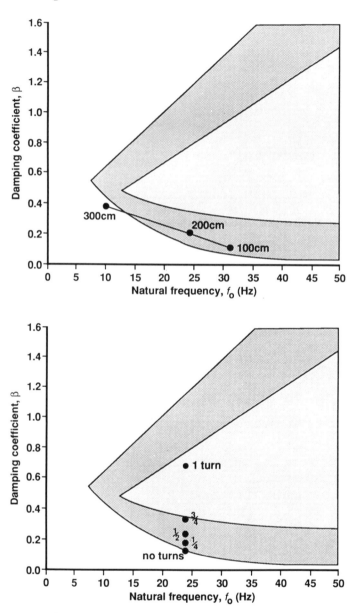

Figure 3.2 Beneficial effects of using shorter tubing and of adjusting the needle valve of the Accudynamic on the dynamic characteristics of a typical pressure monitoring system. (From Allan *et al.*, 1988.)

Occasionally systems become overdamped, usually by the introduction of large air bubbles or clot formation on the catheter, and waveforms become flattened.

Waveform Display

It must be possible to display pressure waveforms at all times, and calibration on-screen should be possible, with the ability to freeze waveforms or obtain hard copy for review. Digital-only displays have serious limitations when pressures are being measured. The numerical display reflects integration over a finite time and may produce erroneous readings, due especially to respiratory variability (Maran, 1980; Raper & Sibbald, 1986).

In the example shown in Fig. 3.3a (Raper & Sibbald, 1986) the marked inspiratory swings in pulmonary artery occlusion pressure are interpreted by the algorithm as part of the pressure wave. Although the true end-expiratory pressure is 20 mm Hg, integration of the pressure signal occurs over a set time period leading to erroneously low values on the digital display, indicated by the dotted line.

The ability to freeze waveforms is especially important when assessing the true end-expiratory point following pulmonary artery occlusion. The sophisticated algorithms built into modern monitors are remarkably good at determining the end-expiratory point, often by sensing the point at which least change in pressure is occurring. This is usually the end-expiratory pause period, but these algorithms may be fooled during spontaneous breathing and reversed I:E ratio ventilation.

In the example shown in Fig. 3.3b of a wedged tracing in a patient on reversed I:E ratio ventilation, the upper dashed line at about 20 mm Hg is where the monitor has determined end expiration to be. This is actually end inspiration, and the lower dotted line indicates the clinicians preferred choice at 14 mm Hg. Other methods of determining end expiration such as measurement of airway pressure or airway thermistors are not in routine clinical use.

Patient Factors

The recording system must not unduly interfere with blood flow or dissipate the pressure generated within the circulation. Mean aortic pressure is the perfusion pressure to the vital organs and is best assessed by having the tip of the arterial catheter in a large artery such as the femoral or brachial. This site also gives optimum waveforms for analysis since distal arteries, such as the radial and dorsalis pedis, overestimate systolic pressure, although mean pressure is accurate (Carroll, 1988). Problems can, however, arise with use of the femoral artery when there is severe atheroma of the aortoiliac vessels. Passage of the Seldinger wire may be impeded and femoral artery pressure may underestimate aortic root pressure, although it may perhaps reflect splanchnic and renal perfusion pressure. The ease of insertion via the femoral artery in shocked patients more than offsets any perceived problems with infection and embolization at this site.

Use of the Pulmonary Artery Flotation Catheter

A legion of complications have been described with the use of the pulmonary artery flotation catheter (PAFC) (Putterman, 1989) (Table 3.1), yet in experienced hands their use is associated with little morbidity and virtually no mortality (Shah *et al.*, 1984).

Table 3.1 Complications associated with pulmonary artery flotation catheters

Associated with venous access
    Pneumothorax
    Air embolization
    Arterial puncture
    Nerve injury
    Thoracic duct injury
    Sepsis
    Thrombosis
Associated with passage of catheter
    Arrhythmias
    Knotting
    Malposition
Associated with the catheter itself
    Balloon rupture
    Catheter disintegration
    Intracardiac trauma
    Pulmonary artery rupture
    Pulmonary infarction
Problems with cardiac output estimations
    Arrhythmias with injection

Insertion of the PAFC

The preferred site of insertion is the right internal jugular vein using a middle or high approach which reduces the risk of pneumothorax and thoracic duct damage, and enables pressure to be applied if there is inadvertent arterial puncture. Bleeding from the subclavian artery is not easily controlled, making subclavian vein puncture by any route a less attractive choice in the critically ill patient. Attempts at bilateral subclavian cannulations are a recipe for disaster.

Insertion of a PAFC is a sterile procedure and a strict aseptic technique must be followed. The skin should be prepared with antiseptic from the mastoid process to the tip of the chin, down the mid-line to the level of the

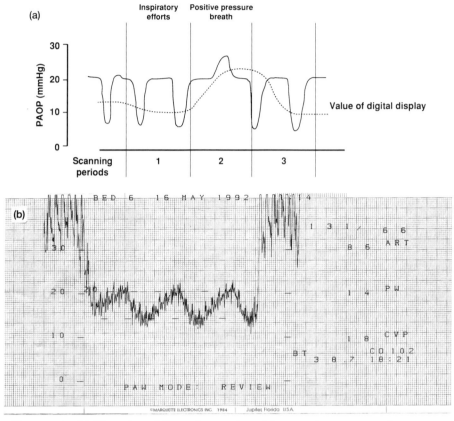

Figure 3.3 (a) The value of direct observation of the waveform compared to acceptance of computer assessment. (Adapted from Raper & Sibbald, 1986.) (b) An example of an actual printout.

nipples and across the chest to the upper arm. If there is failure to obtain access at the preferred site, it is then possible to use another site on the same side. The use of a transparent drape may improve provision of a sterile field.

The pressure monitoring system should be assembled for use as described above. The ECG and digital, if not visual, display of the arterial pressure should be on screen at all times.

Following skin preparation and draping, the PAFC and vascular access kit should be checked. All unused lumens of the PAFC and the side arm of the introducer sheath should have stopcocks attached and be flushed with heparinized saline. A transducer should be connected to the distal lumen and the tip of the catheter placed approximately at heart level to confirm a visible trace and that zeroing is correct. Shaking the catheter up and down should cause the waveform to oscillate rapidly. Take care here to ensure that the waveform on screen is from the distal lumen and not inadvertently a proximal one. Check the balloon inflates before threading it through the concertina sheath, and again afterwards (Fig. 3.4).

Place the patient head down to distend the venous system and reduce the possibility of air embolism. After infiltration of the puncture site with local anaesthetic, locate the internal jugular vein with a small-gauge seeker needle and then perform venepuncture with the introducer needle (some authorities recommend the use of a plastic cannula over needle technique). Venepuncture may be easier when the vein is distended by a positive pressure breath. After venepuncture is confirmed (blood is dark, non-pulsatile and slow flowing, compare PO_2 to arterial sample or transduce the pressure if in doubt), pass the J-shaped guide wire approximately 20 cm. There may be a few ectopic beats if the wire is passed too far but these are rarely troublesome and stop when the wire is pulled back. Remove the introducer needle, leaving the wire in place. Making a stab incision along the track of the wire with a No. 11 scalpel blade to allow the dilator and sheath assembly to be introduced over the wire and into the vein, after which the wire and dilator are removed.

The side arm of the introducer sheath should be aspirated to confirm intravenous placement and then flushed with heparinized saline. Return the patient to the horizontal position for insertion of the PAFC so that accurate pressures will be recorded. The catheter should be passed through

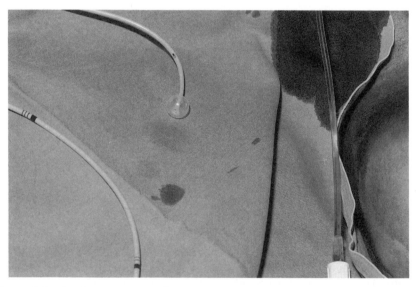

Figure 3.4 A pulmonary artery flotation catheter with ideal balloon inflation characteristics – concentric balloon, patent distal lumen and balloon protecting catheter tip.

the self-sealing membrane in the introducer sheath and far enough to protrude from the sheath, typically 20 cm. The balloon is now fully inflated with the recommended volume of air, usually 1.5 ml. A central venous waveform should be visible on screen with respiratory excursions confirming intrathoracic placement. Continue to feed the catheter until the right ventricle is entered, usually by 25 cm using the right internal jugular approach. If difficulty is experienced in floating the catheter into the right ventricle because of tricuspid regurgitation, then filling the balloon with saline may help (Venus & Mathreu, 1982). No more than 15 cm of catheter should be inserted after entering the right ventricle before a pulmonary artery trace is obtained, otherwise coiling and knotting may occur. This period is frequently associated with ventricular ectopics, but these are seldom serious and rarely require treatment. With the balloon still fully inflated, the catheter is advanced until a wedged trace is obtained, usually before the 50 cm mark on the catheter. The balloon should now be deflated and a pulmonary artery trace should return immediately. If difficulty in entering the pulmonary artery is experienced, then placing the patient in the head up and right lateral position to ensure the pulmonary outflow trace is uppermost may be helpful.

Tighten the self-sealing valve of the introducer sheath to grip the catheter lightly (the concertina sheath on some systems can be tightly secured onto the catheter at its proximal end). The proximal end of the catheter should be taped to the patient to prevent tension developing and any possibility of accidental catheter withdrawal. A chest X-ray must be ordered immediately to confirm the position of the catheter and to rule out a pneumothorax. If necessary, a lateral X-ray may be taken to confirm West zone III conditions as described later (West et al., 1964).

Misinterpretation of Pulmonary Artery Pressure Measurements

Pulmonary artery occlusion pressure (PAOP) monitoring is designed to obtain an indirect estimate of left ventricular (LV) end-diastolic pressure and hence end-diastolic volume. There are numerous assumptions and possible confounding factors which need to be taken into account before this is possible (O'Quin & Marini, 1983; Nadeau & Noble, 1986).

With a balloon occluding a branch of the pulmonary artery, then at the end of diastole when both the aortic and pulmonary valves are closed but the mitral valve is open, there is a continuous uninterrupted column of blood from the left ventricle to the tip of the PAFC. If diastolic time is adequate and there is no impedance to flow, there will be equilibrium of pressures and flow will cease. With the balloon inflated, the tip of the catheter is isolated from fluctuations on the right side of the heart and therefore reflects pulmonary venous pressure. This is assumed to reflect left atrial pressure (LAP) and hence LV end-diastolic pressure.

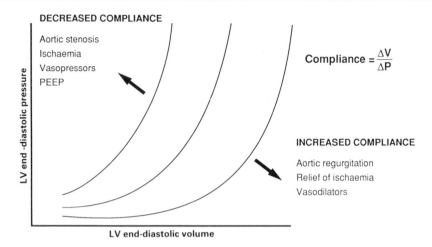

Figure 3.5   Relationship between left ventricular end-diastolic pressure and left ventricular end-diastolic volume.

However, the curvilinear relationship of LV end-diastolic pressure to LV end-diastolic volume is altered by numerous factors in the critically ill patient which alter LV compliance (see Fig. 3.5). LV end-diastolic pressure, does not, therefore, have a constant relationship with LV end-diastolic volume, which is better assessed at the bedside by echocardiography (Raper & Sibbald, 1986).

Use of the pulmonary artery (PA) end-diastolic pressure is rarely acceptable as an index of LV end-diastolic pressure. If diastolic time is short, for instance when there is a tachycardia, full equilibrium of pressures cannot take place and PA end-diastolic pressure tends to increase although LV end-diastolic pressure may fall. If right bundle branch block is present, right ventricular (RV) systole is delayed although pulmonary artery pressure continues to fall during the × descent of the LAP trace as the left atrium relaxes and PA end-diastolic pressure may dip below mean LAP.

Factors such as sepsis, hypercarbia, hypoxia, embolism and chronic lung disease make elevated pulmonary vascular resistance common in ICU patients. The resistance to flow may prolong the time needed for equilibrium, and PA end-diastolic pressure will tend to be greater than LAP. This, of course, will be aggravated by any degree of tachycardia.

Fibrotic, obstructive or neoplastic processes can compress or obliterate pulmonary veins and cause pulmonary artery occlusion pressure (PAOP) to exceed LAP by reducing equilibration time. Remember that wedge pressure reflects pulmonary venous pressure not capillary pressure, and that if equilibration does occur there can still be a high capillary pressure despite a normal wedge pressure if pulmonary venous resistance is elevated.

Local variations in the pulmonary circulation have been described in patients with chronic lung disease (Henriquez *et al.*, 1988). If an unexpectedly abnormal value is found, this may reflect an abnormal area of circulation and wedging at a different site should be attempted.

Any condition which reduces flow through the mitral valve such as stenosis, presence of artificial valves or left atrial myxoma will delay the equilibration of pressures and PAOP will overestimate LV end-diastolic pressure.

Mitral regurgitation may also lead to misrepresentation of LV end-diastolic pressure. The *v* wave of the left atrial trace is produced during LV contraction. In mitral regurgitation, large *v* waves may occur and these may actually appear on the pulmonary artery trace as a second hump. During wedging, the pulmonary artery contour is lost but the large *v* wave may remain visible, as demonstrated in Fig. 3.6. If this is not recognized as an atrial waveform, it may appear that wedging has not occurred and predispose to pulmonary artery rupture. In these circumstances, LV end-diastolic pressure is most accurately estimated by the height of the *a* wave, not the mean PAOP or height of the *v* wave, since atrial ejection into a stiff left ventricle can significantly raise LV end-diastolic pressure. It is precisely in this type of circumstance that visual confirmation of waveforms is so essential.

Although mitral regurgitation is the commonest cause of *v* waves greater than 10 mm Hg, these are neither sensitive nor specific for the presence of severe mitral regurgitation (Fuchs *et al.*, 1982). The presence of *v* waves is related to the compliance of the left atrium, its volume at the start of atrial filling, and the volume of blood entering the atrium during the period of filling. An increase in pulmonary venous inflow, as seen with large left to

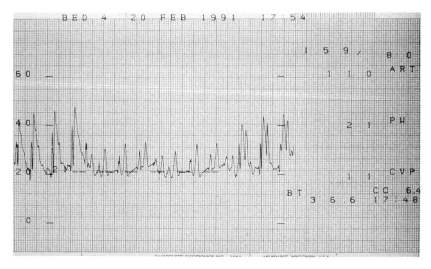

Figure 3.6 Example of giant *v* during wedging of pulmonary artery flotation catheter.

right shunts, may lead to v waves. Mitral stenosis may lead to poor atrial compliance and predispose to large v waves, although angiographic evidence of mitral regurgitation may be absent. Overdamping may prevent recognition of large v waves on the wedge trace, or may lead to the misinterpretation of the damped pulmonary arterial trace for a wedged trace.

LV end-diastolic pressure can be higher than PAOP when there is regurgitant flow from the aorta into the left ventricle. The regurgitant flow causes premature closure of the mitral valve but further ventricular filling continues from the aorta and LV end-diastolic pressure increases. This pressure, however, is not transmitted back to the pulmonary vascular bed since the mitral valve is closed.

Pulmonary Artery Occlusion Pressure and Ventilation

The lungs can be divided arbitrarily into three zones as shown in Fig. 3.7a (West *et al.*, 1964). Even under skilled supervision pulmonary artery flotation catheters may not be placed in the optimum position (Fig. 3.7b) as shown in the following clinical situations (Fig. 3.7c–f). In zone I, alveolar pressure is greater than both pulmonary arterial and venous pressure, a catheter wedged in zone I will reflect alveolar pressure. In zone II, pulmonary arterial pressure is greater than alveolar pressure, but alveolar pressure is greater than pulmonary venous pressure. Again the measured wedge pressure will not reflect LAP since alveolar pressure will collapse the surrounding vessels at some point between their arterial and venous ends, the so-called 'Starling resistor'. Only in zone III, where pulmonary artery and pulmonary venous pressures are greater than alveolar pressure will an uninterrupted column of blood be present between the tip of the catheter and the left atrium. Only zone III conditions are suitable for measurement of pulmonary artery wedge pressure (see Table 3.2). If there is any doubt as to the position of the PAFC, a lateral chest X-ray can be taken to confirm that

Table 3.2   Criteria to ensure zone III conditions

1   The wedged tracing should demonstrate *a* and *v* waves.
2   Atrials waves should disappear promptly with balloon deflation to show a pulmonary arterial trace.
3   Excessive respiratory swings should not be present.
4   Mean PAOP must be less than or equal to PA end-diastolic pressure, and less than mean pulmonary artery pressure. (Remember the presence of large *v* waves may elevate the PĀP.)
5   Catheter tip obstruction should be excluded by a fast flush and easy aspiration of blood.
6   In the wedged position, aspiration of highly oxygenated blood should be obtained with no less than 10 mm Hg (1.3 kPa) difference between wedged PO_2 and arterial PO_2. However, incomplete arterialization of the sample may occur when the catheter tip is in a low $\dot{V}/\dot{Q}$ area.

the tip is at or below the level of the left atrium in the supine position. Fluorscopy may be preferable since the tip of the PAFC may move during wedging.

Since the pulmonary artery catheter is flow-directed it normally wedges in zone III, usually at the right base. However, zone III can be converted into zone II or even zone I conditions by positional changes, hypovolaemia, and ventilator therapy especially if positive end-expiratory pressure (PEEP) is used or intrinsic PEEP (Pepe and Marini, 1982) develops. An aid to whether zone I or II conditions are present can be obtained by review of the pulmonary artery and wedge pressure traces. Respiratory swings are normally

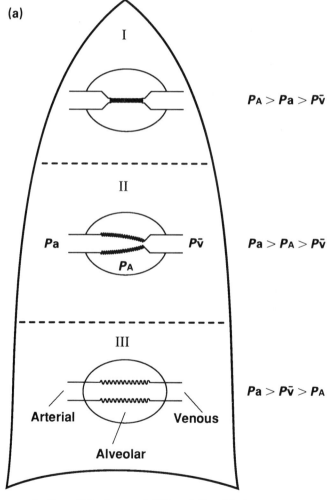

(a)

I

$P_A > Pa > P\bar{v}$

II

Pa $P\bar{v}$

P_A

$Pa > P_A > P\bar{v}$

III

$Pa > P\bar{v} > P_A$

Arterial   Venous

Alveolar

Figure 3.7 (a) Demonstration of West zones I–III in relationship to measurement of pulmonary artery wedge pressure. (b) Chest X-ray of catheter in correct position. (c)–(f) Incorrect positions of pulmonary artery flotation catheters.

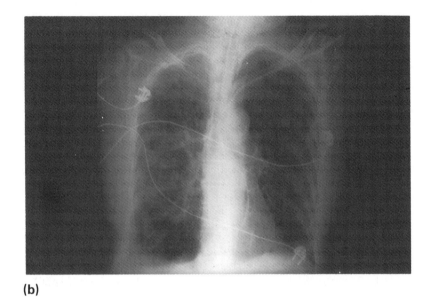

(b)

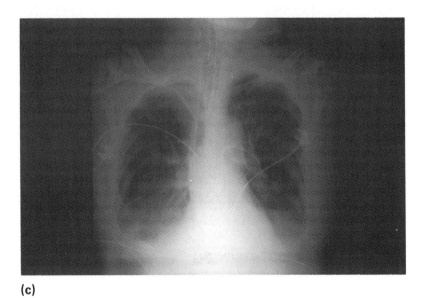

(c)

Figure 3.7   Continued.

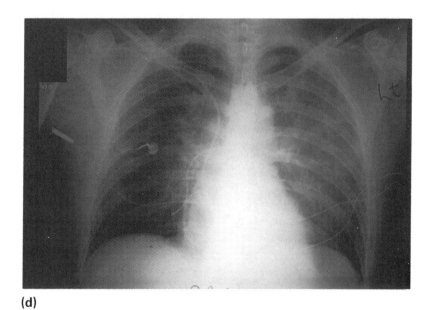

(d)

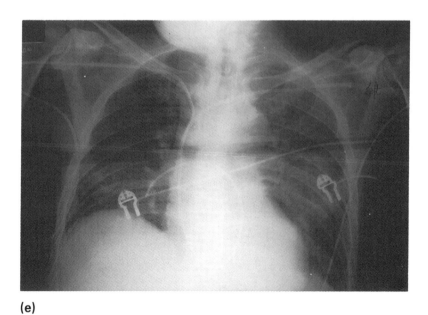

(e)

Figure 3.7 Continued.

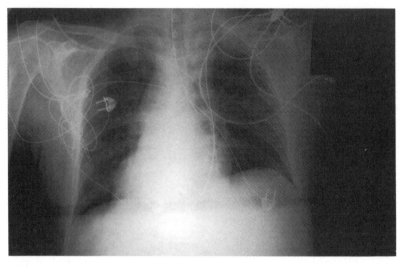

(f)

Figure 3.7 Continued.

seen on the pulmonary artery trace during positive pressure ventilation. If the height of the respiratory swing on the wedged trace is greater than on the pulmonary artery trace then zone III conditions are unlikely (Teboul *et al.*, 1992).

Figure 3.8 shows marked positive pressure fluctuations in the wedged trace, compared to the minimal respiratory swing on the pulmonary artery trace, in an asthmatic patient with a high level of intrinsic PEEP.

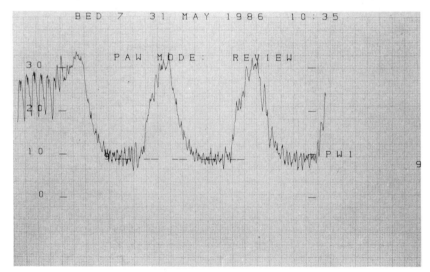

Figure 3.8 A clinical example of wide variations in wedge pressure of a patient being mechanically ventilated.

Wedge pressures should be taken at end expiration in both spontaneously breathing and mechanically ventilated patients. It is generally recommended that PEEP is not removed since cardiorespiratory status may be altered by the sudden decrease in mean intrathoracic pressure. Hypervolaemia may occur in the central vessels, and there may be deleterious effects on oxygenation. However, the effect of a short disconnect during wedging to determine the effect of PEEP on the wedge pressure has been described (Carter et al., 1985). The nadir pressure was reached within 2 s. In post-operative patients (Pinsky et al., 1991), there were no deleterious effects on oxygenation, and although this technique can be criticized we have occasionally found it useful.

Although intravascular pressures are usually measured with reference to atmospheric pressure, true intravascular pressure is the difference between the intravascular pressure and surrounding tissues, the transmural pressure. Extravascular pressure is often assumed to equal pleural pressure, but only if pleural pressure equals atmospheric at end expiration will a true intravascular pressure be obtained. Because of the presence of intrinsic PEEP (Pepe and Marini, 1982), which is rarely measured routinely, and applied PEEP, which has a variable degree of transmission to the pulmonary vascular bed, it is not possible to say that airway pressure at end expiration is an accurate reflection of pleural pressure. Pleural pressure can be measured by inserting catheters into the pleural space and oesophagus although pleural catheters are not in routine use because of the potential hazards, and oesophageal balloons have been only considered reliable in the lateral position. It is possible to get accurate estimates of pleural pressure by varying the oesophageal balloon position and use of an occlusion test (Higgs et al., 1983) but in clinical practice it is frequently not possible to assess true transmural pressure, and patient management must be guided by intravascular wedge pressure measurements with an appreciation of their limitations.

Although PEEP can alter cardiac transmural pressure, the degree of transmission of pleural pressure to the heart will depend critically on lung compliance. In severe adult respiratory distress syndrome (ARDS), PEEP may not necessarily affect PAOP estimation or LV end-diastolic pressure measurements (Teboul et al., 1989). Zapol and co-workers found that PEEP up to 30 cm H_2O did not affect vascular pressure measurements in patients with ARDS and very poor lung compliance (Zapol & Snider, 1977). If the tip of the PAFC is not below the left atrium, then PEEP, especially if associated with hypovolaemia, will frequently lead to non-zone III conditions (Shasby et al., 1980). In normal lungs, if the wedge pressure increases more than half of the applied increment of PEEP, then zone III conditions are unlikely (O'Quin & Marini, 1983), but simple formulae such as this may be unreliable in lung injury and disease because of regional variations in lung compliance.

A major problem, often not appreciated by clinicians, is that cardiac filling pressures bear virtually no relationship to blood volume, except at the extremes, as shown in Fig. 3.9 (Shippy et al., 1984).

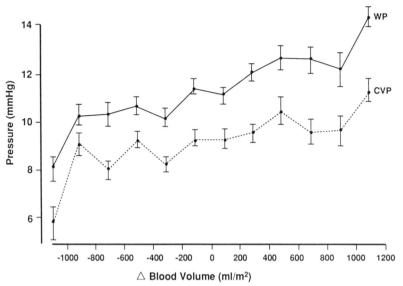

Figure 3.9   Relationship between circulating blood volume and cardiac filling pressures.

Estimation of Cardiac Output

The accurate and reproducible measurement of cardiac output by the thermodilution technique forms the basis of the routine application of oxygen transport principles in the ICU. Although the direct Fick method is often referred to as the gold standard, in clinical practice there is no such thing (Taylor & Silke, 1988) since the conditions under which this method is accurate are difficult to achieve.

Thermodilution techniques applied to flow-directed pulmonary artery catheters with thermistors (Ganz *et al.*, 1971) allowed the use of cold water as the indicator and revolutionized the clinical application of cardiac output measurement. Only by an adequate understanding of the theory and assumptions behind the measurements can potential problems be recognized and averted. The Stewart–Hamilton equation is used to calculate cardiac output by the thermodilution technique:

$$\text{cardiac output} = Vi \times \frac{(Tb - Ti)}{\int_0^\infty \Delta Tb(t)\,dt} \times \frac{(Si \times Ci)}{(Sb \times Cb)} \times 60 \times k$$

where Vi = volume injected; Tb = temperature of blood; Ti = temperature of injectate; Si = specific gravity of injectate; Sb = specific gravity of blood; Ci = specific heat of injectate; Cb = specific heat of blood; and k = correction factor for loss of indicator during transit. The error associated with the manufacturers' calibration is $< 5\%$.

For constant injectate type, catheter type and length, rate of injection plus correction for other variables such as haematocrit and protein concentration, the equation can be simplified to:

$$\text{cardiac output} = K \times Vi \times \frac{(Tb - Ti)}{\text{AUC}}$$

where K = constant provided by the manufacturer and AUC = the area under the temperature curve.

It can be seen that a small curve will indicate a high cardiac output and vice versa. The Stewart–Hamilton equation can also be rearranged into the following form:

$$\text{cardiac output} = k' \times \frac{(Ti - Tb)}{\int_{0}^{\infty}(Tt - Tb)dt}$$

where k' = a constant and Tt = catheter tip temperature over time.

If the injectate is at room temperature, then there will be little loss of thermal indicator, but reference to the equation shows that the signal-to-noise ratio will be much greater if the injectate temperature is maximally separated from the blood temperature. This will reduce variability in cardiac output measurements which may be important if cardiac output is high. It can also be seen that any variation in the baseline blood temperature, Tb, will predominantly affect the value of the denominator of the equation since Tt and Tb are similar, whilst the value of Ti is further from Tb. This assumes importance since even small fluctuations in blood temperature, for instance due to rapid fluid infusion, may affect the accuracy of cardiac output estimations (Wetzel & Latson, 1985). Variations in cardiac output due to this cause will not be apparent unless the baseline temperature is displayed and cardiac output computers should warn if the baseline is unstable.

Accurate and reproducible cardiac output estimations require the patient to be in a relatively steady state. There are numerous potential problems in clinical practice. Arousal, due to pain, discomfort or from interventions such as physiotherapy, can alter tissue oxygen demand and hence cardiac output.

Alterations in cardiac rhythm such as atrial fibrillation or multiple ectopic beats will lead to variations in cardiac output over short periods.

In tricuspid regurgitation, the curve is splayed and cardiac output may read low or not record adequately. Although some authors have not found tricuspid regurgitation to be a major problem (Kashtan et al., 1987), it may lead to problems with measurement of right ventricular ejection fraction (Spinale et al., 1992).

Intracardiac shunts alter thermodilution cardiac output readings, with overestimation of cardiac output when there are left-to-right shunts, and underestimation when there are right-to-left shunts.

In practice, inject at a steady rate to ensure the ratio of volume of indicator to volume of blood is relatively constant. For a volume of 10 ml, the injection should be completed in 4 s or less, 5 ml in 3 s and 3 ml in 1 s. Automated systems are available but not in routine widespread use. Inject as near to the patient as possible to minimize indicator loss. The use of an in-line probe will ensure that the true indicator temperature is recorded; do not assume the iced injectate is at 0°C. Studies where volume and temperature of injectate have been varied show that compared to 10 ml of iced injectate at 0°C, the use of 10 ml at room temperature or 5 ml at 0°C gives comparable reproducibility. Use of 5 ml at room temperature and 3 ml at 0°C produced unacceptable variability, although overall the errors introduced were small (Pearl et al., 1986).

In patients of short stature, the use of a standard sized introducer sheath may mean that the injectate port lies within the sheath. This will lead to a spuriously high central venous pressure and inaccurate cardiac output estimations (Stoller et al., 1986). Shorter introducer sheaths are available from some manufacturers.

Cardiac output curves should be rejected if there is any inflection on the down slope, any obvious baseline drift or respiratory or cardiac perturbations. Approximately 10% of curves will be found to be unsatisfactory; this emphasizes the need for a graphical display and review of the curve. Curves which are broad with a slow upstroke may represent tricuspid incompetence, and those with a prolonged downstroke may represent rapid recirculation or left-to-right shunts. Some recirculation will, of course, occur via the coronary arteries and may account for the usual underestimation of thermodilution cardiac output by about 7% compared to dye dilution cardiac output.

Always remember that equipment set-up errors, such as selecting the wrong catheter size or injectate volume, can lead to varying degrees of inaccuracy.

The effect of respiratory efforts on cardiac function can be complex. If ventilator asynchrony exists, then loading conditions on the heart will vary on a breath by breath basis and make interpretation of individual cardiac output recordings difficult. Respiratory variation in pulmonary blood flow is not a problem when using indocyanine green as an indicator, since the lungs have a capacitive effect and sampling is from a systemic artery over more than one respiratory cycle. Thermodilution cardiac output computers calculate over much shorter periods, typically less than one respiratory cycle, and show marked respiratory variability (Jansen et al., 1990). Injections started at peak inspiration or end expiration gave results with the least variability (Stevens et al., 1985). Random injections spaced evenly throughout the respiratory cycle would give a truer integrated cardiac output but are technically more demanding. Cardiac output estimations would have greater than 10% variability, but the values should not be discarded if the curve is acceptable, since they probably reflect real changes. For a complete assessment of the integrated cardiac output, four injections spread equally over the respiratory cycle are recommended (Jansen & Versprille, 1986). In practice, most clinicians have concentrated on improving reproducibility and utilize end-expiratory calculations by starting the injections at the end of inspiration, although others inject at the end of expiration. Whichever technique is chosen, consistency between operators is important. Generally the random error of a single measurement should be no more than 5–8%.

Calculation of Derived Variables

The most frequent calculations are those of stroke volume index (SVI), left and right ventricular stroke work index (SWI), and systemic vascular resistance (SVR). Calculation of pulmonary vascular resistance (PVR) has an unsound physiological basis since the pulmonary circulation is distensible, recruitable, and flow is predominantly pulsatile.

Haemodynamic and oxygen transport variables are indexed to body surface area (BSA) which should be accurately determined from the patient's height, using a tape measure, and weight, by use of a weigh bed or sling assembly. Standard formulae exist to calculate BSA which is usually done automatically by the monitor. Errors can be introduced even at this stage and the BSA calculation should be confirmed as feasible before derived variables are reviewed.

All of the more common equations used for cardio respiratory calculations are given in Appendix 2.

It can be seen that errors in central venous pressure (CVP) measurement affect calculated SVR and RVSWI, and that errors in PAOP measurement will affect calculated PVR and LVSWI. Errors in cardiac output measurement will affect calculations of SVI, SVR, PVR, RVSWI and LVSWI.

When perusing a set of measured and derived haemodynamic data, obvious errors in derived variables can alert one to basic errors. For instance, in Table 3.3 RVSWI in set 1 is negative, an obvious error due to false measurements of the direct variables. Since RVSWI involves mean pulmonary artery pressure (P̄AP), CVP and cardiac output measurements, we should look at these. Indeed we see that the CVP is high due to the rapid administration of fluids through the PAFC introducer sheath (note also the low calculated SVR). When the infusion was stopped, the CVP fell to 21 mm Hg and the erroneous RVSWI and SVR calculations were corrected, set 2.

Although the equation for SVR includes CVP, this can lead to nonsensical values when CVP is high and mean arterial pressure (M̄AP) is low. In right ventricular infarction with shock, if M̄AP is 50 mm Hg and CVP is 20 mm Hg when cardiac output is 3 litres min^{-1}, then calculated SVR = 800 dynes s cm^{-5} implying vasodilation, unlikely in cardiogenic shock. This emphasizes that measured variables, not derived ones, should be the target of therapeutic interventions.

Another common problem that produces errors is flushing of pressure lines during calculations performed by the bedside monitor.

The SVR is frequently quoted as an index of left ventricular afterload. Afterload may be defined as impedance to flow and depends upon the mass

Table 3.3 An example of artifactual errors in the calculation of derived variables (possibly one of the most common traps for the intensivist)

	Set 1	Set 2
Directly measured values		
Cardiac output	9.2	9.2
Mean arterial pressure	101	99
Heart rate	82	83
Central venous pressure	46	21
PAM	37	37
PAW	18	18
Indirectly calculated values		
Cardiac index	4.5	4.5
Stroke volume	112	111
Stroke volume index	55	54
Systemic vascular resistance	478	678
Pulmonary vascular resistance	165	165
Left ventricular stroke work index	62	60
Right ventricular stroke work index	−6	12

Definitions of the values and the calculations can be found in the appendices at the end of the book.

and viscosity of the blood ejected, the distensibility of the great vessels and peripheral arteriolar tone. True left ventricular afterload is represented by end-systolic wall stress. As well as reflecting peripheral loading conditions, end-systolic wall stress depends on ventricular chamber pressure, dimensions and wall thickness. The SVR at best gives some estimate of peripheral arterial tone. In canine experiments where haemodynamic changes were induced by vasoactive agents, SVR underestimated changes in left ventricular end-systolic wall stress by up to 54%. With infusion of noradrenaline, SVR increased by 21% but left ventricular end-systolic wall stress fell by 9%, confirming the important contribution of geometric changes in the left ventricle (Lang *et al.*, 1986).

Blood-Gas Measurements

Quality assurance programmes in the ICU satellite laboratory ensure calibration and maintenance procedures are performed, and monitor accuracy and reproducibility of measurements (Clausen & Murray, 1985). It is essential that accurate measurements of PaO_2 and $PaCO_2$ are obtained for calculation of respiratory and oxygen transport variables. An acceptable limit for reproducibility of PO_2 and PCO_2 measurements is ± 3 mm Hg (0.4 kPa). Precision of measurements is more difficult to establish. Many quality control solutions are unsuitable for clinical practice, especially PO_2 standards because the low oxygen content and buffering ability make them susceptible to contamination and temperature changes. Accepted limits for precision are 3% for PCO_2 and 4% for PO_2.

Blood Sampling and Transport of Specimens

Accurate estimation of blood gases and haemoglobin requires careful attention to sampling procedure. All dead space must be removed from the system. Typically this will be 4 ml for an arterial line (Clapham *et al.*, 1987) and 5 ml for samples taken through the distal port of the PAFC. In view of the potential blood loss from repeated samples, take no more than is necessary for analysis; typically 2 ml will be sufficient for the various bedside analysers to be found in the ICU. Sampling from the PAFC should be done over 30 s to minimize arterialization of the specimen which would give a spuriously high $S\bar{v}O_2$ and calculated shunt fraction. Ensure there is a pulmonary artery trace before and after sampling. If the $P\bar{v}CO_2$ is $\leq PaCO_2$ then contamination by pulmonary capillary blood should be suspected (Shapiro *et al.*, 1974).

Heparin added to a syringe should not comprise more than 10% of the final volume. Dilution of blood samples with heparin leads to reductions in PCO_2 and calculated bicarbonate, although there is little change in PO_2 and pH until 40% of the sample volume is heparin (Hutchinson *et al.*, 1983). Avoid excess heparin by use of preheparinized syringes, otherwise use heparin 1000 iu ml^{-1} to lubricate the syringe and expel as much as possible. With a 2-ml syringe this will leave 0.1 ml in the dead space (5% of sample volume and final concentration of 50 iu ml^{-1}).

Remove any froth and large air bubbles to reduce diffusion in or out of the sample, then seal the syringe. A large bubble or froth will lead to a significant change of PO_2 within 2 min and of PCO_2 within 3 min. Requirements for pH are less exacting, no significant change was seen after 5 min (Biswas *et al.*, 1982).

Samples for blood-gas analysis should be assayed on the ICU immediately (Biswas *et al.*, 1982). If a delay of 10 min or more is expected the samples should be stored on ice to reduce metabolism by blood components. PO_2 can change significantly within 20 min in samples kept at room temperature but does not change significantly for up to 30 min if kept at 0°C by surrounding with crushed ice. However, in patients with extremely high white cell counts ($> 50\,000$) this will not prevent a fall in PO_2 unless metabolism is arrested totally (Fox *et al.*, 1979).

The pH, PCO_2 and calculated bicarbonate did not change significantly for up to 30 min at room temperature in one study (Biswas *et al.*, 1982).

Since oxygen can diffuse through plastic, glass syringes are recommended if blood samples are small, if PO_2 is very high or very low, and especially if haemoglobin is low since buffering capacity is reduced.

Clinicians are notoriously optimistic about the fractional percentage of oxygen that they believe patients are receiving. Since calculation of alveolar PO_2 depends on the FiO_2, and oxygenation indices utilizing PaO_2 are in clinical use, this is not merely academic. With a standard type of face mask and a fresh gas glow of 15 litres min^{-1} it is unusual to exceed 50% inspired oxygen in a patient who is dyspnoeic (Gibson *et al.*, 1976).

The Use of the Cooximeter

Arterial and mixed venous oxygen contents may be measured directly or calculated from measurements of haemoglobin and oxyhaemoglobin saturation (Willis & Clapham, 1985). Direct measurement of oxygen content is not usual clinically, but would avoid problems caused by changes in the shape of the oxyhaemoglobin dissociation curve, which are common in the critically ill, or by debates over which value should be used for the Hufner factor (millilitres of oxygen combining with 1 g of haemoglobin, typically 1.39).

Saturation may be measured, or estimated from the oxygen tension. Because of marked variability in the shape of the oxyhaemoglobin dissociation curve in ICU patients, saturations estimated from oxygen tensions, even when temperature, CO_2 and pH compensated, can be inaccurate (Willis & Clapham, 1985) since there is no compensation for 2,3-diphosphoglycerate level. Estimation of oxygen content from calculated saturation can be extremely inaccurate on the mixed venous sample which lies on the steep part of the oxyhaemoglobin dissociation curve and only measured saturations should be used to calculate oxygen content.

Measurement of oxyhaemoglobin saturation should use a spectrophotometric method with multiple wavelengths so that the presence of abnormal haemoglobin species can be detected. These must be taken into account during calculation of oxygen contents. When arterial and mixed venous blood samples are inserted into modern blood-gas analysers which incorporate or interface with cooximeters, indices of pulmonary function such as cardiac shunt fraction ($\dot{Q}s/\dot{Q}T$) may be calculated. Failure of the equations used to derive end-capillary oxygen content to account for all haemoglobin species may lead to erroneous estimations of shunt fraction. The cooximeter data should be checked to ensure a normal distribution of haemoglobin species before the cardaic shunt fraction is accepted.

Haemoglobin levels must be close on both arterial and mixed venous samples or else errors from calculated oxygen contents will occur. A common problem is failure to agitate the samples between analyses. Sedimentation occurs with streaming during aspiration of the sample, leading to variability in haemoglobin levels.

The mixed venous sample must be taken from the pulmonary artery. Although the oxyhaemoglobin saturation of samples taken from the vena cavae and right atrium may correlate with those taken from the pulmonary artery, the 95% confidence limits are so wide that these sites should not be used for calculation of mixed venous oxygen content. The normal relationship of saturations between these sites also changes in seriously ill patients (Lee et al., 1972).

Summary and Recommendations

With careful attention to measurement procedures, haemoglobin levels and oxyhaemoglobin saturation can be used to estimate arterial and mixed venous oxygen content accurately.

Similarly, systemic and pulmonary arterial pressures, cardiac filling pressures, thermodilution cardiac output and derived haemodynamic variables can be obtained accurately enough for clinical use.

Furthermore, these measurements can be used to estimate $\dot{D}O_2$ and $\dot{V}O_2$ and to allow rational manipulation of oxygen transport variables. These should, however, be interpreted carefully in the light of the known limitations of the estimations.

References

Allan MWB, Gray WM & Asbury AJ (1988) Measurement of arterial pressure using catheter-transducer systems. Improvement using the Accudynamic. *Br. J. Anaesth.* **60:** 413–18.

Bennett D, Boldt J, Brochard L *et al.* (1991) The use of the pulmonary artery catheter. *Intensive Care Med.* **17:** I–VIII.

Biswas CK, Ramos JM, Agroyannis B & Kerr DNS (1982) Blood gas analysis: effect of air bubbles in syringe and delay in estimation. *Br Med. J.* **284:** 923–7.

Carroll GC (1988) Blood pressure monitoring. *Crit. Care Clin.* **4:** 411–34.

Carter RS, Snyder JV & Pinsky MR (1985) LV filling pressure during PEEP measured by nadir wedge pressure after airway disconnection. *Am. J. Physiol.* **249** (*Heart Circ. Physiol.* 18)**:** 770–6.

Clapham MCC, Willis N & Mapleson WW (1987) Minimum volume of discard for valid blood sampling from indwelling arterial cannulae. *Br. J. Anaesth.* **59:** 232–5.

Clausen JL & Murray KM (1985) Clinical applications of arterial blood gases: How much accuracy do we need? *J. Med. Technol.* **2:** 19–21.

Fox MJ, Brody JS, Weintraub LR *et al.* (1979) Leukocyte larceny: A cause of spurious hypoxemia. *Am. J. Med.* **67:** 742–6.

Fuchs RM, Heuser RR, Yin FCP & Brinker JA (1982) Limitations of pulmonary wedge v waves in diagnosing mitral regurgitation. *Am. J. Cardiol.* **49:** 849–954.

Ganz W, Donoso R, Marcus HS *et al.* (1971) A new technique for measurement of cardiac output by thermodilution in man. *Am. J. Cardiol.* **27:** 392–6.

Gardner RM (1981) Direct blood pressure measurement – dynamic response requirements. *Anesthesiology* **54:** 227–36.

Gardner RM (1986) Hemodynamic monitoring: From catheter to display. *Acute Care* **12:** 3–33.

Gibson RL, Comer PB, Beckham RW & McGraw CP (1976) Actual tracheal oxygen concentrations with commonly used oxygen equipment. *Anesthesiology* **44:** 71–3.

Henriquez AH, Schrijen FV, Redondo J & Delorme N (1988) Local variations of pulmonary arterial wedge pressure and wedge angiograms in patients with chronic lung disease. *Chest* **94**: 491–5.

Herbert WH (1970) Pulmonary artery and left heart end-diastolic pressure relations. *Br. Heart J.* **32**: 774–8.

Higgs BD, Behrakis PK, Bevan DR & Milic-Emili J (1983) Measurement of pleural pressure with esophageal balloon in anesthetized humans. *Anesthesiology* **59**: 340–3.

Hutchinson AS, Ralston SH, Dryburgh FJ *et al.* (1983) Too much heparin: possible source of error in blood gas analysis. *Br. Med. J.* **287**: 1131–2.

Jansen JRC & Versprille A (1986) Improvement of cardiac output estimation by the thermodilution method during mechanical ventilation. *Intensive Care Med.* **12**: 71–9.

Jansen JRC, Schreuder JJ, Settels JJ *et al.* (1990) An adequate strategy for the thermodilution technique in patients during mechanical ventilation. *Intensive Care Med.* **16**: 422–5.

Kashtan HI, Maitland A, Salerno TA *et al.* (1987) Effects of tricuspid regurgitation on thermodilution cardiac output: studies in an animal model. *Can. J. Anaesth.* **34**: 246–51.

Lang RM, Borow KM, Neumann A & Janzen D (1986) Systemic vascular resistance: an unreliable index of left ventricular afterload. *Circulation* **74**: 1114–23.

Lee J, Wright F, Barber R & Stanley L (1972) Central venous oxygen saturations in shock: a study in man. *Anesthesiology* **36**: 472–8.

Maran AG (1980) Variables in pulmonary capillary wedge pressure: variation with intrathoracic pressure, graphic and digital recorders. *Crit. Care Med.* **8**: 102–5.

Nadeau S & Noble WH (1986) Misinterpretation of pressure measurements from the pulmonary artery catheter. *Can. Anaesth. Soc. J.* **33**: 352–63.

O'Quin R & Marini JJ (1983) Pulmonary artery occlusion pressure: Clinical physiology, measurement, and interpretation. *Am. Rev. Respiratory Dis.* **128**: 319–26.

Pearl RG, Rosenthal MH, Nielson *et al.* (1986) Effect of injectate volume and temperature on thermodilution cardiac output determination *Anesthesiology* **64**: 798–801.

Pepe PE & Marini JJ (1982) Occult positive end-expiratory pressure in mechanically ventilated patients with airflow obstruction. *Am. Rev. Respiratory Dis.* **126**: 166–70.

Pinsky M, Vincent J-L & De Smet J-M (1991) Estimating left ventricular filling pressure during positive end-expiratory pressure in humans. *Am. Rev. Respiratory Dis.* **143**: 25–31.

Putterman C (1989) The Swan–Ganz catheter: a decade of hemodynamic monitoring *J. Crit. Care* **4**: 127–46.

Raper R & Sibbald WJ (1986) Misled by the wedge? The Swan–Ganz catheter and left ventricular preload. *Chest* **89**: 427–34.

Shah KB, Rao TLK, Laughlin S & El-Etr AA (1984) A review of pulmonary artery catheterization in 6,245 patients. *Anesthesiology* **61**: 271–5.

Shapiro HM, Smith G, Pribble AH *et al*. (1974) Errors in sampling pulmonary arterial blood with a Swan–Ganz catheter. *Anesthesiology* **40:** 291–5.

Shasby DM, Dauber IM, Pfister S *et al*. (1980) Swan–Ganz catheter location and left atrial pressure determine the accuracy of the wedge pressure when positive end-expiratory pressure is used. *Chest* **80:** 666–70.

Shippy CR, Appel PL & Shoemaker WC (1984) Reliability of clinical monitoring to assess blood volume in critically ill patients. *Crit. Care Med.* **12:** 107–12.

Spinale FG, Mukherjee R, Tanaka R & Zile MR (1992) The effects of valvular regurgitation on thermodilution ejection fraction measurements. *Chest* **101:** 723–31.

Stevens JH, Raffin TA, Mihm FG *et al*. (1985) Thermodilution cardiac output measurement. Effects of the respiratory cycle on its reproducibility. *J. Am. Med. Assoc.* **253:** 2240–2.

Stoller JK, Herbst TJ, Hurford W & Rie MA (1986) Spuriously high cardiac output from injecting thermal indicator through an ensheathed port. *Crit. Care Med.* **14:** 1064–5.

Taylor SH & Silke B (1988) Is the measurement of cardiac output useful in clinical practice? *Br. J. Anaesth.* **60:** 90S–8S.

Teboul J-L, Zapol WM, Brun-Buisson C *et al*. (1989) A comparison of pulmonary artery occlusion pressure and left ventricular end-diastolic pressure during mechanical ventilation with PEEP in patients with severe ARDS. *Anesthesiology* **70:** 261–6.

Teboul J-L, Besbes M, Andrivet P *et al*. (1992) A bedside index assessing the reliability of pulmonary artery occlusion pressure measurements during mechanical ventilation with positive end-expiratory pressure. *J. Crit. Care* **7:** 22–9.

Venus B & Mathreu M (1982) A maneuver for bedside pulmonary artery catheterization in patients with right heart failure. *Chest* **6:** 803–4.

West JB, Dollery CT & Naimark A (1964) Distribution of blood flow in isolated lung: relation to vascular and alveolar pressures. *J. Appl. Physiol.* **19:** 713–24.

Wetzel RC & Latson TW (1985) Major errors in thermodilution cardiac output measurement during rapid volume infusion. *Anesthesiology* **62:** 684–7.

Willis N & Clapham M (1985) The validity of oxygen content calculations. *Clin. Chim. Acta* **150:** 213–20.

Zapol WM & Snider MT (1977) Pulmonary hypertension in severe acute respiratory failure. *New Engl. J. Med.* **296:** 476–80.

4 Haemodynamic and Oxygen Transport Patterns in Shock: Pathophysiology, Monitoring, Outcome Prediction and Therapy

William C. Shoemaker

Introduction

Problems in Diagnosis

Shock, which is a syndrome or symptom complex, is recognized clinically by subjective symptoms and signs such as cold clammy skin, altered mental status, weak thready pulse, and unstable vital signs. Unfortunately, therapeutic management is also based on these subjective and imprecise evaluations.

Traditionally, shock is classified by aetiology, such as haemorrhagic, cardiogenic, traumatic and septic shock syndromes. These aetiologic categories are described by clinical signs and symptoms, laboratory findings and primary pathophysiologic derangements; therapy based on this approach has been developed for each aetiology of shock. This approach is simple, easily understood and generally accepted, but seriously misleading. The real problem is that this one-dimensional approach proposes simplistic one-dimensional therapy for complex problems.

In practice, each primary aetiologic event does not begin and end with a single pathophysiologic defect that when therapeutically corrected leads to survival. Rather, the primary precipitating event of each aetiologic type of shock stimulates neurohormonal compensatory reactions as well as numerous cascades that activate various biochemical mediators and inflammatory responses. Irrespective of the initiating event, there are concomitant interacting circulatory changes in volume, pressure, flow and oxygen transport that lead to tissue hypoxia, organ failure and death. The sequential pattern of changes is key to the separation of primary events from secondary reactions and their consequences (Wiggers, 1940; Cournand *et al.*, 1943; Clowes & Del Guercio, 1960; Heilbrunn & Allbritten, 1960; Del Guercio *et al.*, 1964; Wilson *et al.*, 1965; Shoemaker *et al.*, 1967, 1971, 1973, 1979, 1985, 1988a,b, 1992; Siegel *et al.*, 1971; Lowe & Ernst, 1981; Bland & Shoemaker, 1985a,b; Bland *et al.*, 1985; Shoemaker, 1987, 1989).

Problems in Developing a Therapeutic Plan

The conventional approach consists of a search for specific defects, their documentation, and then their correction. This one-at-a-time search for defects followed by their normalization unfortunately leads to fragmented, episodic patient care. Therapy based on this approach may not be maximally effective. Since shock is recognized clinically by hypotension tachycardia, and oliguria, these superficial manifestations are often treated with vasopressors and diuretics. However, the underlying physiologic problem may remain uncorrected.

Although most patients eventually get the therapy they need, it is not necessarily at the right time, in the right amount, or in the right order. Ideally, therapy of shock, irrespective of the precipitating event, should address the major circulatory components: heart, lungs and tissue perfusion.

Physiologic Description of Shock Syndromes

It is crucial to develop a coherent organized therapeutic plan based on pathophysiology for the high-risk, critically ill patient. Therapy intuitively based on simplistic notions, inadequate models, or anecdotal information is likely to be suboptimal. If the pathophysiology is not understood or monitoring is not appropriate, death will be attributed to the patient's disease rather than to inappropriate therapy.

The physiologic natural histories of various types of clinical shock produced by haemorrhage, accidental or surgical trauma, sepsis, cardiac problems and various combinations of these were described beginning from the time of the precipitating aetiologic event. These descriptions were based on serial measurements obtained during periods remote from therapy, i.e. before therapy was begun or after the immediate direct effects of therapy were over. The distinctive haemodynamic and oxygen transport patterns of survivors and non-survivors of the various clinical aetiologies have been characterized. Physiologic mechanisms are best observed by comparison of survivor and non-survivor patterns. Therapeutic strategies then may be based on circulatory mechanisms that determine survival.

Monitoring with systemic arterial and pulmonary arterial catheters provides frequent measurements of arterial and venous pressures in the systemic and pulmonary circulations, cardiac output, arterial and mixed venous gases, pH and saturations, core temperature, haemoglobin (Hb), and haematocrit (Hct) (Bland et al., 1985). Several haemodynamic values may be derived from these, including cardiac index (CI), systemic (SVRI) and pulmonary (PVRI) vascular resistance index, left (LVSWI) and right (RVSWI) ventricular stroke work index, and left (LCWI) and right (RCWI) cardiac work index. Arterial and mixed venous gases, saturation and haemoglobin content (Hb) are measured simultaneously with cardiac output; they are used to calculate oxygen delivery ($\dot{D}O_2$), oxygen consumption ($\dot{V}O_2$), oxygen extraction, pulmonary venous admixture or shunting ($\dot{Q}s/\dot{Q}T$), and alveolar–arterial oxygen gradient ($P(A-a)O_2$). Flow and volume-related variables are indexed according to body surface area. The variables, abbreviations, units, formulae, normal values, and optimal values are shown in Table 4.1 (Shoemaker *et al.*, 1973, 1988b; Bland *et al.*, 1985; Shoemaker, 1989).

Haemodynamic and Oxygen Transport Patterns of Survivors and Non-survivors of Surgical Trauma

Surgical trauma provides a unique opportunity to describe and analyse the temporal patterns of shock, because the exact times of the precipitating aetiologic event, i.e. the start and end of the operation, are known. This allows physiologic measurements to be obtained in a pre-illness baseline control period, before and during the haemodynamic crisis, and throughout the subsequent recovery periods of survivors and those who die during their present hospitalization. The survivor pattern reflects the effects of trauma and compensatory responses, while the non-survivor patterns reflect the effects of trauma, which may be overwhelming or have inadequate compensations. This approach to sequential physiologic events of post-operative shock provides a conceptual model for other aetiologic types of shock.

Circulatory patterns in several large series of critically ill surgical patients were observed over their temporal course in the peri-operative periods to characterize the effects of surgical trauma in terms of the actual time elapsed since the beginning or end of the surgical operation (Shoemaker *et al.*, 1988b). Many pre-operative conditions including age, sepsis, accidental trauma, stress, hypovolaemia, cirrhosis, and cardiac failure affect these patterns (Bland & Shoemaker, 1985a). More importantly, the vigorousness and extensiveness of therapy may also affect these patterns.

The physiologic pattern of the survivors compared with the pattern of those who died provide the basis for evaluating the nature and biological importance of circulatory compensations. Changes from the normal range may indicate expected compensatory responses that have survival value, or the effect of overwhelming trauma, inadequate compensations, complications, and cardiorespiratory deterioration of the patient.

In order to characterize the circulatory effects of operative trauma *per se*, circulatory patterns were observed in critically ill patients who had normal

Table 4.1 Cardiorespiratory variables: abbreviations, units, calculations, normal values, optimal values and predictive capacity

	Abbreviations	Units	Measurements or calculations	Normal values	Optimal values	Per cent correct
Volume-related variables						
Mean arterial pressure	$M\bar{A}P$	mm Hg	Direct measurement	82–102	>84	76
Central venous pressure	CVP	cm H_2O	Direct measurement	1–9	>12	62
Stroke volume index	SVI	ml m^{-2}	SVI = CI ÷ HR	30–50	>48	67
Haemoglobin	Hb	g dl^{-1}	Direct measurement	12–16	>12	66
Mean pulmonary artery pressure	$P\bar{A}P$	mm Hg	Direct measurement	11–15	<19	68
Wedge pressure	PCWP	mm Hg	Direct measurement	0–12	>9.5	70
Blood volume	BV	ml m^{-2}	BV = PV ÷ (1-Hct)[a] × surf. area	Men 2.74 Women 2.37	>3.0 >2.7	76
Red cell mass	RCM	ml m^{-2}	RCM = BV – PV	Men 1.1 Women 0.95	>1.1 >0.95	85
Flow-related variables						
Cardiac index	CI	litres min^{-1} m^{-2}	Direct measurement	2.8–3.6	>4.5	70
Left ventricular stroke work index	LVSWI	min^{-1} m^{-2}	LVSWI = SVI × $M\bar{A}P$ × 0.0144	44–68	>55	74
Left cardiac work index	LCWI	min^{-1} m^{-2}	LCWI = CI × $M\bar{A}P$ × 0.0144	3–4.6	>5	76
Right ventricular stroke work index	RVSWI	min^{-1} m^{-2}	RVSWI = SVI × $P\bar{A}P$ × 0.0144	4–8	>13	70
Right cardiac work index	RCWI	min^{-1} m^{-2}	RCWI = CI × $P\bar{A}P$ × 0.0144	0.4–0.6	>1.1	69
Stress-related variables						
Systemic vascular resistance index	SVRI	dyne s cm^{-5} m^{-2}	SVRI = 79.92 ($M\bar{A}P$-CVP)[b] ÷ CI	1760–2600	<1450	62
Pulmonary vascular resistance index	PVRI	dyne s cm^{-5} m^{-2}	PVRI = 79.92 ($P\bar{A}P$ – WP)[b] ÷ CI	45–225	<226	77
Heart rate	HR	beats min^{-1}	Direct measurement	72–88	<100	60
Rectal temperature	temp	°C	Direct measurement	36.5–37	>38	64
Oxygen-related variables						
Hb saturation	SaO_2	%	Direct measurement	95–99	>95	67
Arterial CO_2 tension	$PaCO_2$	mm Hg	Direct measurement	36–44	>30	69
Arterial pH	pH		Direct measurement	7.36–7.44	>7.47	74
Mixed venous O_2 tension	$P\bar{v}O_2$	mm Hg	Direct measurement	33–53	>36	68
Arterial–mixed venous O_2 content difference	$C(a-\bar{v})O_2$	ml dl^{-1}	$C(a-\bar{v})O_2 = CaO_2 - C\bar{v}O_2$	4–5.5	<3.5	68
O_2 delivery	$\dot{D}O_2$	ml min^{-1} m^{-2}	$\dot{D}O_2 = CaO_2 × CI × 10$	520–720	>600	76
O_2 consumption	$\dot{V}O_2$	ml min^{-1} m^{-2}	$\dot{V}O_2 = C(a-\bar{v})O_2 × CI × 10$	100–180	>167	69
O_2 extraction rate	OER	%	OER = $(CaO_2 - C\bar{v}O_2) ÷ CaO_2$	22–30	<31	69

[a] Hct corrected for packing fraction and large vessel haematocrit/total body haematocrit ratio.
[b] Venous pressures expressed in mm Hg.

cardiac output pre-operatively and no evidence of associated medical conditions (Fig. 4.1). Intra-operatively, the mean CI, $\dot{D}O_2$ and $\dot{V}O_2$ values fell from normal pre-operative values in both survivors and non-survivors, but this fall was greater in the non-survivors.

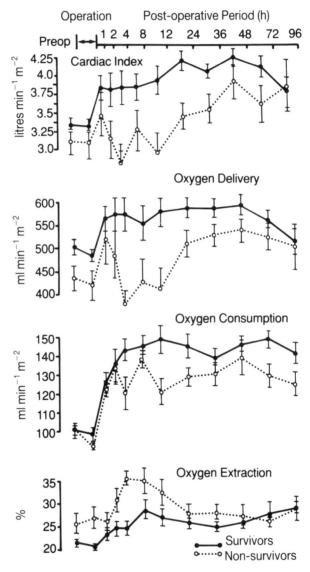

Figure 4.1 Temporal patterns of cardiac index, oxygen delivery and oxygen consumption and oxygen extraction for survivors and non-survivors in the pre-operative control period, intra-operative period and at various time intervals in the post-operative period. Dots represent mean values; vertical bars represent SEM.

Post-operatively, there were minimal variations in the routine vital signs of both groups, but in survivors, the mean CI, $\dot{D}O_2$, $\dot{V}O_2$, and oxygen extraction increased during the first 12 post-operative hours. The median post-operative values reached at their peaks were CI 4.5 litres $min^{-1} m^{-2}$, $\dot{D}O_2$ 500 ml $min^{-1} m^{-2}$, and $\dot{V}O_2$ 170 ml $min^{-1} m^{-2}$. The non-survivors maintained normal, or near normal cardiac function; their $\dot{D}O_2$ and $\dot{V}O_2$ values were also normal, but significantly below those of the survivors, and their oxygen extraction ratios rose in partial compensation. Despite normal blood gases, the non-survivors' $\dot{Q}s/\dot{Q}T$ and $P(A-a)O_2$ values increased intra-operatively and post-operatively (Shoemaker et al., 1988b).

Patients with low pre-operative cardiac output (elderly, cardiac failure, haemorrhagic shock) developed post-operative stress responses that were similar, but less intense than those with normal pre-operative values. That is, the survivors' CI, $\dot{D}O_2$, $\dot{V}O_2$ values increased in the post-operative period from their low pre-operative baseline values, while the non-survivors maintained lower post-operative CI, $\dot{D}O_2$, $\dot{V}O_2$ values despite high wedge pressure (WP). The non-survivors also had significantly greater increases in PVR and $\dot{Q}s/\dot{Q}T$ (Bland & Shoemaker, 1985a).

High pre-operative CI values in patients with sepses, trauma, and advanced cirrhosis suggest pre-operative compensatory circulatory responses. The mean CI, $\dot{D}O_2$, $\dot{V}O_2$ values increased post-operatively above their pre-operative baseline values; these increases also were greater in the survivors than in the non-survivors, while the WP, PVRI and $\dot{Q}s/\dot{Q}T$ values were higher in the non-survivors. Both groups maintained their mean intravascular pressures and other nonflow-related variables in relatively normal ranges or in their pre-operative ranges (Bland & Shoemaker, 1985a; Shoemaker et al., 1988b).

Sequential Patterns of Survivors and Non-survivors in Shock of Various Aetiologies

Most reports in the literature have described haemodynamic and oxygen transport variables in various aetiologic types of shock in terms of their mean values and SD or SEM (Wiggers, 1940; Cournand et al., 1943; Clowes & Del Guercio, 1960; Heilbrunn & Allbritten, 1960; Del Guercio et al., 1964; Wilson et al., 1965). These are expressed as sets of data unrelated to their temporal sequence or the progression of the syndrome. Occasionally reference is made to values obtained in the early or late stages, but only rarely are sequential patterns presented for survivors and non-survivors. Part of this problem is the difficulty in identifying the time of onset of shock in sepsis, occult haemorrhage, accidental injury as well as the rate of progression in septic, haemorrhagic, cardiogenic, traumatic, and post-operative shock syndromes. Even if the time of onset of shock (or the time of the precipitating event) could be identified and this time were used as a 'zero' time, the subsequent time course would not necessarily be in phase with progression of the syndrome because shock may develop rapidly or slowly. Neverthe-less, initial low-point of mean arterial pressure (MĀP) values of the series have been used to identify an early time point of the syndrome (Shoemaker *et al.*, 1973). Similarly, the highest CI, $\dot{D}O_2$ or $\dot{V}O_2$ values during or immediately after resuscitation represents another identifiable point. The initial low and the subsequent high CI values define two points that partially describe a time frame for the syndrome. This is roughly similar to the concept of the 'peak and trough' levels for antibiotics.

Haemorrhagic Shock

With rapid blood loss (>4 h), the pattern of haemorrhagic shock is reduced blood pressure, cardiac index, central venous pressure (CVP), WP, $S\bar{v}O_2$, pH, Hct, Hb, $\dot{D}O_2$ and $\dot{V}O_2$, commitment with increased SVR and O_2 extraction rate. PaO_2 values are usually well-maintained with moderate degrees of hypovolaemia, but hyperpnoea and tachypnoea (air hunger) occurring with severe hypovolaemia may slightly raise PaO_2 and pH and lower $PaCO_2$, indicating initial respiratory alkalosis. When shock is pro-longed, poor tissue perfusion and oxygenation lead to acidosis with low pH, increased lactate levels, and base deficits.

Compensatory responses include increased heat rate that increases CI by neural and neurohormonal mechanisms, increased SVRI that tends to main-tain arterial pressures in the face of decreasing flow, and increased oxygen extraction ratios that improve tissue oxygenation when blood flow is reduced.

When blood loss was slow (>4 h), the haemorrhagic shock pattern showed greater reductions in haematocrit with lesser reductions in MĀP, CI, $\dot{D}O_2$ and $\dot{V}O_2$. However, the reduced rate of $\dot{V}O_2$ was less quantitatively, but more prolonged than after rapid losses of comparable quantities of blood.

After the haemorrhage was stopped and blood volume was restored with appropriate fluids, the recovery period was characterized by increased (supranormal) values for CI, $\dot{D}O_2$ and $\dot{V}O_2$.

Shock After Accidental Trauma

The haemodynamic and oxygen transport patterns after accidental trauma were similar to those described after surgical trauma, except there were wide variations after accidental injuries because of differences in the amount and location of injuries, associated blood loss, organ injury, and the time delays until complete resuscitation occurred. Non-survivors were shown to have greater initial reductions in MĀP, CI, $\dot{D}O_2$ and $\dot{V}O_2$ and lesser elevations in these parameters in the early period of resuscitation. However, after 3 or 5 days, septic complications and organ failures led to higher $\dot{V}O_2$ values, particularly in the preterminal stage (Shoemaker *et al.*, 1971, 1988b; Bishop *et al.*, 1993a,b).

In 65 severe shock trauma patients with blood loss >3000 ml, Bishop *et al.* (1993a,b) observed that when the accumulated delays from the time of injury through the Emergency Department, definitive surgical correction of the injury to the time post-operatively that the optimal supranormal values was <24 h the mortality was 12%, but when these accumulated delays were >24 h, the mortality was 40%.

Sepsis and Septic Shock

Hypovolaemia after haemorrhagic shock is a rather straightforward event that is at least recognizable and measurable. Sepsis, by contrast, is often a more subtle disorder whose time relationships are obscure and whose progress from localized infection to generalized infection to the septic shock syndrome may be so gradual that its progression is not recognized until far advanced. On the other hand, fulminating sepsis may lead to a cataclysmic deterioration and rapid demise.

Septic shock is also difficult to understand because of the heterogenous groups of patients who are affected; that is, there are widely different clinical manifestations in post-operative, post-trauma, urological, respiratory distress, and general internal medical patients. Sepsis may be the primary disorder or it may be a complication. Sepsis also may be the expected consequence of patients with obstruction to the normal flow of biologic fluids (urine, bile, or GI fluids), immunocompromised patients, and those with carcinomatosis or other late-stage malignancies.

The usual physiologic picture of septic shock has been that of increased CI, $\dot{D}O_2$ and, to a lesser extent, $\dot{V}O_2$ unless the patient is dehydrated or terminal. However, there were wide variations in the magnitude of these changes depending on associated medical conditions, blood volume status, degree of hypotension, and stage of shock.

Hankeln *et al.* (1987) confirmed that in their series of post-operative and cardiac patients with adult respiratory distress syndrome (ARDS), those who survived had supranormal CI and $\dot{D}O_2$, but the non-survivors had lower values than the survivors. Others also observed increases in CI, $\dot{D}O_2$ and $\dot{V}O_2$ in septic patients (Abraham *et al.*, 1984; Haupt *et al.*, 1985; Gilbert *et al.*, 1986; Russell *et al.*, 1988). Abraham *et al.* (1984) demonstrated additional $\dot{D}O_2$ and $\dot{V}O_2$ increases after fluid loading with colloids in septic patients with peritonitis. Others have corroborated the increased CI, $\dot{D}O_2$ and $\dot{V}O_2$ in septic patients given fluids or inotropes (Packman & Rackow, 1983; Astiz *et al.*, 1987; Rackow *et al.*, 1987; Tuchschmidt *et al.*, 1989). Edwards *et al.* (1988, 1989) took the concept one step further by driving $\dot{D}O_2$ and $\dot{V}O_2$ to optimal supranormal values with fluids and dobutamine; they demonstrated improved survival rates in severely ill septic patients with this approach. In prospective randomized studies on medical patients with septic shock, Tuchschmidt *et al.* (1991) showed marked reduction in mortality when CI 6 litres $min^{-1} m^{-2}$ was used as the therapeutic goal.

Cardiogenic Shock

Traditionally, the Starling myocardial performance curve and an arbitrary WP of 18 or 20 mm Hg are used to evaluate cardiogenic shock. Four quadrants defined by this Starling curve and WP identify the physiologic impairment and suggest therapy appropriate to these observed conditions (Forrester et al., 1977).

Chronic congestive cardiac failure and acute circulatory failure in chronic cardiac patients have been extensively studied; reduced CI and MĀP with high WP and SVRI were commonly found. Although numerous studies have documented these CI–venous pressure relationships, there have been only two studies of cardiogenic shock after acute myocardial infarction that have reported the fundamental relationship of CI to tissue perfusion and oxygenation as measured by $\dot{D}O_2$ and $\dot{V}O_2$. DaLuz et al. (1975) reported oxygen transport data in seven patients, but all had received adrenergic drugs before the studies were made. Creamer et al. (1990) reported on 19 post-myocardial infarction patients in cardiogenic shock before therapy. There were 14 patients with CI of 1.3 ± 0.5 litres min^{-1} m^{-2} before therapy, who in response to therapy developed CI of 2.5 ± 0.4 associated with marked increases in $\dot{D}O_2$ from 230 ± 69 ml min^{-1} m^{-2} to 397 ± 60 ml min^{-1} m^{-2} and $\dot{V}O_2$ from 103 ± 31 ml min^{-1} m^{-2} to 124 ± 22 ml min^{-1} m^{-2}; 13 of these 14 patients survived. Two other patients with mean CI of 0.9 ± 0.4 litres min^{-1} m^{-2} died before therapy could be given and three other patients spontaneously recovered (Creamer et al., 1990). They concluded that in cardiogenic shock, supply-dependent $\dot{V}O_2$, while not as dramatic as that of septic shock, was nevertheless an important component of therapy. Other goals of therapy included $\dot{D}O_2$ 300–400 ml min^{-1} m^{-2}, O_2 extraction ratio reduced to about 30%, and $S\bar{v}O_2$ increased to approximately 70% (Edwards, 1991).

Haemodynamic and Oxygen Transport Patterns in Relation to Oxygen Debt in Critically Ill Post-operative Patients

Since $\dot{V}O_2$ measures the rate at which oxygen is utilized, not the rate that is required, it is necessary to estimate the rate of oxygen need independently to evaluate potential oxygen debts in high-risk surgical patients. The $\dot{V}O_2$ need may be estimated from the patient's own pre-operative values under normal steady-state conditions, then correction terms used to estimate the $\dot{V}O_2$ need under anaesthesia and with temperature changes. Lowe and Ernst (1981) reported $\dot{V}O_2$ under anaesthesia in healthy elective patients, $\dot{V}O_2$ (anaesth) $= 10 \times \text{kg}^{0.72}$. This $\dot{V}O_2$ (anaesth) value was then corrected for the effects of temperature and this derived value was used to estimate the $\dot{V}O_2$ need during the time the patient underwent general anaesthesia. This was approximately 100 ml min^{-1} m^{-2}. The temperature correction term assumed metabolic activity increased or decreased at the rate of 7% per degree Fahrenheit (Shoemaker *et al.*, 1988a). The $\dot{V}O_2$ need after recovery from anaesthesia in the post-operative period was estimated from the patient's own pre-operative baseline $\dot{V}O_2$ corrected for the effects of temperature. After the anaesthetic was reversed in the post-operative period, the temperature-corrected baseline pre-operative $\dot{V}O_2$ was used as the $\dot{V}O_2$ need. Thus, the net cumulative amount of intra- and post-operative oxygen deficit was calculated from the measured $\dot{V}O_2$ minus the $\dot{V}O_2$ need estimated from the patient's own resting pre-operative control values, corrected for both temperature and anaesthesia and integrated over time.

Figure 4.2 shows the patterns of selected haemodynamic and oxygen transport variables in a series of 253 consecutively monitored surviving and non-surviving high-risk surgical patients in the pre-operative, intra-operative and immediate post-operative period (Shoemaker *et al.*, 1992). Cardiac index, oxygen delivery, and $\dot{V}O_2$ of survivors without organ failure were highest, those who survived with organ failure were intermediate, while the values of those who subsequently died were lowest. The mean non-survivor values, however, were within the normal range. The magnitude and duration of the calculated $\dot{V}O_2$ deficit was greatest with non-survivors, somewhat less in survivors with organ failure, and least in survivors without organ failure.

The oxygen debt was also calculated in the prospective randomized study testing the effect of supranormal values empirically observed in survivors of critically ill surgical patients (Shoemaker *et al.*, 1992). There were significantly smaller oxygen debts in protocol patients who had supranormal oxygen transport values as therapeutic goals compared with the control group who had normal values as therapeutic goals.

Specific Organ Failures and Their Times of Onset

Table 4.2 details the number of type and organ failures in non-survivors and survivors. There were 1.72 organ failures per non-survivor, and 1.42 organ failures per survivor with organ failure, or 0.28 organ failures per all survivors.

The average time of appearance of each organ failure is listed in Table 4.2. Although there were wide ranges in the time of appearance of each organ failure, pulmonary failure often occurred first, followed by cardiac failure, renal failure, disseminated intravascular coagulation (DIC), sepsis and CNS failures. However, the order of appearance varied widely. The average time of appearance for all organ failures occurred 5.5 ± 4.2 days post-operatively, the first organ failure occurred 2.3 ± 1.9 days post-operatively; this was later than the oxygen debt which began intra-operatively and reached maximum values in 10.1 h post-operatively for survivors and 17.3 h for non-survivors. Organ failures usually became clinically apparent after the maximum cumulative oxygen debt was reached, but before the debt had been entirely corrected.

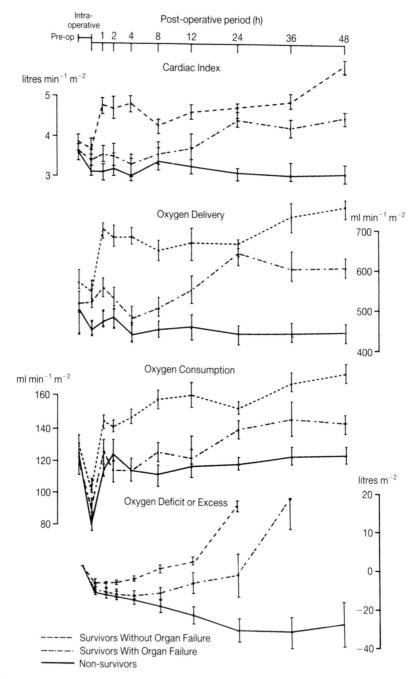

Figure 4.2 Serial measurements of cardiac index, oxygen delivery, oxygen consumption and net cumulative $\dot{V}O_2$ deficit for survivors without organ failure, survivors with organ failure and non-survivors, calculated for the intra-operative period and successive time periods post-operatively. (Modified from Shoemaker *et al.* 1992.)

Table 4.2 Organ failures

	Non-survivors (N = 64)	Survivors with organ failure (N = 31)	Total with organ failure (N = 95)	Time of appearance (days postoperative) (mean ± SD)
Lung: $PaO_2/FIO_2 < 250$, $\dot{Q}s/\dot{Q}t > 20\%$	30 (47%)	19 (61%)	49 (52%)	3.6 ± 3.1
Sepsis: positive cultures, white blood cell count > 13 000, temperature > 38.9°C	28 (44%)	11 (35%)	39 (41%)	7.4 ± 4.9
Heart: CI < 2.5 L/per min·m², WP > 20 mm Hg	26 (41%)	3 (10%)	29 (30%)	4.3 ± 4.8
Kidney: blood urea nitrogen > 50 mg per dl, creatinine > 3 mg per dl	18 (28%)	7 (23%)	25 (26%)	5.9 ± 4.1
DIC: platelets < 75 000, prothrombin time > 18/12 s, partial thromboplastin time > 2× normal, fibrin split products	7 (11%)	3 (10%)	10 (11%)	6.2 ± 5.6
CNS: coma	1 (1%)	1 (3%)	2 (2%)	11

[a] Number of organ failures and the percentage of patients with this organ failure.
Organ failures per non-surviving (110/64) patients = 1.72.
Organ failures per survivors with organ failure (44/31) = 1.42.
Organ failures per all survivors (44/158) = 0.28.

Relationship of Oxygen Debt to Tissue Hypoxia, Organ Failure and Death

The data demonstrate a strong relationship of the magnitude and duration of the $\dot{V}O_2$ deficit with the subsequent appearance of organ failure and death. There were greater tissue oxygen debts in surviving patients who subsequently developed multiple organ failure than in surviving patients without organ failure. The oxygen deficits were greater in magnitude and duration in non-survivors than in those who survived with organ failure. Moreover, the early appearance of oxygen debt suggested that reduced tissue oxygenation is the primary event, while organ failure and death are the result of this antecedent physiologic event. This is supported by prospective clinical trials that demonstrated reduced morbidity and mortality when increased $\dot{V}O_2$ had been maintained at supranormal values. Thus, evidence suggests that the early circulatory mechanism producing organ failure and death is reduced tissue oxygenation from maldistributed or inadequate tissue perfusion, especially in the face of increased metabolic needs. Persistently reduced $\dot{V}O_2$ produces a cumulative tissue oxygen debt that must be repaid by compensatory increases during the immediate post-operative period for survival to occur. The greater the initial reduction in $\dot{V}O_2$, the greater must be the compensatory $\dot{V}O_2$ increases (Shoemaker *et al.*, 1993).

Physiologic Considerations

The relevant circulatory physiology may be summarized as: (a) the transport of blood constituents, particularly oxygen, is the major function of the circulation; (b) oxygen which has the highest extraction ratio and the greatest A–V gradient is the easiest blood constituent to measure; (c) since oxygen cannot be stored, the rate at which oxygen is transported across the alveolar capillary membrane in steady-state conditions is equivalent to the rate at which oxygen is consumed by the tissues; (d) the overall circulatory function is best evaluated in terms of the bulk transport of oxygen; (e) the rate of oxygen utilization ($\dot{V}O_2$) reflects the sum of all oxidative metabolic reactions and measures the body's overall metabolic state; and (f) $\dot{V}O_2$ may be rate-limited by hypovolaemia, reduced $\dot{D}O_2$, or flow maldistributions produced by accidental trauma, surgical operations, anaesthetic agents, sepsis, post-operative states, endocrine and metabolic disorders, and capillary leak.

Pathophysiologic Significance of Haemodynamic and Oxygen Transport Patterns

$\dot{D}O_2$ and $\dot{V}O_2$ provide the best available measure of the functional adequacy of both circulation and metabolism. As such, the patterns of these two oxygen transport variables provide the means to evaluate abnormalities in both circulatory and metabolic functions as well as changes due to therapy. In the early period of acute circulatory problems, insufficient $\dot{D}O_2$, the supply side of the equation, may limit $\dot{V}O_2$. Inadequate $\dot{V}O_2$ is not just associated with shock, it is the major pathogenic mechanism of shock syndromes as well as a major determinant of outcome (Shoemaker, 1987, 1989; Shoemaker et al., 1988a,b).

Inadequate $\dot{V}O_2$ is produced by low cardiac output from haemorrhage or other causes of hypovolaemia and by maldistribution of flow from uneven vasoconstriction, mediator-induced responses, and increased metabolic demands after trauma, burns and sepsis. Thus, the basic physiologic problem of shock is tissue hypoxia from inadequate transport of oxygen (and other nutrients) relative to the increased metabolic needs.

The major determinants of outcome are the degree of tissue hypoxia from inadequate blood volume or flow and the patients' inability to compensate with increased CI and $\dot{D}O_2$ in response to increased tissue requirements for $\dot{V}O_2$ (Shoemaker et al., 1992). Uneven local vascular tone leads to uneven distribution of flow that compromises local tissue perfusion and tissue metabolism. Hypovolaemia produced by haemorrhage or by leakage of plasma volume from the intravascular to the interstitial compartment limits the cardiac capacity to compensate with increased CI and $\dot{D}O_2$. Anaesthesia also affects the cardiovascular system; inhalation anaesthetics depress myocardial function, neural control of peripheral vascular tone, cellular function, and body metabolism; these effects may be manifested by reduced $\dot{V}O_2$.

Surgical patients with pre-operative hypovolaemia, associated medical illnesses, or other cardiorespiratory problems may have altered pre-operative values. However, their post-operative biphasic haemodynamic and oxygen transport patterns are similar, except that they begin from different pre-operative baselines. In essence, haemorrhagic and cardiac hypovolaemic patients begin with low baseline CI values and septic patients start with high baseline values. Although both survivors and non-survivors have compensatory responses, survivors have smaller $\dot{V}O_2$ reductions and greater $\dot{V}O_2$ increases, while non-survivors have greater $\dot{V}O_2$ reductions and smaller compensatory increases.

Blood Volume and Fluid Status

The first and most important therapeutic goal for haemorrhagic, traumatic and septic shock is to restore blood volume. Conventional criteria for this are tachycardia and reduced MĀP, CVP, PCWP and Hct values based on observations immediately after clinical evidence of sudden acute haemorrhage. Unfortunately, these values, including PCWP, do not reflect the actual blood volume status in the subsequent post-resuscitation course. In critically ill post-operative patients, these commonly used criteria were unreliable compared with careful measurements of blood volume (Shippy et al., 1984).

Surgeons are often accused of overly aggressive fluid administration in patients with surgical or accidental trauma. Medical patients, especially those with chronic cardiac, renal, pulmonary and hepatic disorders, usually have too much salt or water and require diuretics with fluid restriction. Furthermore, fluid therapy controversies frequently arise from a failure to differentiate between extracellular water and plasma volume excesses or deficits. For example, the patient with peripheral oedema obviously has too much total body water, but also may have hypovolaemia. Frequently, patients have maldistributed flow with contracted plasma volume, but expanded interstitial water. Therapy should be aimed at improving circulatory function by restoring plasma volume, not overloading an already expanded interstitial space with crystalloids.

Since the most important correctable therapeutic problem in acute circulatory shock is restoration of blood volume, it is essential to have a reliable means to assess this volume. Measurement of plasma volume by ^{125}I-labelled albumin or red cell mass by [55]Cr-labelled red cells are time-consuming, expensive, and usually used only in research centres. The CVP and WP, which can be repeated at frequent intervals or monitored continuously, were thought to have the needed accuracy, and have largely replaced blood volume measurements in most clinical conditions. CVP and WP rapidly decrease with acute haemorrhage and increase immediately after fluid therapy. High venous pressures are associated with both acute

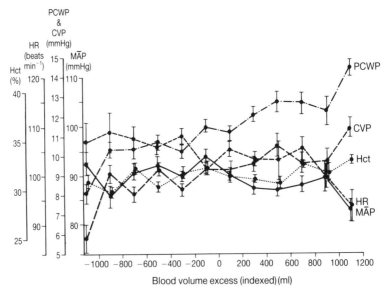

Figure 4.3   Blood volume index values plotted against commonly monitored variables on the *y*-axis. —— Mean arterial pressure (MĀP); – – – pulmonary capillary wedge pressure (PCWP); —·—· central venous pressure (CVP); – – – – heart rate (HR); .... haematocrit (Hct). Blood volume values are expressed as millilitres excess (+) or deficit (−) from the patient's predicted norm indexed to BSA. Note the very poor correlation of the commonly monitored variables. (From Shippy *et al.*, 1984, with permission.)

blood volume overload and cardiac failure. However, venous pressures as well as haematocrit, MĀP and heart rate (HR) are notably unreliable indicators of blood volume status in ICU patients because of venous wall compliance changes (Fig. 4.3). In the post-operative ICU period, venous pressures accommodate to either high or low blood volumes with values which usually remain in the range of 8–12 mm Hg (Shippy *et al.*, 1984). Figure 4.4 illustrates the scatter of blood volume deficit or excess relative to their corresponding CVP values.

CVP and WP values reflect venous pressures but do not accurately reflect blood volume in most ICU patients. They are useful to titrate fluid therapy to prevent acute volume overload during rapid fluid restoration. Thus, venous pressures reflect the capacity of the vascular system to accept more volume without producing pulmonary oedema. However, pulmonary oedema may result from massive crystalloid infusions that expand the interstitial space without fully restoring plasma volume or exceeding 'safe' venous pressures (Shippy *et al.*, 1984).

Daily weight and fluid balance measurement are used to monitor fluid management, but these both are limited because they reflect body water or changes in body water, not blood volume. The distribution of body water between the plasma, interstitium and intracellular compartments can be definitely measured only by isotopic body composition studies.

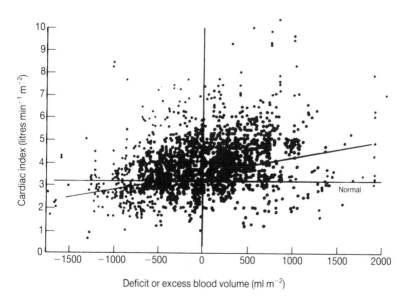

Figure 4.4 Blood volume index values plotted against their simultaneously measured cardiac index values. (From Shippy *et al.*, 1984, with permission.)

Prediction of Outcome as a Measure of Severity of Illness

Relative Importance of Haemodynamic and Oxygen Transport Variables as Outcome Predictors

Non-parametric statistical analyses have been used to predict outcome early in the post-operative period (Shoemaker *et al.*, 1979, 1985; Bland & Shoemaker, 1985b). These analyses also provide an objective, physiologic basis for therapeutic decisions. The sole criterion of this type of empiric physiologic analysis is survival. More importantly, predictors objectively reflect severity of illness and express this in quantitative terms. The biologic importance of each monitored variable may be evaluated by its ability to predict outcome. Similarly, this predictive ability is also the best criterion of its usefulness in making clinical decisions. If a variable is not related to outcome, it should not be relevant to therapy. However, if it does predict outcome, it may reflect important pathophysiology and, therefore, provide a useful criterion for therapeutic decisions.

The percentages of correctly predicted outcomes for each monitored variables were calculated at each stage and for all stages in a series of post-operative patients (Table 4.1) (Shoemaker *et al.*, 1979, 1985, 1988b, 1992; Bland & Shoemaker, 1985a). The commonly monitored variables were the poorest predictors. By contrast, oxygen transport-related variables were good outcome predictors and, therefore, are clinically important. This concept has been corroborated in both surgical and medical patients (Hankeln *et al.*, 1987; Edwards *et al.*, 1989).

Subsequently, a modified predictor was also prospectively tested in a fresh series of patients and found to be 94% correct. Figure 4.5 shows significant separation between survivors and non-survivors in the prospective series beginning 2–4 h post-operatively (Bland & Shoemaker, 1985b).

These predictors objectively analyse the complex physiologic problems with no preconceptions and minimal assumptions. The criteria are determined solely by the observed values of critically ill surgical patients who survived as compared with the values of those who subsequently died.

THERAPY

Therapeutic Goals

Optimal therapeutic goals for high-risk post-operative patients were defined by outcome predictors and the values of survivors of life-threatening critical illnesses. Criteria from two large retrospective series (Shoemaker *et al.*, 1973; Bland & Shoemaker, 1985b) and several prospective

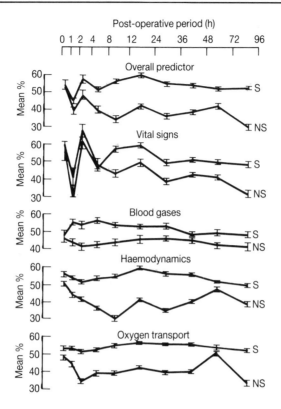

Figure 4.5 Upper section: overall prediction for survivors (S) and non-survivors (NS) at each time interval post-operatively. Second section: Predictions calculated from the vital signs variables for S and NS. Third section: Predictions calculated from the blood–gas variables for S and NS. Fourth section: Predictions calculated from the haemodynamic variables for S and NS. Lowest section: Predictions calculated from the oxygen transport variables for S and NS. Dots represent mean values, vertical bars SEM. (From Bland & Shoemaker, 1985b.)

series (Low & Ernst, 1981; Bland & Shoemaker, 1985b; Bland et al., 1985; Shoemaker et al., 1992) include: (a) CI 50% greater than normal (4.5 litres $\text{min}^{-1}\,\text{m}^{-2}$); (b) DO_2 somewhat greater than normal (600 ml $\text{min}^{-1}\,\text{m}^{-2}$); (c) $\dot{V}O_2$ about 30% greater than normal (170 ml $\text{min}^{-1}\,\text{m}^{-2}$); and (d) blood volume 500 ml in excess of the norm, i.e. 3.2 litres m^{-2} for males, 2.8 litres m^{-2} for females (Shoemaker et al., 1973, 1985, 1992; Bland & Shoemaker, 1985a; Bland et al., 1985; Shoemaker, 1989). These increased values are needed to overcome poorly distributed blood volume and blood flow as well as to supply the increased metabolism associated with wound healing, fever, and the accumulated oxygen debt. Severely traumatized, stressed, septic, cirrhotic and burn patients may require even higher values (Bland & Shoemaker, 1985a; Bland et al., 1985; Shoemaker et al., 1985).

Outcome prediction for each haemodynamic and oxygen transport variable varies from stage to stage as the shock syndromes evolve. Predictors are stage-specific: DO_2 and PVRI are good early predictors, but are not good in the late stage. MĀP is a poor early predictor, but a good late predictor. Most variables predict outcome well in the late stage, but clinical judgement is also excellent and the usefulness of predictors is minimal at this time (Shoemaker, 1989).

Physiologic Compensations and Their Therapeutic Implications

Physiologic compensatory responses maintain circulatory function and integrity after trauma, haemorrhage, sepsis, cardiogenic and other types of shock. Increased cardiac output may compensate for reduced haematocrit, low PaO_2, or uneven flow, all of which produce inadequate tissue oxygenation. Organ failures occur when these responses fail to compensate adequately (Shoemaker et al., 1988a). Therapy should be directed toward augmenting compensatory flow increases that have survival value. The use of β-blockers to reduce high cardiac output values or tachycardia in patients with traumatic or septic shock may lead to circulatory and metabolic deterioration. If the physiology is misunderstood and monitoring is inappropriate, death will be attributed to the patient's disease rather than to inappropriate therapy.

It is assumed for the purpose of this haemodynamic review that airway management and mechanical ventilation will have been provided as part of the ABCs of resuscitation. This is, indeed, routine in the trauma victim and in post-operative patients, who are usually already intubated. The present review will, therefore, focus on the haemodynamics and oxygen transport aspects of shock and therapy of these circulatory deficiencies.

Conventional Approach to Therapy

The standard conventional approach to therapy is to search for specific defects, document their presence, and then correct them. This one-at-a-time search for each abnormality and then correction, results in a fragmented, episodic plan. An alternative approach is to base therapy on survivor patterns in order to prevent complications and death. The hypothesis is that the survivor pattern reflects successful compensations to trauma and, therefore, represents the appropriate therapeutic goals. This hypotheses has been tested in several prospective clinical trials (Shoemaker et al., 1988b, 1992).

A Therapeutic Plan Using a Branched-Chain Decision Tree for Post-operative Patients

Strategies for achieving therapeutic goals were determined empirically by evaluating the relative effectiveness of each therapy to produce the desired goals. Decision rules generated from survivor or non-survivor patterns and responses to specific therapeutic interventions were used to develop a branched-chain decision tree (Fig. 4.6). A branched-chain decision tree helps to achieve therapeutic goals expeditiously by providing an organized management plan. The plan aims to prophylactically maintain the patient in the optimal haemodynamic state in order to prevent the development of tissue hypoxia from deficits in blood volume, maldistributed flow and inadequate oxygen transport. It is not necessary to wait for patients to develop tissue hypoxia from an oxygen debt before initiating therapy. Therapy should be started promptly to optimize the CI, $\dot{D}O_2$ and $\dot{V}O_2$ as soon as possible, preferably within the first few hours after the onset of accidental trauma or before, during and immediately after surgery in the high-risk elective patient.

Volume Therapy

Vigorous and rapid volume loading without exceeding PCWP values greater than 18–20 mm Hg is the first and most important therapy. It is easier to achieve the therapeutic goals in the initial resuscitation and in the early phase of shock with colloids because they expand the plasma volume without overexpansion of the interstitial water. Plasma volume restoration cannot be assumed in patients with peripheral oedema who have received large volumes of crystalloids because hypovolaemia frequently occurs in the presence of expanded interstitial water. In these conditions, we prefer to give concentrated (25%) albumin, which expands plasma volume by shifting interstitial water back into the plasma volume. This may be followed by furosemide, if PCWP exceeds 20 mm Hg.

Inotropic Agents

After the maximum effect of fluids on oxygen transport has been obtained, an inotropic agent such as dobutamine may be started at about $5 \,\mu g \, min^{-1} kg^{-1}$ until the appropriate dose is obtained by titration to achieve the optimal CI, $\dot{D}O_2$ and $\dot{V}O_2$ goals. Dobutamine produced marked and significant increases in CI and stroke index, cardiac and stroke work, HR, $\dot{D}O_2$, and $\dot{V}O_2$ as well as decreases in systemic and pulmonary vascular resistances and intravascular pressures including $\overline{MAP}$, $\overline{PAP}$, CVP and WP.

The effects of dobutamine at various doses are summarized in Fig. 4.7. The data show pronounced changes at the $2.5 \,\mu g \, kg^{-1} min^{-1}$ dose, but individual patients sometimes responded with greater flow effects with doses as high as $100 \,\mu g \, kg^{-1} min^{-1}$.

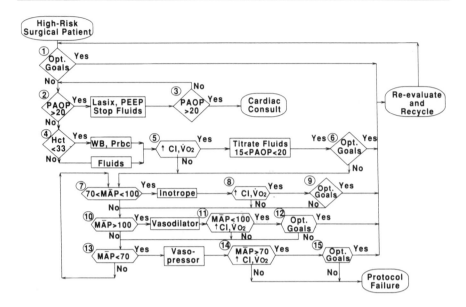

Figure 4.6   Branched-chain decision tree for post-operative ICU patients. Preliminary evaluation of high-risk critically ill patients by routine ICU work-up that includes arterial blood gases, chest X-ray, routine blood chemistries, ECG and coagulation studies. These tests should be either performed or in process and the observed defects corrected. *Step 1:* Measure CI, $\dot{D}O_2$, $\dot{V}O_2$ and blood volume (BV) to determine if the patient has reached the optimal goals. If CI <4.5 litres min^{-1} m^{-2}, $\dot{D}O_2$ <600 ml min^{-1} m^{-2}, $\dot{V}O_2$ <170 ml min^{-1} m^{-2}, or BV <3 litres m^{-2} for men or <2.7 litres m^{-2} for women, proceed to step 2, but if the goals are reached, the objective of the algorithm has been achieved; re-evaluate and recycle at intervals to maintain these goals. *Step 2:* Take pulmonary capillary wedge pressure (PCWP). If >20 mm Hg, proceed to step 3; if <20, proceed to step 4. *Step 3:* If PCWP >20 mm Hg, give furosemide i.v. at increasing dose levels (20, 40, 80, 160 mg) if there is clinical or X-ray evidence of salt and water overload or clinical findings of pulmonary congestion. If not, consider vasodilators, nitroprusside or nitroglycerin if MÃP > 80 and systolic pressure > 120 mm Hg. Recycle to titrate the dose as needed to reduce PCWP < 15 mm Hg but maintain MÃP > 80 mm Hg. If unsuccessful, place on cardiac protocol. *Step 4:* If Hct $<33\%$, give 1 unit of whole blood (WB) or 2 units of packed red blood cells (Prbc). If Hct $>33\%$, give a fluid load (volume challenge) consisting of one of the following (depending on clinical indications of plasma volume deficit or hydration state): 500 ml of 5% plasma protein factor; 500 ml of 5% albumin; 100 ml of 25% albumin (25 g); 500 ml of 6% hydroxyethylstarch; 500 ml of 6% dextran 60; or 1000 ml of lactated Ringer's solution or normal saline. *Step 5:* If the blood or fluid load improved any of the optimal therapeutic goals defined in step 1, proceed to step 6; if none is improved, proceed to step 7. *Step 6:* If goals are not reached, recycle steps 2–6 until these goals are met or WP > 20 mm Hg. *Step 7:* If MÃP > 70 and <100 mm Hg, give dobutamine by constant i.v. infusion in doses to increase CI, $\dot{D}O_2$ and $\dot{V}O_2$. *Step 8:* Titrate dobutamine beginning with 2 µg kg^{-1} min^{-1} and gradually increasing doses up to 20 µg kg^{-1} min^{-1} or more provided there is improvement in CI, $\dot{D}O_2$, or $\dot{V}O_2$ until goals are met. *Step 9:* If goals are reached, re-evaluate and recycle. If goals are not reached or it becomes evident that higher doses of the drug are not more effective or that they produce hypotension and tachycardia, continue dobutamine at its most effective

The effects of dobutamine were observed in a small group of patients before and after a fluid load consisting of 500 or 1000 ml of 5% albumin; there were greater flow effects with no hypertension and tachycardia when blood volume had been increased. Hypovolaemic patients are more sensitive to vasodilators and blocking agents; additional fluids must be given with other vasodilators. Inotropic stimulation of the tired heart may be therapeutically effective, but stimulation of the tired empty heart may be disastrous. Sudden hypotension after dobutamine or any blocking agent may be reversed with rapid administration of fluids, principally colloids.

Vasodilator Therapy

If the patient has normal or high MĀP with high systemic vascular resistance index (SVRI), vasodilation with nitroglycerine, nitroprusside, labetalol, or prostaglandin (PGE_1) may be considered. The optimal dose is obtained by titration to achieve improved cardiac index without producing hypotension (i.e. MĀP >80 mm Hg, systolic arterial pressure (SAP) >100 mm Hg). Blood volume must be restored prior to the administration of vasodilation or blocking agents.

Vasopressors

If fluids, inotropic agents and vasodilators fail to achieve optimal goals, vasopressors such as dopamine may be given at the lowest dose needed to

---

dose range. *Step 10:* If MĀP >100 mm Hg give vasodilator such as sodium nitroprusside, nitroglycerine, labetalol, prostaglandin E_1, etc. in gradually increasing doses provided there is improvement in CI, DO_2, or VO_2. *Step 11:* Titrate vasodilators to decrease MĀP and increase CI, DO_2 and VO_2. If there is no improvement in CI, DO_2, or VO_2 with the vasodilator, or if hypotension (MĀP <70 mm Hg, SAP <110 mm Hg) ensues, discontinue the vasodilator. If there is improvement in CI, DO_2, or VO_2, titrate the vasodilator to its maximum effect consistent with satisfactory arterial pressures. *Step 12:* If optimal goals are reached, re-evaluate and recycle at intervals. *Step 13:* If these goals are not reached and MĀP <70 mm Hg and SAP <110 mm Hg, give dopamine or other vasopressor. *Step 14:* Titrate doses of vasopressor in the lowest doses possible to maintain arterial pressures, MĀP >80 mm Hg, SAP >110 mm Hg and CI, DO_2 and VO_2 to their optimal values. If the goals and pressures cannot be maintained, the patient is considered to be a protocol failure. *Step 15:* If goals are reached, re-evaluate and recycle. Consider additional therapy to further increase CI, DO_2 and VO_2, assuming greater than expected tissue hypoxia from poor tissue perfusion. (From Shoemaker *et al.* (40) with permission.)

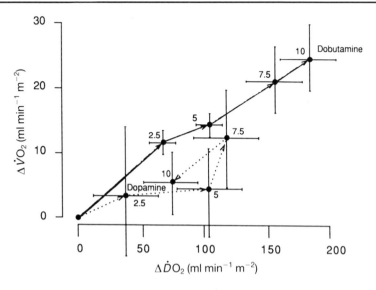

Figure 4.7   Comparison of oxygen delivery ($\dot{D}O_2$) and oxygen consumption ($\dot{V}O_2$) effects of dobutamine and dopamine at infusion rates of 0, 2.5, 5, 7.5, and 10 μg kg^{-1} min^{-1}. (From Shoemaker *et al.* with permission.)

maintain MAP >80 mm Hg and SAP >110 mm Hg in patients with normal pre-illness values. Vasopressors are given as a last resort because they increase venous pressures, pulmonary and systemic shunts, and lactic acidaemia. Moreover, the increased venous pressure produced by vaso-pressors may limit optimal fluid administration.

Prospective Clinical Trials

In two prospective studies, we tested the hypothesis that if the CI, $\dot{D}O_2$ and $\dot{V}O_2$ values of post-operative patients are promptly brought up to the 'optimal' values empirically determined by survivors, mortality and mor-bidity will be reduced. The therapeutic plan that used the survivors' values as therapeutic goals was prospectively tested in clinical trials against a control group which used normal values as the therapeutic goals (Shoe-maker *et al.*, 1988b, 1992). Both protocol and control groups had the same availability of X-rays and laboratory tests, monitoring, nursing care, ancil-lary facilities and therapy. In the first study, patients whose critical illnesses were specified by pre-arranged criteria were prospectively allocated to con-trol or protocol services. The results of this study demonstrated marked reduction in morbidity and mortality in the protocol patients; however, about one third of these patients entered the trial at various times post-operatively (Shoemaker *et al.*, 1988b). In a second study, this hypothesis was more rigorously tested by identifying high-risk patients pre-operatively with predetermined criteria and randomizing them to one of these therapeutic regimens: (a) CVP catheter with values available by this catheter brought to their normal range, (b) pulmonary artery catheter with values available by this catheter brought to their normal range as goals, and (c) pulmonary artery catheter with optimal values of CI, $\dot{D}O_2$ and $\dot{V}O_2$ as goals of therapy (Shoemaker *et al.*, 1992). The eligible high-risk patients were strictly randomized to one of the three monitoring/therapeutic approaches.

The results showed no statistically significant difference between the mortality of patients managed with a CVP catheter (23%) and those with the pulmonary artery catheter with normal values as therapeutic goals (33%). However, use of supranormal goals with the pulmonary artery catheter led to significantly reduced (4%) mortality. Moreover, the numbers of complications, hospital days, ICU days, ventilator days and hospital costs were also significantly reduced. The supranormal values were achieved with fluid, principally colloids in about two-thirds of the patients and with dobutamine in the remainder; vasodilators were needed in 6%. The goals were achieved in the first 8–12 h post-operatively.

A number of investigators (Packman & Rackow, 1983; Abraham *et al.*, 1984; Haupt *et al.*, 1985; Gilbert *et al.*, 1986; Astiz *et al.*, 1987; Rackow *et al.*, 1987; Edwards *et al.*, 1988, 1989; Russell *et al.*, 1988; Tuchschmidt *et al.*, 1989, 1991) have confirmed that survivors of post-operative states, trauma, sepsis, cardiogenic states and ARDS have higher CI. $\dot{D}O_2$ and $\dot{V}O_2$ values than do non-survivors in comparable conditions. Furthermore, prospective trials have demonstrated efficacy with regimens that further increased $\dot{D}O_2$ and $\dot{V}O_2$ (Edwards *et al.*, 1989; Creamer *et al.*, 1990; Tuchschmidt *et al.*, 1991; Bishop *et al.*, 1993a,b). These prospective clinical trials suggest that most post-operative deaths are due to physiologic problems that can be identified, described, predicted and prevented, and that therapeutic goals for critically ill post-operative patients should be defined by physiologic criteria of survivors and implemented prophylactically and promptly, i.e. within the first 8–12 h.

Treatment of Other Aetiologic Types of Shock

Similar underlying physiologic alterations occur in haemorrhage, severe accidental trauma, cardiac conditions and sepsis, but the optimal goals are not quantitatively the same as those of post-operative patients. The metabolic requirements in patients with severe trauma, burns, stress, sepsis and other hypercatabolic states are greater in magnitude, but more variable than those of elective surgical patients. The underlying physiologic defects may be qualitatively similar, but their greater metabolic requirements or oxygen debts will require more aggressive therapy. However, greater than normal metabolism should not be interpreted to mean that all metabolic needs have been met as there may still be an oxygen debt.

The optimal values after haemorrhage, severe accidental trauma, and sepsis cannot be defined precisely nor determined directly because of the widely varying degrees of oxygen debt and increases in body metabolism. The answer to this dilemma is an operational definition for therapy. Volume is given as long as this improves CI, $\dot{D}O_2$ and $\dot{V}O_2$, or until PCWP reaches 18 or 20 mm Hg. In this approach, PCWP is not used as a measure of blood volume because it clearly does not reflect blood volume (Hankeln *et al.*, 1987). Rather, PCWP is used as an upper limit for volume therapy in order to avoid pulmonary oedema. Then, continue to give each therapy as long as it improves CI, $\dot{D}O_2$, and $\dot{V}O_2$, unless limited by PCWP >20 mm Hg in the case of fluid loading, tachycardia >140 beats per min in the case of inotropic agents, and hypotension <80 mm Hg $\overline{M}AP$ or SAP <110 mm Hg in the case of vasodilators. Thus, tissue oxygen demand is inferred indirectly by an empirical trial of therapy. If therapy increases CI, $\dot{D}O_2$, and $\dot{V}O_2$, it may be assumed that the therapy may have opened up additional microcirculatory channels that perfused relatively hypoxic tissue which then extracted more oxygen. Since tissues cannot take up more oxygen than they use, the increased $\dot{V}O_2$ after therapy indicates the presence of an oxygen debt and suggests that this debt was at least partially satisfied.

Vasopressors are used as a last resort to maintain sufficient $\overline{M}AP$ to provide for coronary and cerebral perfusion after achieving the maximum effects of fluids, inotropes and vasodilators. The haemodynamic effectiveness of each agent given separately should be established before combining agents. The most important principles in these complex clinical conditions are to: (a) document baseline haemodynamic and oxygen transport variables; (b) measure changes with each appropriate agent; (c) give the agent that most effectively improved tissue perfusion; and (d) titrate the dose to achieve optimal values as determined by $\dot{D}O_2$ and $\dot{V}O_2$ measurements.

Elderly and cardiac patients have considerably different physiologic problems and more limited compensatory capacities compared with post-operative patients with normal cardiac function and multiple vital organ failures. The heart is the weak link in the cardiac patient, but oxygen transport functions and tissue perfusion are more likely to limit survival in the septic, traumatic or post-operative patient. An appropriate strategy in cardiac patients may be to improve cardiac function with inotropic agents and to reduce cardiac work by afterload reduction with vasodilators; preload may be augmented, but overdilation should be avoided.

The strategy in each case is to try to open up unevenly vasoconstricted metarteriolar–capillary networks by vigorous volume loading and by increasing flow with inotropic agents and subsequently by vasodilators.

Summary

Physiologic variables in surgical patients have been serially measured in the pre-operative period, during the haemodynamic crises, and during the subsequent periods leading to recovery or death from shock and its sequelae. The empirically observed sequential patterns of survivors and non-survivors of surgical shock provide a basis for physiologic analysis, definition of therapeutic goals, outcome predictions and clinical trials. These studies may also serve as a model for other shock syndromes where time relationships are not as easily defined.

Five basic physiologic concepts define the therapeutic problem of shock. First, inadequate $\dot{V}O_2$ leading to tissue hypoxia is the primary pathogenic mechanism for the shock syndromes. Second, the basic function of the circulation is the transport of gases, nutrients and other blood constituents; the overall circulatory function, therefore, is best tracked by $\dot{D}O_2$, the bulk movement of oxygen. The third concept is that $\dot{D}O_2$ may limit $\dot{V}O_2$ either by low flow which occurs with haemorrhagic and cardiogenic shock, or unevenly distributed flow and increased metabolic need which occur with trauma and sepsis. Fourth, $\dot{V}O_2$ represents the sum of all oxidative reactions and therefore reflects the body's oxidative metabolic activity; when $\dot{V}O_2$ is not rate-limited by blood flow, it is a measure of metabolic demand. Fifth, in acute circulatory insufficiency, $\dot{V}O_2$ is the regulatory mechanism of circulatory failure; reductions in $\dot{V}O_2$ below what is needed stimulate compensations including increased heart rate, myocardial contractility, cardiac output and respiratory functions. In the traditional approach, the objective is to restore commonly monitored $\overline{MAP}$, HR, CVP and urine output to normal as soon as abnormalities are discovered. Normal values are appropriate for normal, unstressed, resting subjects, but the empirically determined patterns of surviving patients are the appropriate goals of therapy for patients with shock and critical illness.

Therapy directed toward increasing $\dot{D}O_2$ and $\dot{V}O_2$ to the range of survivors of life-threatening shock was shown to improve outcome in prospective clinical trials. A branched-chain decision developed from decision rules based on physiologic data from survivors expedites fluid and pharmacologic management of critically ill post-operative surgical patients. This approach to post-operative shock may also serve as a point of departure for patients with prior associated medical problems who must undergo surgery as well as for patients with haemorrhagic, traumatic, septic and other types of shock. The improved mortality in prospective studies supports the hypothesis that compensatory responses of the survivors are major determinants of outcome because therapy that augments the compensations of the survivors, clearly improves survival rates. Prospective studies confirm the usefulness of an organized coherent algorithmic approach.

The need for this proposed approach is clear: more than 28 million major surgical operations are performed annually in the United States, with an estimated annual mortality of about 450 000. Studies indicating sharply reduced mortality and morbidity for a university-run county hospital suggest the possiblity that comparably improved outcome could occur nationwide with the application of these principles.

References

Abraham E, Bland RD, Cobo JC & Shoemaker WC (1984) Sequential cardiorespiratory patterns associated with outcome in septic shock. *Chest* **85**: 75.

Astiz ME, Rackow EC, Falk JL *et al.* (1987) Oxygen delivery and consumption in patients with hyperdynamic septic shock. *Crit. Care Med.* **15**: 26.

Bishop MH, Shoemaker WC, Appel PL *et al.* (1993a) Influence of time and optimal circulatory resuscitation in high risk trauma. *Crit. Care Med.* (in press).

Bishop MH, Shoemaker WC, Fleming AW *et al.* (1993b) Relationship between ARDS, hemodynamics, fluid balance and pulmonary infiltration in critically ill surgical patients. *Am. Surg.* **57**: 785.

Bland RD & Shoemaker WC (1985a) Common physiologic patterns in general surgical patients. Hemodynamic and oxygen transport changes during and after operation in patients with and without associated medical problems. *Surg. Clin. North Am.* **65**: 793.

Bland RD & Shoemaker WC (1985b) Probability of survival as a prognostic and severity of illness score in critically ill surgical patients. *Crit. Care Med.* **13**: 91.

Bland RD, Shoemaker WC, Abraham E *et al.* (1985) Hemodynamic and oxygen transport patterns in surviving and nonsurviving postoperative patients. *Crit. Care Med.* **13**: 85.

Clowes GHA Jr & Del Guercio LRM (1960) Circulatory response to trauma of surgical operations. *Metabolism* **9**: 67.

Cournand A, Riley RL, Bradley SE *et al.* (1943) Studies of the circulation in clinical shock. *Surgery* **13**: 964.

Creamer J, Edward JD & Nightingale P (1990) Hemodynamic and oxygen transport, variables in cardiogenic shock following acute myocardial infarction and their response to treatment. *Am. J. Cardiol.* **65**: 1297.

DaLuz P. Cavanilles JM & Michael S (1975) oxygen delivery, anoxic metabolism and hemoglobin P50 in patients with acute myocardial infarction and shock. *Am. J. Cardiol.* **36**: 148.

Del Guercio LRM, Commarswamy RF, Feins NR *et al.* (1964) Pulmonary arteriovenous admixture and the hyperdynamic state in surgery for portal hypertension. *Surgery* **56**: 57.

Edwards JD (1991) Oxygen transport in cardiogenic and septic shock. *Crit. Care Med.* **19**: 658.

Edwards JD, Redmond AD, Nightingale P *et al.* (1988) Oxygen consumption following trauma. *Br. J. Surg.* **75**: 690.

Edwards JD, Brown GCS, Nightingale P *et al.* (1989) Use of survivors' cardiorespiratory values as therapeutic goals in septic shock. *Crit. Care Med.* **17**: 1098.

Forrester JS, Diamond GA & Swan HJC (1977) Correlation classification of clinical and nemodynamic function after acute myocardial infarction. *Am. J. Cardiol.* **39**: 137.

Gilbert EM, Haupt MT, Mandanas RT *et al.* (1986) The effect of fluid loading blood transfusion, and catacholamine infusion on oxygen delivery and consumption in patients with sepsis. *Am. Rev. Respiratory Dis.* **134**: 873.

Hankeln K, Senker R, Schwarten JM *et al.* (1987) Evaluation of prognostic indices based on hemodynamic and oxygen transport variables in shock patients with adult respiratory distress syndrome. *Crit. Care Med.* **15**: 1.

Haupt MT, Gilbert EM & Carlson RW (1985) Fluid loading increases oxygen delivery and consumption in septic patients with lactic acidosis. *Am. Rev. Respiratory Dis.* **131**: 912.

Heilbrunn A & Allbritten FF (1960) Cardiac output during and following surgical operation. *Ann. Surg.* **152**: 197.

Lowe JG & Ernst EA (1981) *The Quantitiative Practice of Anesthesia: Use of the Closed Circuit*, pp. 146–7. Baltimore: Williams & Wilkins.

Packman MI & Rackow EC (1983) Optimal left heart filling pressure during fluid resuscitation of patients with hypovolemia and septic shock. *Crit. Care Med.* **11**: 165.

Rackow EC, Kaufman BS, Falk JL *et al.* (1987) Hemodynamic response to fluid repletion in patients with septic shock. *Circ. Shock* **22**: 11.

Russell JA, Lockhat D, Belzberg M *et al.* (1988) Oxygen delivery and consumption and ventricular preload are greater in survivors then nonsurvivors of ARDS. *Chest* **94**: 755.

Shippy CR, Appel PL & Shoemaker WC (1984) Reliability of clinical monitoring to assess blood volume in critically ill patients. *Crit. Care Med.* **12**: 107.

Shoemaker WC (1987) Circulatory mechanisms of shock and their mediators. *Crit. Care Med.* **15**: 787.

Shoemaker WC (1989) Shock states: pathophysiology, monitoring, outcome prediction, and therapy. In Shoemaker WC, Ayres SM, Grenvik A, Holbrook PR & Thompson WL (eds), *Textbook of Critical Care* (2nd edition). Philadelphia: W.B. Saunders.

Shoemaker WC, Printen KJ, Amato JJ *et al.* (1967) Hemodynamic patterns after acute anesthetized and unanesthetized trauma. *Arch. Surg.* **95**: 492.

Shoemaker WC, Boyd DR, Kim SI *et al.* (1971) Sequential oxygen transport and acid-base changes after trauma to the unanesthetized patient. *Surg. Gynecol. Ostet.* **132**: 657.

Shoemaker WC, Montgomery ES, Kaplan E *et al.* (1973) Physiologic patterns in surviving and nonsurviving shock patients. *Arch. Surg.* **106**: 630.

Shoemaker WC, Czer L, Chang P *et al.* (1979) Cardiorespiratory monitoring in postoperative patients: I. Prediction of outcome and severity of illness. *Crit. Care Med.* **7**: 237.

Shoemaker WC, Bland RD & Appel PL (1985) Therapy of critically ill postoperative patients based on outcome prediction and prospective clinical trials. *Surg. Clin. North Am.* **65**: 811.

Shoemaker WC, Appel PL & Kram HB (1988a) Tissue organ debt as a determinant of lethal and nonlethal postoperative organ failure. *Crit. Care Med.* **11**: 1123.

Shoemaker WC, Appel PL, Kram HB *et al.* (1988b) Prospective trial of supranormal values of survivors as therapeutic goals in high risk surgical patients. *Chest* **94:** 1176.

Shoemaker WC, Appel PL & Kram HB (1992) Role of oxygen debt in the development of organ failure, sepsis and death in high risk surgical patients. *Chest* **102:** 208.

Shoemaker WC, Printen KJ, Amato JJ *et al.* (1967) Hemodynamic patterns after acute anesthetized and unanesthetized trauma. *Arch. Surg.* **95:** 492.

Siegel J, Goldwyn PM & Friedman HP (1971) Pattern in process in the evolution of human septic shock. *Surgery* **70:** 232.

Tuchschmidt J, Fried J, Swinney R *et al.* (1989) Early hemodynamic correlates of survival in patients with septic shock. *Crit. Care Med.* **17:** 719.

Tuchschmidt J, Fried J, Astiz M *et al.* (1991) Supranormal oxygen delivery improves mortality in septic shock patients. *Crit. Care Med.* **19:** S66.

Wiggers CJ (1940) *Physiology of Shock.* New York: Commonwealth Fund.

Wilson RF, Thal AP, Kinding PH *et al.* (1965) Hemodynamic measurements in shock. *Arch. Surg.* **91:** 124.

5 The Significance of Mixed Venous Oxygen Saturation and Technical Aspects of Continuous Measurement

Aurel C. Cernaianu and Loren D. Nelson

Major problems related to tissue perfusion and oxygenation may be encountered in critically ill patients or in those undergoing surgery and anaesthesia. In order to detect early physiologic deterioration, monitoring of cardiorespiratory dynamics has become standard practice. Generally, therapeutic interventions should be directed toward the assurance of a balance between oxygen demand and oxygen delivery (Snyder & Carroll, 1982). Only recently has the concept that 'oxygen transport patterns provide an objective basis for the assessment of tissue perfusion' gained more attention (Shoemaker, 1991).

The technologic landmark of bedside pulmonary artery (PA) catheterization (Swan *et al.*, 1970) has provided the basis of sophisticated invasive cardiopulmonary monitoring. Yet, despite this technologic revolution, its effectiveness in improving ICU survival rate (Robin, 1983) or the quality of life (Cullen *et al.*, 1976) has been questioned. While the widespread use of flow-directed PA catheters has increased the clinician's ability to assess haemodynamics, there have been reports which question the need for PA catheterization (Robin, 1985) and stress the inherent pitfalls and complications (Morris *et al.*, 1984; Wiedemann *et al.*, 1984). Regardless of the arguments for and against, a PA catheter provides haemodynamic data that may have an impact in therapeutic decisions. Also increasing experience and refinement of PA catheterization technology allows today a minimal incidence of complications (Curling *et al.*, 1984).

With the development of the reflectance fibre-optic oximetry technique and its incorporation into the flow-directed PA catheter, the principle of continuous monitoring of mixed venous oxygen saturation ($S\bar{v}O_2$) has become integrated into the cardiopulmonary monitoring arsenal. Continuous bedside measurement of $S\bar{v}O_2$ and determination of trends have become important elements of continuous cardiopulmonary surveillance as well as means for assessing optimal responses to therapeutic interventions. Although the measurement of $S\bar{v}O_2$ is recognized as a beneficial index of dynamic oxygen transport balance, its accurate application in the clinical setting requires appropriate knowledge of the technology involved, the physiologic basis for the measurement and its correct interpretation in a particular clinical situation. This chapter discusses the principle of continuously monitored $S\bar{v}O_2$ and its clinical applications.

Fibre-Optic Technology for Measurement of $S\bar{v}O_2$

History

The principles underlying continuous venous oximetry were developed decades ago. Early experiments in spectrophotometry performed by Kramer (1934) and Brinkman and Zijstra (1949) coupled with the mathematical principle developed by Rodrigo (1953) culminated with the development of the $S\bar{v}O_2$ reflectance oximeter in 1960 (Polanyi & Hehir, 1960) and its *in vivo* fibre-optic counterpart (Polanyi & Hehir, 1962).

Reflectance spectrophotometry relies upon the absorbance and reflectance characteristics of red blood cells in motion. In transmission spectrophotometry red blood cells are usually lysed to release free haemoglobin in serum. Narrow wavebands of light are passed through the solution and the intensity of the light is measured by photodetectors sensitive to the wavelengths of interest. To measure the oxygen saturation of haemoglobin, wavelengths are chosen that will have absorbance peaks for oxyhaemoglobin and deoxyhaemoglobin. Some very sophisticated oximeters use up to eight wavelengths of light to measure the transmission characteristics of other haemoglobin species (i.e. methaemoglobin, carboxyhaemoglobin, sulphhaemoglobin, etc.).

Reflectance spectrophotometry has an advantage over transmission spectrophotometry in that the red cells do not need to be lysed. Rather, the wavelengths of light are based upon the reflectance characteristics of oxyhaemoglobin and deoxyhaemoglobin within red blood cells (Fig. 5.1). The fractional oxyhaemoglobin saturation is calculated as:

$$\% \text{ Saturation} = \frac{\text{oxyhaemoglobin}}{\substack{\text{oxyhaemoglobin} + \text{deoxyhaemoglobin} \\ + \text{ carboxyhaemoglobin} + \text{methaemoglobin}}} \times 100$$

When two wavelengths of light are used, the other species of haemoglobin which do not readily release oxygen are ignored, yielding what is referred to as the oxygen saturation of *functional* haemoglobin. While traditional oxyhaemoglobin saturation values relate the fractional amount of oxyhaemoglobin to the total haemoglobin concentrations, the saturation of functional haemoglobin relates oxyhaemoglobin to the total of oxyhaemoglobin plus deoxyhaemoglobin:

$$\% \text{ Functional saturation} = \frac{\text{oxyhaemoglobin}}{\text{oxyhaemoglobin} + \text{deoxyhaemoglobin}}$$

or

$$\% \text{ Functional saturation} = \frac{\text{fractional oxyhaemoglobin}}{1-(\text{MetHb} + \text{COHb})}$$

Therefore the functional haemoglobin saturation will always exaggerate the fractional haemoglobin saturation by an amount proportional to the amount of abnormal haemoglobins present.

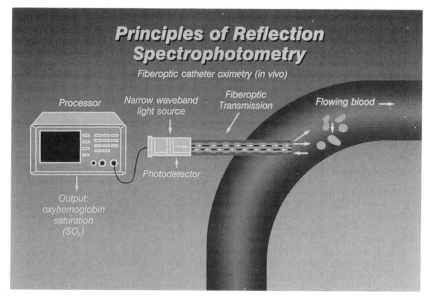

Figure 5.1 Reflectance spectrophotometry. (Reproduced by permission, Abbott Critical Care, Mountain View, CA.)

Acquired haemoglobinopathies such as carboxyhaemoglobinaemia and methaemoglobinaemia will induce differences between functional and fractional oxyhaemoglobin saturation. However, foetal haemoglobin does not influence the $S\bar{v}O_2$ measurement in infants (Wilkinson *et al.*, 1979).

$S\bar{v}O_2$ was first applied clinically by Frommer *et al.* (1965) during cardiac catheterization. Muir *et al.* (1970) first discussed the interdependence between $S\bar{v}O_2$, cardiac output, and survival rate in patients with myocardial infarction. The evolution of the oximetry catheter continued with incorporation of reflectance spectrophotometry into a multiple lumen, two-wavelength central venous fibre-optic catheter (Cole *et al.*, 1972). Martin and associates (1973) presented results using central venous oxygen saturation monitoring during anaesthesia in man. Parr *et al.* (1975) investigated the relationship between $S\bar{v}O_2$ and cardiac output during surgical repair of congenital heart lesions. They were the first associate values of $S\bar{v}O_2$ below 0.60 with reduced survival rates. Studies performed by Kasnitz *et al.* (1976) demonstrated the link between venous desaturation and the appearance of lactic acidosis followed by death. Routine clinical monitoring of venous oxygen saturation in neonates began in the late 1970s using an umbilical artery fibre-optic catheter (Wilkinson *et al.*, 1979).

Early problems related to the catheter design, calibration and transmission of optical signals, vessel wall artifact, loss of light intensity and the effect of varying haemoglobin concentration (Hb) have been elaborated by Reid (1975). Improvements in the quality of the catheter and advancements in computer technology allowed the development in 1981 of the balloon-tipped thermodilution PA catheter by Oximetrix (Mountain View, CA). The flexibility of the catheter was improved a year later and its accuracy and reliability were documented by Baele *et al.* (1982) and by Krouskop *et al.* (1983). The accuracy of the measurement improved with the condition of a third wavelength of light to compensate for changes in the total amount of reflected light (Sperinde & Senelly, 1985). The catheter stiffness was reduced by replacing the glass fibres within the optical system with more flexible plastic fibres.

The $S\bar{v}O_2$ System

Presently, there are three systems available for the continuous measurement of $S\bar{v}O_2$, the Shaw Opticath, Oximetrix 3 (Fig.5.2) (Abbott Critical Care Systems, Mountain View, CA), the Swan–Ganz flow-directed oximetry TD catheter (Fig. 5.3) (American Edwards Laboratories, Irvine, CA), and Spectra-cath (Viggo-Spectramed, Oxnard, CA) (Van Woerkens *et al.*, 1991). All systems continously monitor $S\bar{v}O_2$ using fibre-optic reflectance spectrometry to differentiate between oxygenated and deoxygenated haemoglobin (Schweiss, 1987). Each system consists of a microprocessor capable of *in vitro* calibration and memory storage for retroactive correction *vis-à-vis* a reference calibration. Analysis of the reflected light intensity and calculation of oxy-haemoglobin saturation is achieved by the microprocessor.

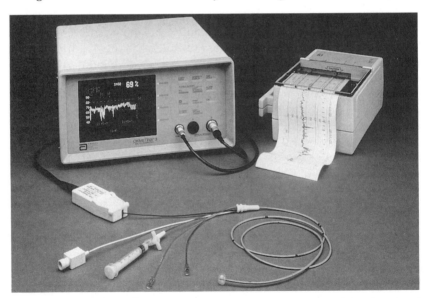

Figure 5.2   The Oximetrix 3 continuous mixed venous oximetry system showing the fibre-optic catheter, the optical module and cable, the processor display unit and a recorder. (Reproduced by permission, Abbott Critical Care, Mountain View, CA.)

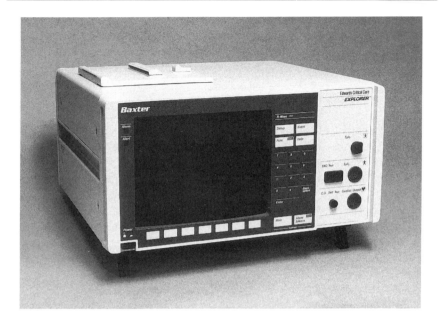

Figure 5.3 The 'Explorer' continuous venous oximeter is the latest multifunction $S\bar{v}O_2$ system introduced. (Reproduced by permission, Edwards Critical Care Division, Baxter International, Inc., Irvine, CA. Baxter is a registered trademark, copyright Baxter International, 1991.)

Two-Wavelength versus Three-Wavelength System

As new systems are introduced there has been much debate related to the accuracy and reliability of the three-wavelength (670, 700 and 800 nm) rather than two-wavelength technology.

Animal studies performed by Gettinger *et al.* (1986, 1987) have shown that values of $S\bar{v}O_2$ measured by the three-wavelength system correlated better with measurements obtained with the reference cooximeter than those measured using two wavelengths. Because of the differences in the Hb disso-ciation curve between man and the canine model, it was suggested that the results obtained from the canine model may not be totally reproducible and/or applicable in humans. Karis and Lumb (1988) studied the accuracy of the two systems in patients undergoing cardiac surgery. Their results showed that measurements of $S\bar{v}O_2$ with the three-wavelength system were closer to con-comitant measurements with the cooximeter than those measured with the two-wavelength system and the percentage error (drift) measured with the latter system increased over time. The three-wavelength technology seems to reflect more accurately the actual $S\bar{v}O_2$ over a longer period of time and under different pathophysiologic conditions. The use of three diodes minimizes drift and artifact interference and compensates for changes in haemoglobin concentration. The most current haemoglobin concentration must be manually entered into the two-wavelength systems to compensate for reflectance changes caused by changes in haemoglobin concentration.

Calibration Pitfalls and Misconceptions

Problems related to the *in vivo* calibration of newer generation of oximeters have resolved with new technology. Presently, all systems have capabilities of *in vitro* and *in vivo* calibration. Most common sources of error are corrected during the *in vitro* calibration process. According to the manufacturer's instructions, the $S\bar{v}O_2$ system should be calibrated *in vitro* prior to insertion of the catheter with the help of a disposable optical reference. This will ensure proper standardization of the catheter. Improper *in vitro* calibration may affect the accuracy and reliability of the system, resulting in an increased need for *in vivo* recalibration. Our practice is to follow the instructions for initial calibration and then to check the calibration once every 24 h after insertion, whenever there are technical problems associated with the connection to the optical module, or whenever the medical staff suspect erroneous values. Recalibration consists of a cross-check for accuracy by measuring the $S\bar{v}O_2$ on a blood sample drawn from the distal port of the PA catheter with a laboratory cooximeter. If the measured value varies by more than 0.04% the system is recalibrated. In contrast to the two-wavelength system, the three-wavelength system does not require additional correction to the actual haemoglobin concentration.

Generally, continuously measured $S\bar{v}O_2$ correlates well ($r = 0.8$–0.9) with laboratory *in vitro* cooximetry results (Karis & Lumb, 1988).

The stiffness of earlier generations of $S\bar{v}O_2$ catheters has led to the misconception that the fibre-optic PA catheters are more difficult to insert. Rajput *et al.* (1989) reported that the insertion of the fibre-optic catheters took longer than the conventional counterparts. McMichan *et al.* (1984) found no special problems related to the insertion of the fibre-optic catheters when compared with the conventional catheters. The fibre-optic catheters may be repositioned more frequently than their traditional counterparts (McMichan *et al.*, 1984; Nelson, unpublished data). This may be related to the fact that the continuous oximetry data alert the medical team immediately if the catheter position is not optimal.

All PA catheters can possibly migrate distally after initial placement. Chest roentgenograms may help to confirm optimal localization of the catheter. A proper proximal catheter tip position will help to ensure accurate measurement of cardiac output by thermodilution and reliable $S\bar{v}O_2$ determinations. The fibre-optic systems are equipped with light intensity or signal quality alarms which indicate distal catheter migration and the need for repositioning. Light intensity alerts can be produced by close proximity of the catheter tip to a vessel wall. In this situation the system will measure tissue light reflectance rather than blood light reflectance. The system is capable of filtering out the vessel wall artifact, eliminating erratic, falsely elevated readings. Fibre-optic integrity and adequacy of signals are also assessed.

An early misconception related to the fibre-optic oximeters was the assumption that $S\bar{v}O_2$ directly correlated with the reflected light intensity. It has been demonstrated not only that this assumption is incorrect but that various changes in the blood pH, haematocrit and blood flow velocity will alter the colour of the blood and change the measured $S\bar{v}O_2$. The oximetry microprocessor integrates the displayed oxygen saturation with light intensity measurements so that many of these artifacts are easily detected and eliminated.

The effect of patient positioning on haemodynamic monitoring and $S\bar{v}O_2$ has been studied recently (Nelson & Anderson, 1989; Briones *et al.*, 1991). In normotensive patients, haemodynamics and $S\bar{v}O_2$ were not significantly different when measured in the supine or lateral position.

Pitfalls of Interpretation of $S\bar{v}O_2$

Invasive monitoring with the fibre-optic PA catheter can establish the basis for early detection of cardiorespiratory abnormalities and evalution of therapy. Successful application of $S\bar{v}O_2$ monitoring depends on consideration of the technical and physiological factors which may affect interpretation of the data. Quite often, the interpretation of the measurement is made without sufficient consideration of the principle involved and the inherent technical limitations.

$S\bar{v}O_2$ is determined by the balance between oxygen delivery (DO_2) and oxygen consumption ($\dot{V}O_2$). This relationship is expressed by the Fick principle (1870) which states that the volume of oxygen consumed by the tissues is equal to the differences between the volume of oxygen delivered from the heart minus the volume of oxygen returned to the heart each minute. DO_2 is equal to cardiac output times arterial oxygen content (CaO_2). Oxygen return to the heart is equal to venous return (which must equal cardiac output) times mixed venous oxygen content ($C\bar{v}O_2$). The descriptions of $S\bar{v}O_2$ calculation and derived oxygen transport parameters have been presented elsewhere (Nelson, 1986a, 1988). According to the Fick equation, when SaO_2 is maintained at high levels, $S\bar{v}O_2$ is inversely related to the oxygen utilization coefficient (OUC) which defines the balance between DO_2 and $\dot{V}O_2$ (Nelson, 1987). The relationship is valid at high SaO_2 when $S\bar{v}O_2$ approximates $C\bar{v}O_2/CaO_2$. In consequence, changes in $S\bar{v}O_2$ reflect changes in the cardiorespiratory components of the Fick equation, i.e. cardiac output, arterial oxygen saturation, haemoglobin concentration and $\dot{V}O_2$. Uncompensated decreases in the factors determining oxygen delivery (SaO_2, haemoglobin and cardiac output) or uncompensated increases in oxygen consumption will decrease $S\bar{v}O_2$.

A common misconception is that changes in $S\bar{v}O_2$ are directly related to changes in cardiac output. This theory was introduced by Boyd *et al.* (1959) and supported by McArthur *et al.* (1962), Kelman *et al.* (1967) and

Krauss *et al.* (1975). More recent studies have continued to look for a strong correlation between the $S\bar{v}O_2$ and cardiac output. Not surprisingly, Richard *et al.* (1989) found a poor relationship between $S\bar{v}O_2$ and cardiac index (CI) in patients suffering from ventricular failure undergoing treatment with angiotensin-converting enzyme inhibitors. Their hypothesis was that a direct relationship between $S\bar{v}O_2$ and CI should exist if the relationship between DO_2 and oxygen extraction ratio was maintained and $\dot{V}O_2$ reached a stable plateau. The belief was that above the critical threshold of DO_2, $\dot{V}O_2$ is constant and independent of DO_2 (Schumaker & Cain 1987).

The key issue in this hypothesis is that critically ill patients are rarely in a steady state (Civetta, 1988a). These patients usually present with physiologic changes and are prone to multiple therapeutic interventions which preclude a steady state. Compensatory mechanisms to balance oxygen transport often increase cardiac output if tissue oxygen requirements increase. However, other mechanisms such as selective redistribution of flow to specific areas with enhanced metabolic activity may also be involved. Our own preliminary data from an ongoing multicentre study of over 300 critically ill patients (Cernaianu, personal communication, 1991) have confirmed results by Nelson (1986a) demonstrating a poor correlation between $S\bar{v}O_2$ and individual determinants of oxygen transport balance (Fig. 5.4a–e) and a high correlation between $S\bar{v}O_2$ and oxygen utilization coefficient (Fig. 5.4f).

Chappel *et al.* (1983) demonstrated that vasodilator therapy in patients with severe left ventricular failure may change the interrelation between $\dot{V}O_2$ and DO_2. Mixed venous blood represents the flow-weighted average of the venous effluents of all perfused vascular beds. Monitoring $S\bar{v}O_2$ reflects the global oxygen transport balance in accordance to all compensatory mechanisms. That is why $S\bar{v}O_2$ has been found to correlate poorly with each individual component of the oxygen transport system (Nelson, 1986a).

However, a relationship between $S\bar{v}O_2$ and CI can be found in groups of patients with stable $\dot{V}O_2$ and haemoglobin concentration. In this case, the ability of $S\bar{v}O_2$ to serve as a therapeutic indicator has been found to be dependent on the baseline $S\bar{v}O_2$ and CI values (Jain *et al.*, 1991). Earlier reports by De La Rocha *et al.* (1978) confirmed that $S\bar{v}O_2$ can correlate with CI ($r = 0.78$) during general anaesthesia in a paediatric population undergoing heart surgery.

Kyff *et al.* (1989) studied 24 adult patients with haemodynamically unstable myocardial infarction. A desaturation of $S\bar{v}O_2$ by 5 and 10% corresponded with a decrease of CI in 45% and 61% respectively. Their survivors had significantly higher mean $S\bar{v}O_2$ and CI values than non-survivors; however, the authors concluded that '$S\bar{v}O_2$ may not be a sensitive measure of cardiac output after myocardial infarction'.

Venous desaturation has been associated with lactic acidosis (Kasnitz *et al.*, 1976). However, Kyff, *et al.* (1989) found no relationship between $S\bar{v}O_2$ level and the arterial blood lactate. While hyperlactaemia has been related to cardiovascular abnormalities accompanied by global cellular hypoxia, it may

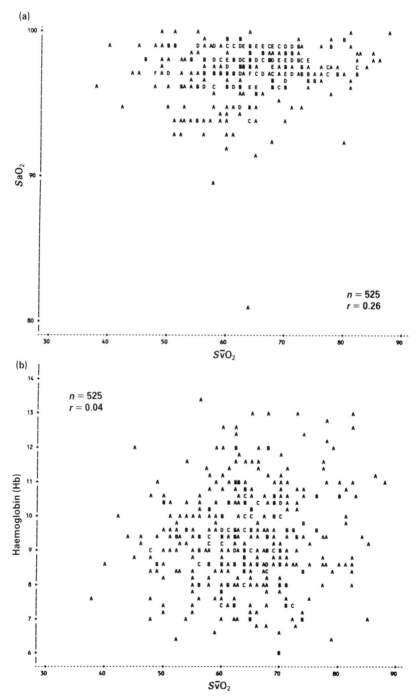

Figure 5.4 The relationship between mixed venous oxygen saturation ($S\bar{v}O_2$) and (a) arterial oxygen saturation (SaO_2), (b) haemoglobin, (c) cardiac output, (d) oxygen delivery, (e) oxygen consumption, and (f) oxygen utilization (delivery) coefficient.

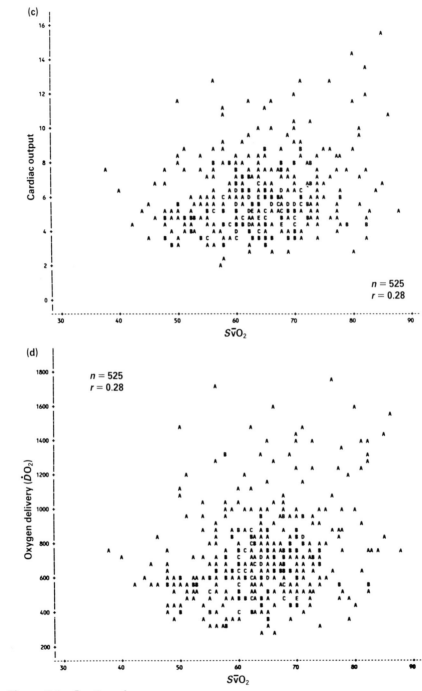

Figure 5.4   Continued.

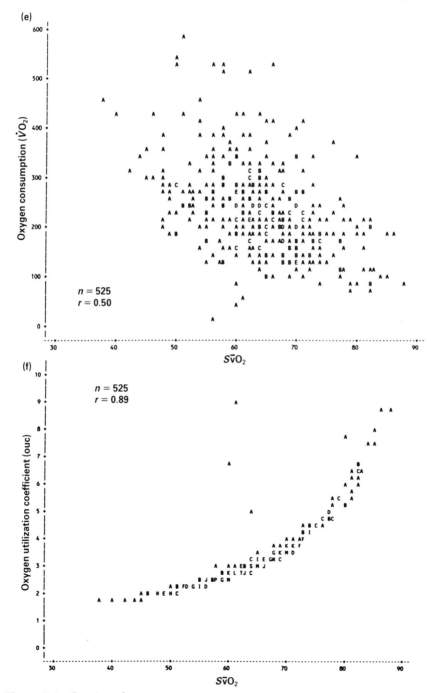

Figure 5.4   Continued.

also occur in vasoderegulated states like sepsis (Rashkin *et al.*, 1985; Groeneveld *et al.*, 1987; Tuchshmidt *et al.*, 1989). The degree of hyperlactaemia is usually related to the magnitude and duration of the ischaemia during the period of oxygen supply–demand imbalance. At $S\bar{v}O_2$ values of less than 0.60, Kyff *et al.* (1989) found that, although not statistically signficant, the level of arterial lactate approached levels that Weil and Afifi (1970) and Forrester *et al.* (1976) described as critical values (2.5 nmol litre^{-1}). In individual patients $S\bar{v}O_2$ does not directly provide information concerning the level of arterial lactate (Benjamin & Iberti 1989) and it should not be seen as a predictor for hyperlactaemia (Rackow *et al.*, 1989).

On the other hand, critically ill patients characterized by loss of vasoregulation may present with paradoxical high $S\bar{v}O_2$ values which may or may not be accompanied by hyperlactaemia due to impaired oxygen uptake. The exact mechanism is poorly understood. Maldistribution of systemic circulation seen in multiorgan system failure due to sepsis has been traditionally represented by high $S\bar{v}O_2$ coupled with lactacidaemia (MacLean *et al.*, 1967; Nishijima *et al.*, 1973; Astiz *et al.*, 1988). In this situation a high $S\bar{v}O_2$ is indicative that global oxygen delivery exceeds oxygen consumption by an amount greater than normal. The increased lactic acid concentration indicates that it is being produced in amounts greater than are being metabolized. This may be the result of localized tissue oxygen demand exceeding oxygen use (consumption) and these tissues operating under (relatively) anaerobic conditions. Alternatively, normal (hepatic) metabolism of lactic acid may be impaired, resulting in lactic acidaemia (Kandel & Aberman, 1983).

Continuously monitored $S\bar{v}O_2$ has been advocated by some investigators as an 'early warning indicator' of cardiorespiratory deregulation (Birman *et al.*, 1984; Divertie & McMichan, 1984). The dependence of $S\bar{v}O_2$ on all oxygen transport components enumerated earlier in this discussion causes speculation that substantial decreases in DO_2 may not trigger significant changes in $S\bar{v}O_2$ due to compensatory mechanisms. Data from our own institution, collected from haemodynamically 'stable' patients post-cardiac surgery have demonstrated that all patients with normal range $S\bar{v}O_2$ (65–75%) had physiologic profiles (haemodynamic and oxygen transport variables) in normal range (Cernaianu *et al.*, 1992). Our results were in agreement with Watson (1983) who stated that 'hemodynamic changes unassociated with derangements in $S\bar{v}O_2$ are not significant when tissue perfusion is adequate'.

The alterations in the management of critically ill patients based on the availability of continuously monitored $S\bar{v}O_2$ has been studied by Boutros and Lee (1986). Unfortunately, the authors studied only 15 critically ill patients; of those, nine died in the ICU due to sepsis. Those may be the cases in which no available management tactics would have changed the outcome. Patients with hyperdynamic states due to sepsis do not obey the 'classical' haemodynamic regulatory mechanisms and paradoxal situations may develop (Vermeij *et al.*, 1991).

Interpretation of $S\bar{v}O_2$ is complicated by the fact that $S\bar{v}O_2$ is measured from blood sampled from the pulmonary artery. $S\bar{v}O_2$ does not reflect the oxygen transport balance of any individual organ (Shibutani, 1983). High-blood-flow, low-oxygen-extraction organs, such as the kidneys, have a greater effect on $S\bar{v}O_2$ than do low-flow, high-extraction organs, such as the myocardium. $S\bar{v}O_2$ is a flow-weighted average of saturation data from all perfused tissues. As long as the vasoregulatory mechanisms are intact, even in the presence of critical illness, readjustment of the distribution of blood flow makes $S\bar{v}O_2$ a useful indicator of oxygen supply–demand balance (Kandel & Aberman, 1983).

Continuous *in vivo* monitoring of $S\bar{v}O_2$ with fibre-optic oximetry raises accuracy questions related to both the PA catheter and the oximetry device. The pitfalls in calibration, measurements and interpretation of data provided by the PA catheter have been reviewed extensively by Tuman *et al.* (1989). The accuracy of the oximetry component is dependent, in part, on proper positioning of the PA catheter. The catheter should be positioned as proximal as possible and yet still be able to float to an occluded waveform position when the catheter balloon is inflated. Generally, this position will allow measurement of the PA occlusion pressure (PAOP, 'wedge') with the full 1.5 ml balloon volume.

Some investigators have questioned the accuracy of the measurement of oxygen transport variables in critically ill patients (Rubin *et al.*, 1982). Non-steady states caused by loss of biologic regulation make the relationship between systemic oxygen transport variables (i.e. $C(a–\bar{v})O_2$, cardiac output and $\dot{V}O_2$) difficult to interpret. Nevertheless, the comparison between measured and Fick-derived values by Iparraguirre *et al.* (1988) demonstrated that in patients with myocardial infarction, oxygen transport variables indirectly calculated by the Fick equation are equivalent to directly measured values by oximetry. This was true despite various degrees of haemodynamic decompensation and/or the effect of applied therapy.

Continuously monitored $S\bar{v}O_2$ correlates with *in vitro* cooximetry. The accuracy of the systems currently available for clinical use has been discussed earlier in this chapter (Baele *et al.*, 1982; Krouskop *et al.*, 1983; Fahey *et al.*, 1984; Divertie & McMichan, 1984; Karis & Lumb, 1988).

Since monitoring of $S\bar{v}O_2$ may provide an assurance of global oxygen transport stability and an early warning to the contrary, confidence in the displayed value of $S\bar{v}O_2$ should be high (Van Woerkens *et al.*, 1991). Mistrust in the measured values encourages unnecessary verification of the components of cardiorespiratory profile (Kyff *et al.*, 1989). In order to gain confidence in the $S\bar{v}O_2$ system, the staff should undergo careful training and be familiar with all aspects of calibration, maintenance and trouble-shooting.

The application of haemodynamic monitoring in the ICU should be related to severity of illness (Swan, 1988). Establishment of ICU 'protocols' for different types of critically ill patients (i.e. cardiac surgical patients) demanding routine verification of cardiopulmonary profiles at regular intervals without specific reasons other than assurance of haemodynamic stability, has proven unnecessary when $S\bar{v}O_2$ is coupled with other standard monitoring techniques (Cernaianu *et al.*, 1992). This, in conjunction with a correct stratification of patients' severity of illness and appropriate utilization of monitoring may lead to improved patient management and decreased cost.

Controversies in $S\bar{v}O_2$ Monitoring

The fibre-optic PA system for assessing $S\bar{v}O_2$ has achieved widespread clinical used in cardiorespiratory monitoring. Increased awareness of the need for cost containment and availability of a multitude of new modes of monitoring have surrounded this expensive and invasive type of monitoring in controversy. A physiologic monitor must accurately measure a clinically useful variable. The information provided should not be readily available by alternative methods. The technique should be safe, convenient, reliable, and the cost of information and risk to the patient must be justified.

Measurement Specificity

Many current monitoring techniques are neither sensitive nor specific. Enderson and Rice (1990) described the ideal monitoring parameter as 'the variable which would be sensitive enough to detect a reduction in perfusion before it adversely affects vital organ function.' One of the limitations of $S\bar{v}O_2$ monitoring is the fact that it is a non-specific indicator of oxygen transport imbalance (Norfleet & Watson, 1985). Changes in the relationship between the oxygen supply and demand can occur without great changes in $S\bar{v}O_2$. The argument is based on the judgement that changes in cardiac output may be compensated for by a rise in oxygen content due to transformations, hyperoxia and/or decreased tissue oxygen consumption. They also emphasize that patients with adequate cardiovascular reserve may have considerable hypoxaemia and not demonstrate an altered $S\bar{v}O_2$ because of the initiation of compensatory cardiovascular reflexes.

Continuously monitored $S\bar{v}O_2$ is a global non-specific cardiorespiratory variable which reflects the oxygen supply–demand balance. The complex configuaration of the oxygen transport system (i.e. the delivery components of arterial oxygen saturation, cardiac output, and haemoglobin concentration) and tissue oxygen consumption interact with various metabolic and local regulatory mechanisms, making the interpretation of the $S\bar{v}O_2$ difficult. For the purpose of simplification, it is considered that augmentation of $S\bar{v}O_2$ reflects an increase in $\dot{D}O_2$ over $\dot{V}O_2$; the opposite trend in $S\bar{v}O_2$ reflects an increase in $\dot{V}O_2$ over $\dot{D}O_2$. As mentioned by Nelson (1986a), $S\bar{v}O_2$ monitoring does not yield specific information regarding any individual oxygen transport variable, however, changes in $S\bar{v}O_2$ give more important information regarding trends in the balance of the entire oxygen transport system.

Changes in non-specificity of $S\bar{v}O_2$ can be due to changes in cardiac output or metabolic demand for oxygen. There are ample data demonstrating that continuously monitored $S\bar{v}O_2$ is a reliable trend indicator of the adequacy of oxygen transport balance during steady or non-steady state and during many therapeutic interventions.

Clinical Importance

The importance of $S\bar{v}O_2$ monitoring remains controversial particularly because of lack of demonstrated clinical significance between the degree of changes in $S\bar{v}O_2$ and other information pertaining to the patient's clinical course. Many patients with circulatory failure may have low $S\bar{v}O_2$. There are situations, mostly theoretical, such as a large right-to-left shunt in which the $S\bar{v}O_2$ is decreased as a result of a decrease in SaO_2, even when the $C(a-\bar{v})O_2$ remains the same. The non-specificity issues addressed earlier in this discussion have been used to argue that continuously monitored $S\bar{v}O_2$ seldom brings new information to change the patient's management. It has been questioned whether transient changes or gradual trends in $S\bar{v}O_2$ should be treated.

Jastremski et al. (1989) studied a group of critically ill patients in which a fibre-optic or a standard PA catheter has been randomly inserted for acute haemodynamic stabilization. They concluded that 'the use of the fibre-optic catheter was not associated with a decrease in potentially adverse hemodynamic events, length of stay in the ICU or mortality rate, and its use does not appear to be beneficial in all patients requiring PA catheterization.'

Closer scrutiny of their data proved that the addition of the $S\bar{v}O_2$ monitoring allowed the diagnosis of haemodynamic derangements which could not be predicted by any other available means in 62% of the cases. Seventy-eight per cent of those patients underwent further laboratory tests resulting in a need for therapeutic interventions in 59% of the cases. Their analysis demonstrated transitory venous desaturations which are characteristic of the patient's severity of illness and the multitude of therapeutic interventions. The lack of differences in outcome is difficult to analyse and blame on the type of the PA catheter used since the patient population and other modalities of treatment are so heterogeneous. The general assessment of 'definitive outcome' of critically ill patients is a difficult task with the currently available criteria (Civetta, 1988b).

It is generally accepted that values of $S\bar{v}O_2$ ranging from 65 to 77% indicate a relative balance between oxygen supply and demand (Jamieson *et al.*, 1982; McMichan, 1983). Higher levels of $S\bar{v}O_2$ may be seen in the presence of hepatitis, major burns, pancreatitis, sepsis, ARDS, increased left-to-right shunt, cyanide toxicity and arterial hyperoxia (Nelson, 1987). $S\bar{v}O_2$ values below normal ranges may be seen in conditions associated with an increase in $\dot{V}O_2$ (shivering, fever, increased activity) or those associated with a decrease in oxygen delivery. It is stated that an increase or decrease in $S\bar{v}O_2$ of more than 10% is clinically significant (Table 5.1).

Table 5.1   Causes of abnormal $S\bar{v}O_2$

High $S\bar{v}O_2$	Low $S\bar{v}O_2$
Reduced oxygen demand	Increased oxygen demand
High oxygen delivery	Inadequate oxygen delivery
Technical error[a]	Technical error[a]

[a] Technical error may be due to incorrect measurement or sampling.

Alternative Monitoring

The amount of monitoring which should be performed in critically ill patients continues to stimulate much controversy. Intermittent measurements of cardiovascular parameters may be inadequate in many critically ill patients. The timing of intermittent evaluations of cardiorespiratory system may not depict periods of unbalanced haemodynamics – time when therapeutic interventions may influence the outcome. Although the trend in the development of future monitoring technologies is toward 'continuous' measurements, currently there are few monitoring devices proven to be as reliable, safe and cost-efficient as the fibre-optic PA catheter. Continuous cardiac output devices, invasive or non-invasive continuous blood-gas analysers, and invasive devices based on the measurements of cardiac volume instead of pressure, have been evaluated on a limited basis with more or less success. The introduction and acceptance in clinical practice of new technologies aimed at monitoring critically ill patients should be seen in relation to the current increasing standards of care and diminishing health care resources.

We are aware of a single prospective randomized study performed by Pearson and associates (1989) in which the authors concluded that post-cardiac surgery patients have no discernible differences in outcome, length of stay in ICU, morbidity or mortality rate when monitored with a CVP catheter alone, a PA catheter or with continuous $S\bar{v}O_2$. The authors' conclusion may be misleading, since CVP pressure monitoring was justified only in 'low-risk' cardiac surgical patients and only when combined with left atrial pressure monitoring. Our conclusion (Cernaianu *et al.*, 1990) is also supported by others (Kupeli & Satwicz, 1989). As mentioned previously, the assessment of severity of disease is important in selecting the appropriate monitoring system. The fibre-optic PA catheter is a unique technology providing information to detect compromise, titrate therapy, and signal physiologic changes.

Cost Efficiency

Fibre-optic PA catheters are more expensive than their standard thermo-dilution counterparts. There are data (Cernaianu et al., 1992) which suggest that, even in an environment with budgetary restrictions and reimburse-ment based on Diagnosis Related Group (DRG) prospective payment, the use of $S\bar{v}O_2$ as an 'on-line' assurance of haemodynamic and oxygen trans-port stability, can eliminate a substantial number of laboratory determin-ations and reduce cost. Continuous $S\bar{v}O_2$ measurement may save an average of 220 min of nursing time (range 90–300) per patient, during an ICU stay of 1½ days. Saving nursing time may not translate directly in cost saving because ICU personnel are still needed. However, in the view of increasing standards of care and decreasing availability of nursing personnel, saved time may be used for other purposes to improve the quality of care.

Larson and Kyff (1989) retrospectively analysed the cost-effectiveness of monitoring with the fibre-optic PA catheter in cardiac surgical patients. Their evalution study could not explain the repeated overuse of haemo-dynamic and laboratory determinations (Cernaianu, 1990). Often mistrust in the haemodynamic indicators and/or the staff's limited knowledge of the interpretation of 'on-line' monitoring technology is responsible for ordering of excessive confirmatory tests.

Cost-effectiveness of $S\bar{v}O_2$ monitoring has been demonstrated (Nelson, 1986b; Orlando, 1986; Jastremsky et al., 1989) when the data are used to enhance clinical decision-making in a goal-oriented manner. In the view of these findings, the initial added cost of the fibre-optic PA catheter is off-set by the savings in intermittent blood-gas analyses and haemodynamic measurements.

$S\bar{v}O_2$ Monitoring and Nursing Care

Cardiovascular monitoring with flow-directed PA catheters impacts on the practice of critical care nursing. The introduction of fibre-optic oximetry adds little additional nursing effort for calibration and maintenance of the system.

The beneficial effects of continuously monitored $S\bar{v}O_2$ on routine nursing care have appeared in the literature (Jaquith, 1985). Since the critical care nurse is instrumental in maintaining monitoring and evaluating the $S\bar{v}O_2$ levels, ample descriptions of the principle of $S\bar{v}O_2$ and the technology are needed (Briones, 1988; Hardy, 1988). The widespread availability of the technology and increased experience with the $S\bar{v}O_2$ system has generated much research to evaluate the effect of nursing technique on oxygen trans-port balance (Stewart, 1988).

Therapeutic nursing interventions in critically ill patients often change $S\bar{v}O_2$. Recently, Clark *et al.* (1990) evaluated the effect of traditional endotracheal suctioning and closed-suctioning combined with hyperoxygenation on $S\bar{v}O_2$ and heart rate in a multihospital setting. Closed-suctioning provided a better method of preserving higher $S\bar{v}O_2$ levels and the authors recommended prophylactic hyperoxygenation before suctioning.

Winslow *et al.* (1990) studied the effect of lateral turning on $S\bar{v}O_2$ and advised that significant transitory changes of up to 9% in $S\bar{v}O_2$ accompanied by significant changes in heart rate may occur with patient positioning. The same kind of impact, although more moderate, has been observed when slow-stroke massage (a manoeuvre designed for providing a patient's comfort and relaxation with minimal cardiovascular stimulation) has been applied to critically ill patients (Tyler *et al.*, 1990).

The appearance of much interest from the nursing point of view demonstrates not only acceptance of $S\bar{v}O_2$ as a valuable tool in the assessment of haemodynamics and oxygen transport, but also confidence in the system's accuracy and reliability. $S\bar{v}O_2$ monitoring can be a valuable estimate of a patient's responses to nursing care.

Clinical Applications of $S\bar{v}O_2$ Monitoring

Cardiothoracic Surgery

This is discussed in Chapter 6.

General Surgery and Trauma

Individual indications in general surgery are given in Chapter 6.

Reports by Rao *et al.* (1983) proved that 'high-risk' patients undergoing anaesthesia and surgery may benefit from early invasive monitoring and treatment of haemodynamic abnormalities, resulting in improvement of mortality and morbidity. The effect of trauma and surgery on $\dot{V}O_2$, acid–base balance, and respiratory function was assessed earlier by Wilson *et al.* (1972). The authors emphasized the prognostic value of oxygen variables in this category of patients. The benefit of continuous $S\bar{v}O_2$ monitoring in patients undergoing general surgery was analysed by Nelson (1986a) and Norwood and Nelson (1986). Their findings suggested that patients who require PA catheterization for determination of cardiopulmonary function and evaluation of therapy receive better monitoring of oxygen transport variable when continuous venous oximetry is used. Orlando (1986) has validated the clinical utility of continuous $S\bar{v}O_2$ for post-operative monitoring and demonstrated cost-effectiveness with its proper use. It is important to emphasize that the cost-effectiveness of the technique is dependent upon how the derived data are used. If the measurements are used to replace repetitive arterial and venous blood-gas analyses, the technique is cost-effective. If the values are ignored or used to trigger frequent confirmatory tests, costs will be increased.

There is probably no better place than the trauma ICU to demonstrate the benefit of continuous $S\bar{v}O_2$ monitoring. Fibre-optic oximetry has been listed among the most important advanced alternatives of assessing the peripheral oxygen delivery in trauma patients (Moore & Haenel, 1988). In our own trauma unit continuous $S\bar{v}O_2$ monitoring is used to assess the adequacy of oxygen transport balance in all patients with combined cardiac and respiratory dysfunction. In addition, the $S\bar{v}O_2$ value is used for the calculation of intrapulmonary shunt fraction ($\dot{Q}s/\dot{Q}t$) as an end-point in the titration of positive end-expiratory pressure (PEEP).

Mixed venous oxygen saturation is also helpful in the assessment of patients with a hyperlactaemia. The elevated lactic acid concentration may be caused by increased production because of *continued* anaerobic metabolism or by decreased clearance of peripheral 'wash-out' of lactate which accumulated in peripheral tissues because of *previous* anaerobic metabolism in ischaemic limbs. A low $S\bar{v}O_2$ suggests continued oxygen transport imbalance and a normal value suggests that the increased lactic acid is due to wash-out or decreased clearance.

Continuous $S\bar{v}O_2$ monitoring has also been used in patients with severe closed head injury who are being dehydrated to lower intracranial pressure. Intravascular volume can be reduced to the point where oxygen transport balance is only minimally affected.

Medical Critically Ill Patients

Most of the data related to the clinical application of the $S\bar{v}O_2$ monitoring in the medical ICU have been already discussed in this chapter. The implementation of venous oximetry has proven to be an efficient tool for both diagnostic and therapeutic interventions in patients with acute myocardial infarction (Birman *et al.*, 1984). A strong correlation ($r = 0.88$) exists between $\dot{D}O_2$ and $S\bar{v}O_2$ in patients with hypoxaemic respiratory failure requiring positive end-expiratory pressure (Fahey *et al.*, 1984). Accuracy and reliability of the fibre-optic oximetry in a heterogeneous group of patients with varying degrees of physiologic disturbances was also demonstrated.

Chappel *et al.* (1983) reported a strong correlation between $\dot{D}O_2$ and $S\bar{v}O_2$ without changes in $\dot{V}O_2$ in patients treated with vasodilators for refractory left ventricular failure. Data from Gore and Sloan (1984) proved that continuous venous oximetry may be used as an indicator of cardiac performance in patients with myocardial infarction. The clinical response to cardioactive or vasodilator therapy was found to match the changes in $S\bar{v}O_2$ level. However, some critics (Richard *et al.*, 1989) advised that $S\bar{v}O_2$ cannot replace CI in the evaluation of haemodynamic effects of cardiovascular therapy. Gilbert (1987) has used $S\bar{v}O_2$ to devise an index of cardiopulmonary performance for cases in which emergent titration of acute interventions (ventilator setting, cardioactive drugs, or fluid administration) is necessary. They showed that $S\bar{v}O_2$ monitoring has potential clinical applications during acute life-threatening crisis in patients with acute respiratory decompensation.

Other Clinical Applications of $S\bar{v}O_2$ Monitoring

When monitored during anaesthesia for cardiothoracic surgery, $S\bar{v}O_2$ decreased significantly when changing from two-lung to one-lung ventilation (Thys et al., 1988). The changes in $S\bar{v}O_2$ strongly correlated with SaO_2 alone but not with CI alone. Multiple regression analysis demonstrated a strong correlation of $S\bar{v}O_2$ with changes in both CI and SaO_2. These data demonstrate that one-lung ventilation induces profound arterial hypoxaemia which can be better monitored with continuous rather than intermittent techniques. The authors attributed the changes in $S\bar{v}O_2$ mainly to hypoxaemia rather than changes in cardiac output.

Continuous venous oximetry has been applied by Yokota et al. (1988) during anaesthesia for major abdominal surgery. They validated catheter accuracy and, demonstrated that in a controlled environment during anaesthesia, a desaturation of $S\bar{v}O_2$ of 5% or more is strongly correlated with CI and oxygen extraction ratio.

$S\bar{v}O_2$ monitoring has been used in selected obstetric cases. Some of the indications for its use are: the administration of massive blood transfusions associated with either oliguria or pulmonary oedema, septic shock, cardiac failure, severe pregnancy-induced hypertension, labour and delivery in patients with significant cardiovascular disease and intra-operative cardiovascular decompensation (Kirshon & Cotton, 1987).

Summary

The present technology for continuously monitored $S\bar{v}O_2$ has been validated with respect to its accuracy, reliability, clinical application and cost-effectiveness. Ample data from both the adult and paediatric population are available. Although still controversial, the concept is widely accepted by both nurses and physicians. There are no additional risks introduced by the continuously measured venous oximetry aside from those already associated with standard PA catheterization. There are no major difficulties in calibration, maintenance or interpretation (reading) of the $S\bar{v}O_2$ monitoring system. The increase in the initial cost of the fibre-optic catheter over the non-oximetry catheter is off-set if the $S\bar{v}O_2$ data are used appropriately. All these qualities, coupled with its unique ability to measure the global adequacy of oxygen transport balance, make the continuous venous oximetry a useful adjunct in the critical care setting.

Cardiovascular monitoring with flow-directed PA catheterization will continue to be one of the invasive options available for assessing critically ill patients. The measurement of $S\bar{v}O_2$ alone or in conjunction with other monitored cardiopulmonary parameters will continue to provide valuable information with regard to the delicate but dynamic oxygen supply–demand balance and the implication of applied therapy upon it. As monitoring technology develops, the use of $S\bar{v}O_2$ will widen progressively in parallel with a broader understanding of the concept of oxygen transport and its evaluation in different clinical settings.

References

Astiz ME, Rackow EC, Kaufman B et al. (1988) Relationship of oxygen delivery and mixed venous oxygenation to lactic acidosis in patients with sepsis and acute myocardial infarction. Crit. Care Med. **16:** 655–8.

Baele PL, McMichan JC, Marsh HM et al. (1982) Continuous monitoring of mixed venous oxygen saturation in critically ill patients. Anesthesia Analgesia **61:** 513–17.

Benjamin E & Iberti TJ (1989) Oxygen delivery and lactic acidosis. Crit. Care Med. **17:** 299.

Birman H, Haz A, Hew E et al. (1984) Continuous monitoring of mixed venous oxygen saturation in hemodynamically unstable patients. Chest **86:** 753–6.

Boutros AR & Lee C (1986) Value of continuous monitoring of mixed venous blood oxygen saturation in the management of critically ill patients. Crit. Care Med. **14:** 132–4.

Boyd AD, Tremblay RE, Spencer FC & Bahanson HT (1959). Estimation of cardiac output soon after intracardiac surgery with cardiopulmonary bypass. Ann. Surg. **150:** 613–26.

Brinkman R & Zijstra WG (1949) Determination and continuous registration of the percentage oxygen saturation in small amounts of blood. Arch. Chir. Neeri **1:** 177–81.

Briones TL (1988) $S\bar{v}O_2$ monitoring: Part I. Clinical case application. Dimens. Crit. Care Nurs. **7:** 70–8.

Briones TL, Dickerson S & Bieberitz R (1991) Effects of positioning on hemodynamics and $S\bar{v}O_2$ Crit. Care Med. **19:** S29.

Cernaianu AC (1990) Cost-effectiveness of Oximetric PAC: A fair evaluation? J. Cardiothor. Anesth. **4:** 300–1.

Cernaianu AC, Moore WA & Posner MA (1990) Invasive monitoring of cardiac surgical patients (letter). Anesthesia Analgesia **70:** 671–2.

Cernaianu AC, DelRossi AJ, Boatman GA et al. (1992) Continuous venous oximetry for hemodynamic and oxygen transport stability post cardiac surgery. J. Cardiovasc. Surg. **33(1):** 14–20.

Chappel TR, Rubin LJ, Markham RV & Firth BG (1983) Independence of oxygen consumption and systemic oxygen transport in patients with either stable pulmonary hypertension or refractory left ventricular failure. Am. Rev. Respatory Dis. **128:** 30–3.

Civetta JM (1988a) The what and when of clinical decision-making. In Civetta JM, Taylor RW & Kirby RR (eds), *Critical Care*, pp. 30–8. Philadelphia: J.B. Lippincott Co.

Civetta JM (1988b) Prediction and definition of outcome in a cost-sensitive era. In Civetta JM, Taylor RW & Kirby RP (eds), *Critical Care*, pp. 1673–97. Philadelphia: J.B. Lippincott Co.

Clark AP, Winslow EH, Tyler DO & White KM (1990) Effects of endotracheal suctioning on mixed venous oxygen saturation and heart rate in critically ill adults. *Heart & Lung* **19**: 552–7.

Cole JS, Martin WE, Cheung PW & Johnson CC (1972) Clinical studies with a solid state fiberoptic catheter. *Am. J. Cardiol.* **29**: 383–8.

Cullen DJ, Ferrar LC, Briggs BA *et al.* (1976) Survival, hospitalization charges, and follow-up results in critically ill patients. *New Engl. J. Med.* **294**: 982–8.

Curling PE, Murphy DA, Kopel M *et al.* (1984) Pulmonary artery catheters: A prospective study of 2070 consecutive patients. *Anesthesiology* **61**: A58.

De La Rocha AG, Edmonds JF, Williams WG *et al.* (1978) Importance of mixed venous oxygen saturation in the care of critically ill patients. *Can. J. Surg.* **21**: 227–9.

Divertie MB & McMichan JC (1984) Continuous monitoring of mixed venous oxygen saturation. *Chest* **85**: 423–8.

Enderson BL & Rice CL (1990) Monitoring. In Moore EE (ed.) *Early Care of the Injured Patient*, pp. 100–6. Philadelphia: B.C. Decker.

Fahey PJ, Harris K & Vanderwarf C (1984) Clinical experience with continuous monitoring of mixed venous oxygen saturation in respiratory failure. *Chest* **86**: 748–52.

Fick A (1870) Uber die Messung des Blutquantums in den Hertzventrikeln. *Sitzungsber. Phys. Med. Ges. Würtzburg* Bd II: XVI.

Forrester JS, Diamond G, Chatterjee K & Swan NJ (1976) Medical therapy of acute myocardial infarction by application of hemodynamic subsets. *New Engl. J. Med.* **295**: 1356–62.

Frommer PL, Ros J, Mason DT *et al.* (1965) Clinical applications of an improved, rapidly responding fiberoptic catheter. *Am. J. Cardiol.* **15**: 672–9.

Gettinger A, Detraglia MC & Glass DD (1986) Accuracy of two mixed venous saturation catheters. *Anesthesiology* **65**: A145.

Gettinger A, Detraglia MC & Glass DD (1987) In vivo comparison of two mixed venous saturation catheters. *Anesthesiology* **66**: 373–5.

Gilbert CC (1987) A continuous monitoring technique for management of acute pulmonary failure. *Chest* **92**: 467–9.

Gore JM & Sloan K (1984) Use of continuous monitoring of mixed venous oxygen saturation in the coronary care unit. *Chest* **86**: 757–61.

Groeneveld ABJ, Kester ADM & Nauta JJP (1987) Relation of arterial blood lactate to oxygen delivery and hemodynamic variables in human shock states. *Circulation Shock* **22**: 35–53.

Guffin A, Girard D & Kaplan JA (1987) Shivering following cardiac surgery: hemodynamic changes and reversal. *J. Cardiothor. Anesth.* **1**: 24–8.

Hardy GR (1988) $S\bar{v}O_2$ continuous monitoring technique. *Dimens. Crit. Care Nurs.* **7**: 8–17.

Iparraguirre HP, Giniger R, Garber VA *et al.* (1988) Comparison between measured and Fick-derived values of hemodynamic and oximetric variables in patients with acute myocardial infarction. *Am. J. Med.* **85:** 349–52.

Jain A, Shroff SG, Janicki JS *et al.* (1991) Relationship between mixed venous oxygen saturation and cardiac index; nonlinearity and normalization for oxygen uptake and hemoglobin. *Chest* **99:** 1403–9.

Jaquith SM (1985) Continuous measurement of $S\bar{v}O_2$: Clinical applications and advantages for critical care nursing. *Crit. Care Nurs.* **5:** 40–4.

Jaquith SM (1987) Continuous monitoring of $S\bar{v}O_2$ following cardiac transplantation. *Crit. Care Nurs.* **7:** 12–19.

Jamieson WRE, Turnbull KW, Larrieu AJ *et al.* (1982) Continuous monitoring of mixed venous saturation in cardiac surgery. *Can. J. Surg.* **25:** 538–43.

Jastremski MS, Chelluri L, Beney KM *et al.* (1989) Analysis of the effect of continuous on-line monitoring of mixed venous oxygen saturation on patient outcome and cost-effectiveness. *Crit. Care Med.* **17:** 148–53.

Kandel G & Aberman A (1983) Mixed venous oxygen saturation: Its role in the assessment of the critically ill patient. *Arch. Intern. Med.* **143:** 1400–2.

Karis JH & Lumb PD (1988) Clinical evaluation of the Edwards Laboratories and Oximetrix mixed venous oxygen saturation catheters. *J. Cardiothor. Anesth.* **2:** 440–4.

Kasnitz P, Druger GI, Yorra F & Simmons DH (1976) Mixed venous oxygen tension and hyperlactemia. *J. Am. Med. Assoc.* **236:** 570–4.

Kelman GR, Nunn JR, Reys-Roberts C & Greenbaum (1967) The influence of cardiac output on arterial oxygenation: Theoretical study. *Br. J. Anesth.* **39:** 450.

Kirshon B & Cotton DB (1987) Invasive hemodynamic monitoring in the obstetric patient. *Clin. Obstet. Gynecol.* **30:** 579–90.

Kramer VK (1934) Ein Verfahren zur fortlaufenden Messung des Sauerstoffgehaltes im stromendum Blute an uneroffneten Gefaben. *Zeitschrift fur Biol.* Bd, pp. 61–75. München: Lehmanns Verlag.

Krauss XH, Verdouw PD, Hugenholtz PZ & Nanta J (1975) On-line monitoring of mixed venous oxygen saturation after cardiothoracic surgery. *Thorax* **30:** 636.

Krouskop RW, Cabatu EE, Chelliah BP *et al.* (1983) Accuracy and clinical utility of an oxygen saturation monitor (arterial in newborns). *Crit. Care Med.* **11:** 744–9.

Kupeli IA & Satwicz PR (1989) Mixed venous oximetry. *Int. Anesth. Clin.* **27:** 176–83.

Kyff JV, Vaughn S, Yang SC *et al.* (1989) Continuous monitoring of mixed venous oxygen saturation in patients with acute myocardial infarction. *Chest* **95:** 607–11.

Larsen LD & Kyff JV (1989) The cost-effectiveness of Oximetrix pulmonary artery catheters in the postoperative care of coronary artery bypass graft patients. *J. Cardiothor. Anesth.* **3:** 276–9.

MacLean LD, Mulligan WB, McLean APH *et al.* (1987). Pattern of septic shock in man – A detailed study of the patient. *Ann. Surg.* **166:** 543–62.

McArthur KT, Clark L, Lyons L & Edwards S (1962) Continuous recording of blood oxygen saturation in open-heart operations. *Surgery* **51:** 121–6.

McMichan JC (1983) Continuous monitoring of mixed venous oxygen saturation: Theory applied to practice. In Schweiss JF (ed.), *Continuous Measurement of Blood Oxygen Saturation in the High Risk Patient*, pp. 27–44. San Diego: Beach International.

McMichan JC, Baele PL & Wignes MW (1984) Insertion of pulmonary artery catheters – A comparison of fiberoptic and nonfiberoptic catheters. *Crit. Care Med.* **12:** 517–19.

Martin WE, Cheung PW, Johnson CE & Wong KC (1973) Continuous monitoring of mixed venous saturation in man. *Anesthesia Analgesia* **52:** 784–93.

Masood RA, Richey HM, Bush BA *et al.* (1989) A comparison between a conventional and a fiberoptic flow-directed thermal dilution pulmonary artery catheter in critical ill patients. *Arch. Intern. Med.* 149: 83–5.

Moore FA & Haenel JB (1988) Advances in oxygen monitoring in trauma patients. *Med. Instrum.* **22:** 135–42.

Morris A, Chapman RH & Gardner RM (1984) Frequency of technical problems mentioned in the measurement of pulmonary artery wedge pressure. *Crit. Care Med.* **12:** 164–70.

Muir AL, Kirby BJ, King AJ & Miller HC (1970) Mixed venous oxygen saturation in relation in cardiac output in myocardial infarction. *Br. Med. J.* **4:** 276–8.

Nelson LD (1986a) Continuous venous oximetry in surgical patients. *Ann. Surg.* **203:** 329–33.

Nelson LD (1986b) Continuous venous oximetry. Part 2. Clinical applications. *Curr. Rev. Respiratory Ther.* **8:** 106–12.

Nelson LD (1987) Venous oximetry. In Snyder JV & Pinski MR (eds) *Oxygen Transport in the Critically Ill Patient*, pp. 235–48. Chicago: Yearbook Medical Publishers.

Nelson LD (1988) Applications of venous saturation monitoring. In Civetta JM, Taylor RW & Kirby RR (eds), *Critical Care*, pp. 327–34. Philadelphia: J.B. Lippincott Co.

Nelson LD & Anderson HB (1989) Physiology effects of steep positioning in the surgical intensive care unit. *Arch. Surg.* **124:** 352–5.

Nishijima H, Weil MH, Shubin H *et al.* (1973) Hemodynamic and metabolic studies in shock associated with gram-negative bacteremia. *Medicine* **52:** 287–94.

Norfleet EA & Watson CB (1985) Continuous mixed venous oxygen saturation measurement: A significant advance in hemodynamic monitoring? *J. Clin. Monit.* **1:** 245–58.

Norwood S & Nelson LD (1986) Continuous monitoring of mixed venous oxygen saturation during aortofemoral bypassing grafting. *Am Surg.* **52:** 114–15.

Orlando R (1986) Continuous mixed venous oximetry in critically ill surgical patients. *Arch. Surg.* **121:** 470–1.

Parr GVS, Blackstone EH & Kirklin JW (1975) Cardiac performance and mortality early after intracardiac surgery in infants and children. *Circulation* **51:** 867–74.

Pearson KS, Gomez MN, Moyers RJ *et al.* (1989) A cost/benefit analysis of randomized invasive monitoring for patients undergoing cardiac surgery. *Anesthesia Analgesia* **69:** 336–41.

Polanyi ML & Hehir RM (1960) New reflection oximeter. *Rev. Sci. Instrum.* **31:** 401.

Polanyi ML & Hehir RM (1962) In vivo oximeter with fast dynamic response. *Rev. Sci. Instrum.* **33:** 1050–4.

Prielipp RC, Butterworth JF, Zaloga JP *et al.* (1991) Effects of Amrinone on cardiac index, venous oxygen saturation and venous admixture in patients recovering from cardiac surgery. *Chest* **99:** 820–5.

Rackow EC, Astiz ME & Weil MH (1989) Cellular oxygen metabolism during sepsis and shock. The relationship of oxygen consumption to oxygen delivery. *J. Am. Med. Assoc.* **259:** 1989–93.

Rao TLK, Jacobs KH & El-Eltr AA (1983) Reinfarction following anesthesia in patients with myocardial infarction. *Anesthesiology* **59:** 499–505.

Rajput MA, Richey HM, Bush BA *et al.* (1989) A comparison between a conventional and a fiberoptic flow-directed thermal dilution pulmonary artery catheter in artificially ill patients. *Arch. Int. Med.* **149:** 83–86.

Rashkin M, Boxkin C & Baughman R (1985) Oxygen delivery in critically ill patients: Relationship to blood lactate and survival. *Chest* **87:** 580–4.

Reid C (1975) The design of fiberoptic oximeters. In Payne JP & Hill DW (eds), *Oxygen Measurements in Biology and Medicine*, pp. 361–8. London and Boston: Butterworths.

Richard C, Thuillez C, Pezzano M *et al.* (1989) Relationship between mixed venous oxygen saturation and cardiac index in patients with chronic congestive heart failure. *Chest* **95:** 1289–94.

Robin ED (1983) A critical look at critical care. *Crit. Care Med.* **11:** 144–8.

Robin ED (1985) The cult of the Swan–Ganz catheter. Over use and abuse of pulmonary flow catheters. *Am. Intern. Med.* **103:** 445–9.

Rodrigo FA (1953) Determination of oxygenation of blood in vitro by using reflected light. *Am. Heart J.* **45:** 809–12.

Rubin SA, Sienienczuk D, Nathan MD *et al.* (1982) Accuracy of cardiac ouput, oxygen uptake, and arteriovenous oxygen difference at rest, during exercise and after vasodilator therapy in patients with severe, chronic heart failure. *Am. J. Cardiol.* **50:** 973–8.

Schumaker PT & Cain SM (1987) The concept of critical oxygen delivery. *Intensive Care Med.* **13:** 223–9.

Schweiss JF (1987) Mixed venous hemoglobin saturation: Theory and application. *Int. Anesth. Clin.* **15:** 113–36.

Shoemaker WC (1991) Tissue perfusion and oxygenation: A primary problem in acute circulatory failure and shock states. *Crit. Care Med.* **9:** 595–6.

Shibutani K (1983) Do mixed venous oxygen saturation and tension adequately reflect tissue oxygenation? *Crit. Care Med.* **3:** 9–13.

Snyder JV & Carroll GC (1982) Tissue oxygenation: A physiologic approach to a clinical problem. *Curr. Probl. Surg.* **19:** 650–719.

Sperinde JM & Senelly KM (1985) The Oximetrix Opticath Oximetrix system: Theory and development. In Fahey PJ (ed.), *Continuous Measurement of Blood Oxygen Saturation in the High Risk Patient. Theory and Practice in Monitoring Mixed Venous Oxygen Saturation*, pp. 59–80. San Diego: Beach International.

Stewart FM (1988) $S\bar{v}O_2$ monitoring. Part II. Nursing research applications. *Dimens. Crit. Care Nurs.* **7:** 79–82.

Swan HJC (1988) Hemodynamic monitoring in the critically ill patient. In Parillo JE (ed.) *Critical Decisions*, pp. 19–25. Philadelphia: B.C. Decker.

Swan HJC, Ganz W, Forrester JS *et al.* (1970) Catheterization of the heart in man with the use of a flow-directed balloon-tipped catheter. *New Engl. J. Med.* **283**: 447–51.

Thys DM, Cohen E & Eisenkraft JB (1988) Mixed venous oxygen saturation during thoracic anesthesia. *Anesthesiology* **69**: 1005–9.

Tuchschmidt J, Fried J, Swinney R & Sharma P (1989) Early hemodynamic correlates of survival in patients with septic shock. *Crit. Care Med.* **17**: 719–23.

Tuman KJ, Carroll GC, Irankovich, AD (1989). Pitfalls in interpretation of pulmonary artery catheter data. *J. Cardiother. Anesth.* **3(5)**: 625–641.

Tyler DO, Winslow EH, Clark AP & White KM (1990) Effect of one-minute back rub on mixed venous saturation and heart rate in critically ill patients. *Heart & Lung* **19**: 562–5.

Van Woerkens E, Trouwborst A & Tenbrink R (1991) Accuracy of a mixed venous saturation catheter during acutely induced changes in hematocrit in humans. *Crit. Care Med.* **19**: 1025–9.

Vermeij CG, Feenstra BWA, Adrichem WJ & Bruining HA (1991) Independent oxygen uptake and oxygen delivery in septic and postoperative patients. *Chest.* **99**: 1438–43.

Waller JL & Kaplan JA (1982) Usefulness of pulmonary artery catheters during aorto-coronary bypass surgery. *Anesthesia Analgesia* **61**: 221–2.

Ware PF, Polanyi ML, Hehir RM *et al.* (1961) A new reflexion oximeter. *J. Thorac. Cardiovasc. Surg.* **42**: 580–8.

Watson CB (1983) The PA catheter as an early warning system. *Anesth. Rev.* **10**: 34–5.

Weil MH & Afifi AA (1970) Experimental and clinical studies on lactate and pyruvate as indicators of the severity of circulatory failure (shock). *Circulation* **41**: 989–1000.

Wiedemann HP, Matthay MA & Matthay RA (1984) Cardiopulmonary monitoring in the intensive care unit (Part 2). *Chest* **85**: 656–68.

Wilkinson AR, Phibbs RH & Gregory GA (1979) Continuous in vivo oxygen saturation in newborn infants with pulmonary disease. *Crit. Care Med.* **7**: 232–6.

Wilson RF, Christensen C & LeBlanc LP (1972) Oxygen consumption in critically ill surgical patients. *Ann. Surg.* **276**: 801–4.

Winslow EH, Clark AP, White KM & Tyler DO (1990) Effects of lateral turn on mixed venous oxygen saturation and heart rate in critically ill patients. *Heart & Lung* **19**: 557–61.

Yokota S, Mizushima M, Kemmotzu O *et al.* (1988) Clinical evaluation of continuous venous oxygen saturation monitoring during anesthesia. *Adv. Exp. Med. Biol.* **222**: 239–43.

Zwichenberger JB (1987) Suppression of shivering decreases oxygen consumption and improve hemodynamic stability during postoperative rewarming. *Ann. Thor. Surg.* **43**: 428–31.

6 Mixed Venous Oxygen Saturation Monitoring in Surgery

Jean-Jacques Lehot & Pierre-Georges Durand

Introduction

The principles of monitoring mixed venous haemoglobin saturation of oxygen ($S\bar{v}O_2$) have been fully explained in the previous chapter. In summary, the oxygen saturation in mixed venous blood ($S\bar{v}O_2$) is a non-specific indicator of the balance between oxygen delivery ($\dot{D}O_2$) and consumption ($\dot{V}O_2$). $S\bar{v}O_2$ is influenced by factors which determine $\dot{D}O_2$: i.e. cardiac output, haemoglobin concentration (Hb), and arterial oxygen saturation (SaO_2), and by the quantity of total body oxygen consumption ($\dot{V}O_2$). As most of these factors are likely to change intra-operatively and post-operatively during major surgery in high-risk patients (Fig. 6.1) $S\bar{v}O_2$ might allow the detection of inadequate or impaired oxygen transport and the monitoring of its correction.

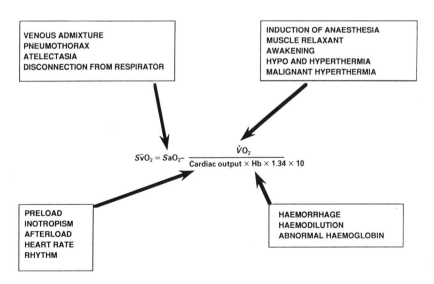

Figure 6.1 Determinants of mixed venous oxygen saturation ($S\bar{v}O_2$) and its major causes of variation intra- and post-operatively. SaO_2 = arterial oxygen saturation; $\dot{V}O_2$ = oxygen consumption; Hb = concentration of haemoglobin (g dl^{-1}).

Intermittent sampling of mixed venous blood in the pulmonary artery is recognized as the single most helpful measurement in evaluating the state of the post-cardiotomy patients (Boyd *et al.*, 1959). Due to usual rapid haemodynamic changes in anaesthesia, intermittent blood samplings are not easy but $S\bar{v}O_2$ pulmonary artery (PA) catheters may provide a unique on-line ability for diagnosing impaired oxygen balance. Three-wavelength systems do not depend on Hb and seem more accurate than two-wavelength systems (Rouby *et al.*, 1990).

Determinants of Mixed Venous Oxygen Saturation

The equation in Fig. 6.1 is derived from the Fick formula. From this equation either an increase in $\dot{V}O_2$ or a decrease in cardiac output, Hb or SaO_2 will produce a decrease in $S\bar{v}O_2$, provided that no change in the other components occur. A stable $S\bar{v}O_2$ indicates that either the determinants of oxygen balance are unchanged or that several factors of this equation change in a compensatory manner. Clinicians sometimes rely on mixed venous oxygen tension ($P\bar{v}O_2$) as an indicator of global tissue perfusion, although this relationship has never been scientifically demonstrated (Miller, 1982). Moreover, the relationship between $S\bar{v}O_2$ and $P\bar{v}O_2$ depends on the haemoglobin dissociation curve. A leftward shift of this curve at constant $P\bar{v}O_2$ increases $S\bar{v}O_2$. For example, a decrease in P_{50} (the PO_2 at 50% saturation under standard conditions) from 25.5 to 19.2 mm Hg (3.39 to 2.55 kPa) increases $S\bar{v}O_2$ from 70 to 80%. This shift can be induced by acute alkalosis, hypocapnia, hypothermia or decrease in red cell 2,3-diphosphoglycerate possibly due to blood transfusion; all these conditions are common during the peri-operative period.

$S\bar{v}O_2$ is more likely to decrease in the face of increased $\dot{V}O_2$ when the patient presents a limitation in cardiorespiratory reserve such as heart failure, valvular stenosis, coronary artery disease or respiratory failure. However, when respiratory distress is not accompanied by circulatory failure, SaO_2 is more likely to decrease first, thus a pulse oximeter may provide earlier information in this setting.

Simultaneous pulse and pulmonary artery oximetry ('dual oximetry') provide real-time values for SaO_2 and $S\bar{v}O_2$ (Rasanen *et al.*, 1987). Dual oximetry allows the calculation of oxygen extraction ratio (OER $= [SaO_2 - S\bar{v}O_2]/SaO_2$) which is highly correlated to oxygen utilization coefficient ($\dot{V}O_2/DO_2$) in abdominal aortic surgery (Zaune *et al.*, 1991) and critically ill surgical patients (Rasanen & Downs, 1988). Zaune *et al.* (1991) suggested OER identifies high-risk patients with compromised oxygen extraction reserve. Moreover, when SaO_2 is likely to approach 100% during elective surgery it can be deduced that:

$$S\bar{v}O_2 = 1 - OER$$

Thus, in these circumstances, $S\bar{v}O_2$ allows an estimate of O_2 extraction reserve.

Interpretation of Changes in $S\bar{v}O_2$

An acute fall of $S\bar{v}O_2$ to 40% or less is usually accompanied by anaerobic metabolism and increased blood lactate levels (Boutros & Lee, 1986; Matsumara *et al.*, 1986). $S\bar{v}O_2$ between 40 and 60% indicates an inadequate $\dot{D}O_2$ to tissues or excessive O_2 demand. In the presence of a low $S\bar{v}O_2$ (Fig. 6.2) a full cardiorespiratory profile (arterial blood gases, haemoglobin concentration, blood lactate level and haemodynamic parameters including cardiac output) should be taken promptly to indicate which intervention is more likely to restore the balance between O_2 supply and demand. An $S\bar{v}O_2$ more than 60% is usually indicative of adequate O_2 transport. However, in patients with hepatic cirrhosis the existence of numerous arterio-venous shunts explains the fact that a high $S\bar{v}O_2$ can accompany inadequate O_2 uptake. Similarly impaired peripheral O_2 utilization during severe sepsis and the adult respiratory distress syndrome (ARDS), acute pancreatitis or extensive burns may lead to $S\bar{v}O_2$ values greater than 85%. Technical errors leading to a falsely high value of $S\bar{v}O_2$ are detailed in the previous chapter. A particularly common cause of a false increase in $S\bar{v}O_2$ is a PA catheter with its tip lying in a distal part of the pulmonary artery; this must be ruled out before any interpretation of $S\bar{v}O_2$ is attempted.

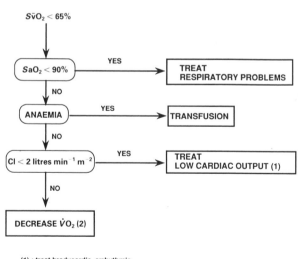

$S\bar{v}O_2 < 65\%$

$SaO_2 < 90\%$ — YES → TREAT RESPIRATORY PROBLEMS

NO

ANAEMIA — YES → TRANSFUSION

NO

$CI < 2$ litres min^{-1} m^{-2} — YES → TREAT LOW CARDIAC OUTPUT (1)

NO

DECREASE $\dot{V}O_2$ (2)

(1) : treat bradycardia, arrhythmia
     optmize preload
     decrease afterload
     increase inotropy
(2) : Treat hyperthermia, stop muscle activity

Figure 6.2 Guidelines for treatment of low $S\bar{v}O_2$ during elective surgery.

General Anaesthesia

$S\bar{v}O_2$ depends on the respective effects of anaesthetic agents on cardiac output and $\dot{V}O_2$. When the decrease in $\dot{V}O_2$ predominates, $S\bar{v}O_2$ increases. Conversely, when the decrease in cardiac output predominates, $S\bar{v}O_2$ will fall. A 28–40% decrease in $\dot{V}O_2$ has been shown both clinically (Schmidt *et al.*, 1982; Brismar *et al.*, 1983; Viale *et al.*, 1988, 1990; Gregoretti *et al.*, 1989) and experimentally (Eichaker *et al.*, 1991; Van der Linden *et al.*, 1991) during anaesthesia. The decrease in $\dot{V}O_2$ is explained by abolition of muscular activity including respiratory muscles during mechanical ventilation and decrease in myocardial and cerebral $\dot{V}O_2$. A decrease in central temperature is seen frequently during anaesthesia, particularly with halothane (Viale *et al.*, 1988) and hypothermia decreases $\dot{V}O_2$ by 7–9% per degree Celsius (Rupp & Severinghaus, 1986). A dose-dependent increase in critical $\dot{D}O_2$ level is shown in dogs by Van der Linden *et al.* (1991) with halothane, enflurane, isoflurane, alfentanil, pentobarbitone but not with ketamine. Thus, most anaesthetic agents may impair oxygen extraction possibly through their peripheral vasodilating effects which alter arteriolar tone (Van der Linden *et al.*, 1991). This deleterious property possibly contributes to the oxygen debt described in some surgical procedures (Waxman *et al.*, 1981, 1982). The decrease in O_2 extraction implies the possibility of tissue hypoxia

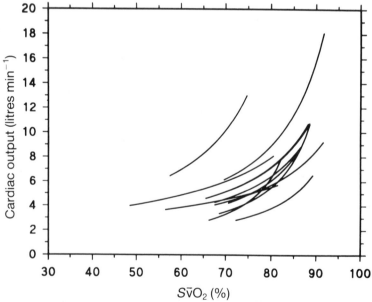

Figure 6.3 Relationship between mixed venous oxygen saturation ($S\bar{v}O_2$) and cardiac output in nine patients during abdominal aortic aneurysm repair under N_2O, isoflurane, fentanyl and atracurium (period of clamping of the aorta was excluded). (With permission from Viale *et al.*, 1991.)

accompanied by relatively high $S\bar{v}O_2$ value. However, this topic is still controversial as Eichaker *et al.* (1991) found that in dogs OER was greater during deep anaesthesia with pentothal as compared to light anaesthesia or awake, and that anaesthesia does not alter mechanisms matching changes in $\dot{D}O_2$ and $\dot{V}O_2$. Interestingly, Mikat *et al.* (1984) showed in dogs that anaesthesia reduces $\dot{V}O_2$ as to compared to awake resting values, but increase $\dot{V}O_2$ as compared to natural sleep. Consequently the starting point in measuring $\dot{V}O_2$ seems important when measuring intraoperative changes in $\dot{V}O_2$.

During stable general anaesthesia $\dot{V}O_2$ is fairly constant as are SaO_2 and Hb, and changes in $S\bar{v}O_2$ are related to changes in cardiac output (Annat *et al.*, 1990). However, the accuracy of changes in $S\bar{v}O_2$ as an indicator of changes in cardiac output depends on the value of $S\bar{v}O_2$ (Fig. 6.3). When $S\bar{v}O_2$ is less than 75%, the accuracy is satisfactory since small changes in cardiac output are associated with large changes in $S\bar{v}O_2$. Above this value, the accuracy decreases, since large changes in cardiac output are required to induce significant changes in $S\bar{v}O_2$ (Annat *et al.*, 1990).

In summary, continuous $S\bar{v}O_2$ monitoring reflects cardiac output during stable anaesthetic and surgical conditions but does not preclude assessment of arterial blood pH and hyperlactaemia in high-risk and long procedures.

Isovolaemic Haemodilution

Trouwborst *et al.* (1990) suggested that $S\bar{v}O_2$ could be used as an indicator of the critical point of haemodilution, i.e. $S\bar{v}O_2$ at which $\dot{V}O_2$ starts to decline during further induced haemodilution. In pigs, the mean critical $S\bar{v}O_2$ was 44% but the inter-individual range was wide (35–55%) corresponding to Hb = $3.6\,g\,dl^{-1}$ (Trouwborst *et al.*, 1990). After extracorporeal circulation for coronary bypass surgery in patients with pre-operative left ventricular ejection fraction greater than 50%, Mathru *et al.* (1990) showed that with Hb as low as $5\,g\,dl^{-1}$, $P\bar{v}O_2$ was significantly lower than with Hb equal to $9.6\,g\,dl^{-1}$. Hb less than $5\,g\,dl^{-1}$ in dogs has been associated with redistribution of coronary flow away from subendocardium (Brazier *et al.*, 1974). During halothane anaesthesia in dogs with a coronary stenosis, regional myocardial dysfunction occurred when haematocrit decreased to 15% (Leone *et al.*, 1990). It is suggested that $S\bar{v}O_2$ may be a global index of haemodilution tolerance but that $S\bar{v}O_2$ reflects poorly the consequences of haemodilution on myocardial regional function.

Recovery from Anaesthesia and Post-operative Period

The post-operative period is accompanied by an abrupt increase in oxygen demand due to thermoregulatory responses, return of pain sensitivity, respiratory work during weaning from mechanical ventilation, payment of intra-operative oxygen debt and corresponding increase in cardiac workload. After abdominal aortic surgery $\dot{V}O_2$ increased by between 74% and 296% (Viale *et al.*, 1991). The increase in oxygen demand is usually satisfied through a mobilization of both cardiac output reserve and O_2 extraction reserve (Fig. 6.4). Thus a moderate decrease in $S\bar{v}O_2$ at this period appears normal in patients with pre-operative left ventricular ejection fraction less than 50% as the cardiac output reserve is limited and the increase in oxygen demand is mostly met by increased oxygen extraction (Viale *et al.*, 1993). During recovery from anaesthesia $S\bar{v}O_2$ allows assessment of the efficacy of treatments aimed at minimizing the increase in oxygen demand:

(1) Henneberg *et al.* (1985) have shown that hot thermal ceiling decreased $\dot{V}O_2$ from 330 to 260 ml min^{-1} during recovery from anaesthesia. Sedation

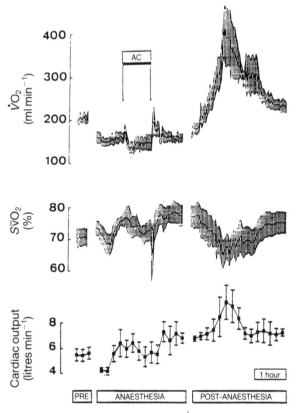

Figure 6.4 Changes in oxygen consumption ($\dot{V}O_2$), mixed venous oxygen saturation ($S\bar{v}O_2$) and cardiac output before (Pre), during (Anaesthesia) and after (post-anaesthesia) anaesthesia for infrarenal aortic aneurysm repair. (With permission from Viale *et al.*, 1991.)

with meperidine i.v. (Pauga *et al.*, 1984; Guffin *et al.*, 1987; Mort *et al.*, 1991) or magnesium sulphate i.v. (Mort *et al.*, 1991) decreased post-operative shivering. Muscle relaxants are very efficient in this regard but they extend the duration of mechanical ventilation (Zwischenberger *et al.*, 1987).

(2) During the first 2 h after major abdominal surgery (Viale *et al.*, 1990) epidural administration of meperidine $0.7 \, \text{mg} \, \text{kg}^{-1}$ slowed the increase in $\dot{V}O_2$ and in central temperature. Clonidine i.v. (5 $\mu\text{g} \, \text{kg}^{-1}$ over 3 h) administered during abdominal surgery reduced the increase in $\dot{V}O_2$ during the first 3 post-operative hours (Quintin *et al.*, 1991).

(3) During weaning from mechanical ventilation the increase in oxygen demand reached 10–20% when pulmonary function was impaired (Armaganidis & Dhainaut, 1989). In patients with limited cardiorespiratory reserve, weaning should be attempted when $S\bar{v}O_2$ is greater than 60% (Armaganidis & Dhainaut, 1989). $S\bar{v}O_2$ may help to select the best mode of weaning (Kanak *et al.*, 1985).

(4) As respiratory weaning can impair left ventricular performance (Coriat *et al.*, 1986; Lemaire *et al.*, 1988) through increased preload, afterload and heart rate, $S\bar{v}O_2$ can decrease during weaning because of a drop in cardiac output and $\dot{D}O_2$. After carotid endarterectomy the decrease in $S\bar{v}O_2$ can be treated by the administration of nifedipine (Godet *et al.*, 1986).

Various Types of Surgery

Thoracic Surgery

$S\bar{v}O_2$ decreased by 11% after collapse of the non-dependent lung in 19 patients out of 26 (Thys *et al.*, 1990). It reflects more the variations of SaO_2 rather than that of cardiac output; $S\bar{v}O_2$ did not change in patients whose $\dot{D}O_2$ was high (Thys *et al.*, 1990). $S\bar{v}O_2$ monitoring must be evaluated in this setting of patients with cardiorespiratory failure. Similar results were observed during unilateral lung transplant (Elman *et al.*, 1990).

Aortic Surgery

$\dot{V}O_2$ decreased by 52%, 49% and 11% respectively during clamping of the descending thoracic (Shenaq *et al.*, 1987), supra-coeliac and infrarenal aorta (Viale *et al.*, 1991), this reduction leading to an increase in $S\bar{v}O_2$. The correlation between $S\bar{v}O_2$ and cardiac output disappeared during aortic clamping (Shenaq *et al.*, 1987; Viale *et al.*, 1991). Aortic unclamping increased $\dot{V}O_2$ and briefly decreased $S\bar{v}O_2$ (Fig. 6.4). Moreover, the lung collapse during thoracic aortic surgery influenced $S\bar{v}O_2$ (Shenaq *et al.*, 1987).

Cardiac Surgery

$S\bar{v}O_2$ changes were shown to reflect cardiac output in some studies (Jamieson et al., 1982; Waller et al., 1982). However, 15 min after completion of cardiopulmonary bypass, $S\bar{v}O_2$ and $\dot{D}O_2$ did not correlate when serum lactate levels were more than 2.5 mmol litre^{-1} (Komatsu et al., 1987). This may be due to impairment of O_2 extraction during and immediately after extracorporeal circulation (Komatsu et al., 1987). During cannulation $S\bar{v}O_2$ decreases but during extracorporeal circulation $S\bar{v}O_2$ is not interpretable because virtually no blood circulates in the pulmonary arteries. Parr et al. (1975) reported that mortality following cardiac surgery in infants was more reliably predicted using cardiac index and $S\bar{v}O_2$ together than one measurement alone. Continuous $S\bar{v}O_2$ monitoring after cardiac surgery has been studied extensively (Jamieson et al., 1982; Schmidt et al., 1982; Gore & Sloan, 1984). Average $S\bar{v}O_2$ was lower after (68%) than during (77%) cardiac surgery due to increased post-operative oxygen demand in the face of virtually unchanged $\dot{D}O_2$ (Schmidt et al., 1982). An absolute fall in $S\bar{v}O_2$ of greater than 10% predicted haemodynamic changes and should prompt haemodynamic evaluation (Jamieson et al., 1982). Comparing the early post-operative period after hypothermic and normothermic cardiopulmonary bypass, $S\bar{v}O_2$ was similar in the two groups in the first post-operative hour (Lehot et al., 1993).

During this period continuous $S\bar{v}O_2$ monitoring was the first indicator of hypovolaemia, showing slight dips in $S\bar{v}O_2$ as long as 15 min before clinicians intervened based on standard monitoring (Hanson & Geer, 1990). Occasionally, a decrease in $S\bar{v}O_2$ has been helpful in delineating otherwise unsuspected cardiac tamponade (Jamieson et al., 1982). Conversely, a rising $S\bar{v}O_2$ over 85% may indicate either elevated cardiac output possibly necessitating β-blocker or calcium-channel inhibitor treatment after coronary artery bypass surgery, or recurrence of left-to-right shunt after interventricular septal defect repair (Bizouarn & Bouyer, 1990).

Schmidt et al. (1982) and Magilligan et al. (1987) found no correlation between cardiac index and $S\bar{v}O_2$, possibly because of post-operative changes in $\dot{V}O_2$. $S\bar{v}O_2$ was not predictive of a cardiac index of less than 2 litres min^{-1} m^{-2}, a level of cardiac performance that indicates low cardiac output syndrome and which requires prompt treatment (Magilligan et al., 1987). Nonetheless, continuous $S\bar{v}O_2$ measurement helped with monitoring of circulatory assistances (Clavey et al., 1990) or selecting between sequential and ventricular pacing (Gore & Sloan, 1984; Divertie & McMichan, 1984).

In a retrospective study Larson and Kyff (1989) could not demonstrate the beneficial effect of $S\bar{v}O_2$ PA catheters on outcome after coronary artery bypass graft surgery and they concluded that these catheters were not cost-effective. Similar results were found in valvular and coronary surgery (Pearson et al., 1989). However, these catheters may be effective in selected high-risk patients for whom prompt peri-operative therapeutic interventions are likely to be required.

Miscellaneous

An experimental study suggested that continuous $S\bar{v}O_2$ monitoring enables early diagnosis of occult bleeding (Scalea *et al.*, 1988). During hepatic transplantation $S\bar{v}O_2$ correlated with cardiac output provided SaO_2 and Hb were maintained within normal limits (Jugan *et al.*, 1990). During neurosurgical sitting procedures air embolism produced a sudden drop in $S\bar{v}O_2$ (Khoury *et al.*, 1990). During abdominal surgery, traction on the mesentery was accompanied by a 10% increase in absolute $S\bar{v}O_2$ value and by a 30% increase in cardiac output, possibly due to decreased systemic vascular resistance (Sagnard *et al.*, 1990).

Summary

Continuous $S\bar{v}O_2$ monitoring allows an early recognition of adverse changes and allows the effectiveness of corrective therapy to be monitored. Consequently, $S\bar{v}O_2$ PA catheters are increasingly being used in high-risk surgical patients and also represent an interesting teaching aid. However, as with ordinary Swan–Ganz catheters, $S\bar{v}O_2$ PA catheters have not been shown to improve morbidity and mortality, possibly because of multiple factors effecting outcome in this type of patient.

References

Annat G, Ravat F, Viale JP *et al.* (1990) Cardiac output is the main factor of variation of mixed venous oxygen saturation during general anesthesia. *Anesthesiology* **73:** 3A–A119.

Armaganidis A & Dhainaut JF (1989) Sevrage de la ventilation articielle: intérêt du monitorage continu de la SvO_2. *Ann. Fr. Anesth. Réanim.* **8:** 708–15.

Bizouarn P & Bouyer L (1990) Monitroage de la SvO_2 et rupture septale. *Ann. Fr. Anesth. Réanim.* **9:** 567–8.

Boutros AR & Lee C (1986) Values of continuous monitoring of mixed venous oxygen saturation in the management of critically ill patients. *Crit. Care Med.* **14:** 134–4.

Boyd AD, Tremblay RE, Spencer FC & Bahnson HT (1959) Estimation of cardiac output soon after intracardiac surgery with cardiopulmonary bypass. *Ann. Surg.* **150:** 613–26.

Brazier J, Cooper N, Maloney JV Jr & Buckberg G (1974) The adequacy of myocardial oxygen delivery in acute nonmovolemic anemia. *Surgery* **75:** 508–13.

Brismar B, Hedenstierna G, Lundh R & Tokics L (1983) Oxygen uptake, plasma catecholamines and cardiac output during neurolept-nitrous oxide and halothane anaesthesia. *Acta Anaesth. Scand.* **26:** 541–9.

Clavey M, Mattei MF, Hubert T *et al.* (1990) Interet de la mesure en continue de la SVO₂ pendant une assistance circulatoire externe. *Ann. Fr. Anesth. Réanim.* **9:** 83–6.

Coriat P, Mundler O, Bousseau D *et al.* (1986) Response of left ventricular ejection fraction to recovery from general anesthesia. *Anesthesia Analgesia* **65:** 593–600.

Divertie MB & McMichan JC (1984) Continuous monitoring of mixed venous oxygen saturation. *Chest* **85:** 423–9.

Eichaker PQ, Waisman Y, Banks SM *et al.* (1991) Effects of pentothal anesthesia on oxygen delivery and consumption in a canine model. *Crit. Care Med.* **19:** 53.

Elman A, Maillard C, Mal H *et al.* (1990) Intérêt de la de Swan–Ganz et mesure de la SvO₂ en continue pendant la transplantation unipulmonaire. *Réanim. Soins, Intens. Med. Urg.* (suppl.) 59.

Godet G, Coriat P, Samama M *et al.* (1986) Treatment of post carotid endacterectomy hypertension with nifedipine: effects on hemodynamic and mixed venous oxygen saturation. *Anesthesiology* **65:** A75.

Gore JM & Sloan K (1984) Use of continuous monitoring of mixed venous oxygen saturation in the coronary care unit. *Chest* **86:** 757–61.

Gregoretti S, Gelman S & Dimick A (1989) Hemodynamic changes and oxygen consumption in burned patients during enflurane or isoflurane anesthesia. *Anesthesia Analgesia* **69:** 431–6.

Guffin A, Girard D & Kaplan JA (1987) Shivering following cardiac surgery: hemodynamic changes and reversal. *J. Cardiothor. Anesth.* **1:** 24–8.

Hanson CW & Geer RT (1990) Mixed venous oximetry in cardiac surgical patients. *Anesthesiology* **73:** A438.

Henneberg S, Eklung A, Jorchimsson PO *et al.* (1985) Effects of a thermal ceiling on postoperative hypothermia. *Acta Anaesth. Scand.* **29:** 602–6.

Jamieson WRE, Turnbull KW, Larrieu AJ *et al.* (1982) Continuous monitoring of mixed venous oxygen saturation in cardiac surgery. *Can. J. Surg.* **25(5):** 583–43.

Jugan E, Albaladejo P, Descorps-Declere A *et al.* (1990) Continuous monitoring of mixed venous oxygen saturation during orthotopic liver transplantation. *Anesthesiology* **73:** A494.

Kanak R, Fahey PJ & Vanderwarf C (1985) Oxygen cost of breathing: Changes dependent upon mode of mechanical ventilation. *Chest* **87:** 126–7.

Khoury A, Cagny Bellet A, Tondriaux A *et al.* (1990) Continuous monitoring of mixed venous oxygen saturation during sitting neurosurgical procedures. *Anesthesiology* **73:** 3A–A184.

Komatsu T, Shibutani K, Okamoto K *et al.* (1987) Critical level of oxygen delivery after cardiopulmonary bypass. *Crit. Care Med.* **15:** 194–7.

Larson Lo & Kyff JV (1989) The cost effectiveness of Oximetrix pulmonary artery catheters in the postoperative care of coronary artery bypass graft patients. *J. Cardiothor. Anesth.* **3:** 276–9.

Lehot JJ, Villard J, Piriz H *et al.* (1992) Hemodynamic and hormonal responses to hypothermic and normothermic cardiopulmonary bypass. *J. Cardiothor. Anesth.* **6:** 132–9.

Lemaire F, Teboul JL, Cinotti L *et al.* (1988) Acute left ventricular dysfunction during unsuccessful weaning from mechanical ventilation. *Anesthesiology* **69:** 171–9.

Leone BJ, Spahn DR, McRae RL & Smith LR (1990) Effects of hemodilution and anesthesia on regional function of compromised myocardium. *Anesthesiology* **73:** A596.

Magilligan DJ, Teasdall R, Eisinminger R & Peterson E (1987) Mixed venous oxygen saturation as a predictor of cardiac output in the postoperative surgical patient. *Ann. Thorac. Surg.* **44:** 260–2.

Mathru M, Kleinman B, Blakeman B *et al.* (1990) Gas exchange during extreme haemodilution in man. *Anesthesiology* **73:** A237.

Matsumura N, Nishijima H, Kojima S *et al.* (1986) Determination of anaerobic threshold for assessment of functional state in patients with chronic heart failure. *Circulation* **68:** 360–7.

Mikat M, Peters J, Zindler M & Arndt J (1984) Whole body oxygen consumption in awake, sleeping and anesthetized dogs. *Anesthesiology* **60:** 220–7.

Miller MJ (1982) Tissue oxygenation in clinical medicine. An historical review. *Anesthesia Analgesia* **61:** 527–35.

Mort T, Rintel T & Altman F (1991) Meperidine vs convection warming vs magnesium sulfate for postcardiac surgery shivering. *Crit. Care Med.* **19 (Suppl):** s83.

Parr GV, Blackstone EH & Kirklin JW (1975) Cardiac performance and mortality early after intracardiac surgery to infants and young children. *Circulation* **51:** 867–74.

Pauga AL, Savage RT, Simpson S & Roy RC (1984) Effect of pethidine, fentanyl and morphine on postoperative shivering in man. *Acta Anaesth. Scand.* **28:** 128–43.

Pearson KS, Gomez MN, Moyers JR *et al.* (1989) A cost benefit analysis of randomized invasive monitoring for patients undergoing cardiac surgery. *Anesthesia Analgesia* **69:** 336–41.

Quintin L, Viale JP, Annat G *et al.* (1991) Oxygen uptake during the postoperative period in patients following major abdominal surgery: effect of clonidine. *Anesthesiology* **76:** 236–41.

Rasanen J & Downs JB (1988) Cardiopulmonary monitoring using dual oximetry. *Anesthesiology* **69:** A319 (abstract).

Rasanen J, Downs JB, Dehaven B & Seidman P (1987) Estimation of oxygen utilization by dual oximetry. *Ann. Surg.* **207:** 621–3.

Rouby JJ, Poete P, Bodin L, Bourgeois JL *et al.* (1990) Three mixed venous saturation catheters in patients with circulatory shock and respiratory failure. *Chest* **98:** 954–8.

Rupp SM & Severinghaus JW (1986) Hypothermia. In Miller RD (ed.), *Anesthesia* (2nd edition), Vol. 3, pp. 1995–2022. New York: Churchill-Livingstone.

Sagnard P, Annat G, Viale JP *et al.* (1990) Consequences hemodynamiques de la traction sur le mesentere: effet du ketoprofene. *Ann. Fr. Anesth. Réanim.* **9 (Suppl.):** R11.

Scalea TM, Holman M, Fuortes M *et al.* (1988) Central venous blood oxygen saturation: an early, accurate measurement of volume during hemorrhage. *J. Trauma* **28:** 725–32.

Shenaq SA, Casar G, Chelly JE *et al.* (1987) Continuous monitoring of mixed venous oxygen saturation during aortic surgery. *Chest* **92**: 796–9.

Schmidt CR, Frank LP, Forsythe SB & Estafanous FG (1984) Continuous $S\bar{v}O_2$ measurement and oxygen transport patterns in cardiac surgery patients. *Crit. Care Med.* **12**: 523–7.

Thys DM, Cohen E & Eisenkraft JB (1990) Mixed venous oxygen saturation during thoracic anesthesia. *Anesthesiology* **69**: 1005–9.

Trouwborst A, Tenbrinck R & Van Woerkens ECSM (1990) Blood gas analysis of mixed venous blood during normoxic acute isovolemic hemodilution in pigs. *Anesthesia Analgesia* **70**: 523–99.

Van der Linden P, Gilbart E, Engelman E *et al.* (1991) Effects of anesthetic agents on systemic critical O_2 delivery. *J. Appl. Physiol.* **71**: 83–93.

Viale JP, Annat GJ, Bertrand O *et al.* (1988) Continuous measurement of pulmonary gas exchange during general anaesthesia in man. *Acta Anaesth. Scand.* **32**: 691–7.

Viale JP, Annat GJ, Tissot SM *et al.* (1990) Mass spectrometric measurements of oxygen uptake during epidural analgesia combined with general anesthesia. *Anesthesia Analgesia* **70**: 559–93.

Viale JP, Annat G, Ravat F *et al.* (1991) Oxygen uptake and mixed venous oxygen saturation during aortic surgery and the first three operative hours. *Anesthesia Analgesia* **73**: 530–35.

Waller JL, Kaplan JA, Bauman DI & Craver JM (1982) Clinical evaluation of a new fiberoptic catheter oximeter during cardiac surgery. *Anesthesia Analgesia* **61**: 676–9.

Waxman K, Lazrove S & Shoemaker WC (1981) Physiologic responses to operation in high risk surgical patients. *Surg. Gynecol. Obstet.* **152**: 633–8.

Waxman K, Nolan LS & Shoemaker WC (1982) Sequential perioperative lactate determination. Physiological and clinical implications. *Crit. Care Med.* **10**: 96–9.

Zaune U, Spies C, Pauli HMF *et al.* (1991) Monitoring of the oxygen utilization by dual oximetry during aortic surgery. *Anesthesiology* **72**: S333.

Zwischenberger JB, Kirsh MM, Dechert RE *et al.* (1987) Suppression of shivering decreases oxygen consumption and improves hemodynamic stability during postoperative rewarming. *Ann. Thorac. Surg.* **43**: 428–31.

Part Two

Practice

7 Therapy: Mechanical Ventilation, Future Trends

J. Denis Edwards

Introduction

To optimize oxygen delivery even to normal values necessitates the manipulation of some or all of the variables in Eqn (7.1). These are, in therapeutic terms, an increase in arterial haemoglobin saturation which is produced by an increase in alveolar concentration of oxygen. Of course, the first manoeuvre would be to ensure an adequate airway and then to ensure an adequate arterial partial pressure or tension of oxygen (PaO_2). This may well entail the use of artificial or so-called mechanical ventilation.

The ideal goals of therapy, including the use of mechanical ventilation, can be deduced from the basic principles of oxygen transport physiology. The equation for calculation of oxygen delivery ($\dot{D}O_2$) is repeatedly given in this book:

$$\dot{D}O_2 = \text{cardiac output} \times CaO_2 \ 10 \, \text{ml min}^{-1} \, \text{m}^{-2} \qquad (7.1)$$

There are two methods of measuring oxygen consumption ($\dot{V}O_2$). One entails the measurement of exhaled gases and uses certain assumptions (described in Chapter 16). However, more conveniently in the patient who has a pulmonary artery flotation catheter (PAFC) *in situ*, the $\dot{V}O_2$ can be calculated from

$$\dot{V}O_2 = \text{cardiac output} \times (CaO_2 - C\bar{v}O_2) \times 10 \, \text{ml min}^{-1} \, \text{m}^{-2} \qquad (7.2)$$

This is an important method of calculation, as other methods using calculations and assumptions from measurements of inspired and exhaled gases may be unreliable at FiO_2 levels of greater than 0.5.

In clinical practice these values are indexed to the patient's body surface area, calculated from direct measurements of height and weight.

Shoemaker is widely quoted on the use of so-called supranormal values as end-points or goals of therapy (Shoemaker *et al.*, 1982, 1988; Bland *et al.*, 1985). However, the consideration of the mythical normal patient with a 95% haemoglobin saturation, a haemoglobin concentration of 15 g dl^{-1}, and a cardiac output of 5.0 litres min^{-1} will show that if the patient has a normal body surface area the oxygen delivery will be approximately 580 ml min^{-1} m^{-2}. Thus the much quoted 'supranormal' value of oxygen delivery is, in reality, the normal resting value. It is not a supranormal value but the values achieved by survivors of acute surgical illness. Healthy individuals lie at rest with a $\dot{D}O_2$ approaching 600 ml min^{-1} m^{-2}. It is, therefore, not unrealistic or illogical that such a level should be a goal of therapy given the added demands of, for instance, sepsis, surgical or accidental trauma (Stoner, 1987).

The minimum requirements for an adequate $\dot{D}O_2$ are (1) mixed venous saturation >70%, and (2) normal arterial blood lactate. The simplistic approach for this situation is that $\dot{D}O_2$ should be increased to a level that produces a levelling out or plateau of $\dot{V}O_2$. This may apply during early phases of resuscitation but, as shown in Figs. 7.1 and 7.2, the relationship between $\dot{D}O_2$ and $\dot{V}O_2$ in patients with acute respiratory distress syndrome (ARDS) can be quite complex with no clear definition of a plateau (Clarke *et al.*, 1991).

This presumably relates to changes in oxygen demand which may relate to repair of injuries, resolution or development of sepsis. In this particular study (Clarke *et al.*, 1991) all patients were well-sedated and paralysed when the measurements were taken, thus obviating the metabolic demands of anxiety, fear or attempts at spontaneous ventilation.

However, to simplify the interpretation of the effects of therapeutic interventions (especially that of the use of the most important intervention in intensive care therapy, i.e. the decision to use mechanical ventilation in an

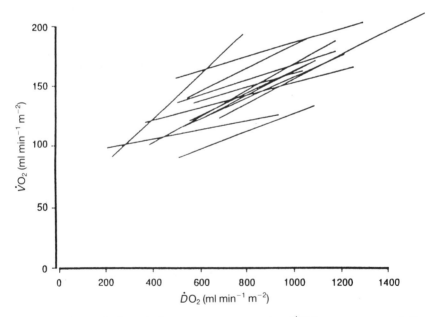

Figure 7.1   Lines for best fit for oxygen consumption ($\dot{V}O_2$) versus oxygen delivery ($\dot{D}O_2$) as determined by simple linear regression in 13 patients.

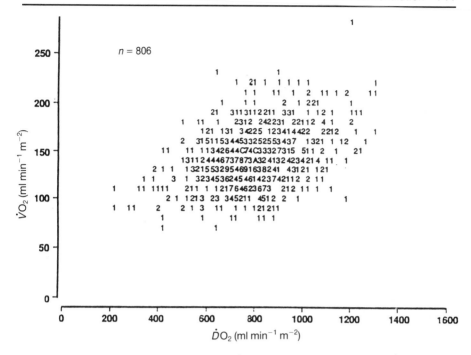

Figure 7.2 Plot of oxygen consumption ($\dot{V}O_2$) against oxygen delivery ($\dot{D}O_2$) for the combined patient data. Frequencies and symbols: (1) 1 data point; (2) 2; (3) 3; (4) 4; (5) 5; (6) 6; (7) 7; (8) 8; (9) 9; (A) 10; (B) 11; (C) 12.

attempt to improve oxygen delivery), the hypothesis of the use of mechanical ventilation is that oxygen delivery will be improved. This is a reaffirmation of the fact that in critically ill patients the delivery of oxygen should be adequate, not necessarily increased to an arbitrary figure (Edwards *et al.*, 1989). To re-emphasize the basic physiology the determinants of oxygen transport, given in Eqn (7.1) above, are

(1) The arterial partial pressure or tension of oxygen, i.e. PaO_2.
(2) The content of fully oxygenated haemoglobin and the saturation of haemoglobin in the arterial circulation. This includes the possible effects of abnormal haemoglobin ligands such as carboxyhaemoglobin and methaemoglobin.

In the calculation of arterial oxygen content values these variables must be recognized, measured and assessed. To ensure the quality of these calculations the primary functions of the blood-gas machine used should be familiar to the clinician. It is possible that there may be variations in the calculations of 'desaturated'. or 'reduced' haemoglobin. A typical example of the results available from a modern blood-gas machine is shown in Fig. 7.3.

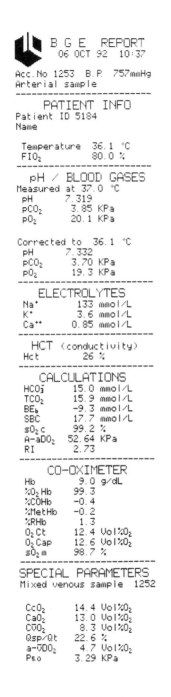

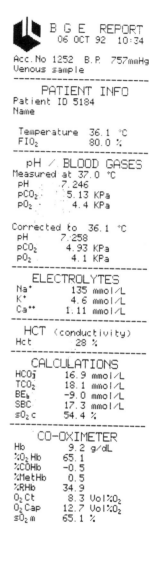

Figure 7.3   Typical blood-gas printout.

The clinician involved should also be aware that some of these variables are measured directly and some are calculated. On occasions, the calculations are based on assumptions that might apply to patients with normal respiratory and cardiac function but do not apply to the patient who is critically ill with the combination of respiratory and circulatory failure so frequently seen on the intensive care unit. Also, of course, there is the added consideration of acute or chronic multisystem organ failures, especially that of the kidney.

Cardiac Output Measurements

The modern thermodilution technique of cardiac output estimation uses the original Stewart–Hamilton equation, and assumes that using a temperature change is the equivalent of a reduction in concentration of a dye or colour indicator. The Stewart–Hamilton gives cardiac output as:

$$\text{cardiac output} = Vi \times \frac{(Tb - Ti)}{\int_0^\infty \Delta Tb(t)\, dt} \times \frac{(Si \times Ci)}{(Sb \times Cb)} \times 60 \times k$$

where Vi = volume injected; Tb = temperature of blood; Ti = temperature of injectate; Si = specific gravity of injectate; Sb = specific gravity of blood; Ci = specific heat of injectate; Cb = specific heat of blood; and k = correction factor for loss of indictor during transit. The error associated with the manufacturers' calibration is $< 5\%$.

The large number of measured and assumed variables in this equation should be appreciated. At first sight these might preclude the use of this method of estimating cardiac output. However, the clinical use of this technique is validated by inspection of the displayed thermodilution cardiac output curves. Examples of typical curves are given in Fig. 7.4.

Technical errors may contribute to a false measurement of cardiac output. In Fig. 7.5 variations in the shape of curves can be seen which are due to errors on the part of the operator. A change in systemic oxyhaemoglobin arterial saturation of oxygen which is artifactual is quite unusual. Nonetheless, for the present the common clinical practice of peripheral pulse oximetry provides (in technical terms) a completely individual and separate index of peripheral haemoglobin saturation from that derived from the PAFC, particularly in those patients with profound vasoconstriction or vasodilation. In shock states, however, this technique has been incompletely validated as yet in patients with profound hypotension.

Therapy: Mechanical Ventilation

Given all these caveats one has to assess the effects of therapeutic intervention, including the most important step on the intensive care unit which is the

(a)

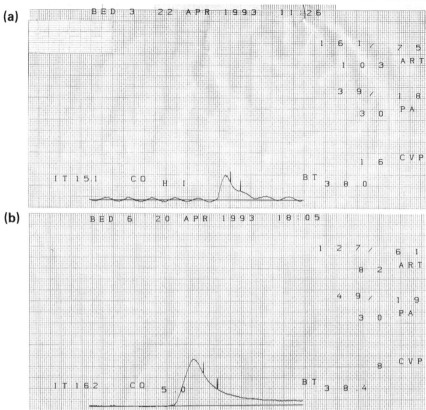

(b)

Figure 7.4   Cardiac output curve measurement showing (a) high cardiac output and (b) low cardiac output.

decision to implement the use of mechanical ventilation. This involves the transition from laboured, distressed and possibly uncomfortable spontaneous ventilation, perhaps with a compromised airway, to controlled ventilation with an artificial airway. In terms of improvement in oxygen transport variables the benefits of mechanical ventilation might seem intuitively obvious. However, there are some potentially deleterious effects (Table 7.1).

Table 7.1   Potential benefits and harmful effects of mechanical ventilation

Potential benefits	Potential harmful effects
Protection of the airway	Difficulties or complications in institu-
Increase in arterial O_2 tension and saturation	tion of ventilation – especially endo-tracheal intubation
Reduction in arterial CO_2 tension	Depression of cardiac output and,
Reduction in the work of breathing	therefore, O_2 delivery to the tissues
Symptomatic relief of respiratory distress	Pulmonary barotrauma
	The need for sedative and relaxant agents

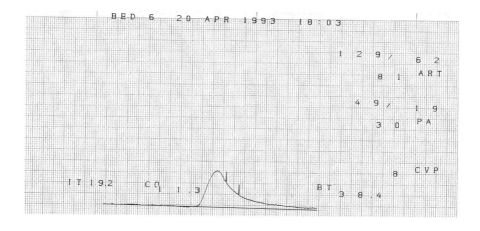

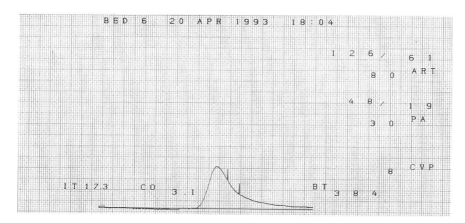

Figure 7.5 Two consecutive curves from cardiac output monitor and printout showing variations in curves due to operator error.

On a conceptional level it might seem that the institution of mechanical ventilation might only improve the arterial tension of oxygen (PaO_2). Also, given the constraints of the minute volume of ventilation it may reduce the arterial concentration and pressure of carbon dioxide ($PaCO_2$).

The relationship between alveolar ventilation and arterial carbon dioxide and oxygen tensions has been repeatedly described with a high degree of reproducibility (Nunn, 1987). The more complex relationship between circulatory shock, muscle fatigue and death is however, poorly appreciated. Respiratory fatigue and diaphragmatic weakness as a cause of shock in hypovolaemia, sepsis and low cardiac output states has been well-described

(Aubier *et al.*, 1981; Edwards *et al.*, 1988a) but unfortunately poorly appreciated. The negative effects of mechanical ventilation have, in fact, been overexaggerated. Cournand *et al.*, (1943) is widely quoted as having demonstrated that intermittent positive pressure ventilation reduces cardiac output. It is salutary to review his original data which were based on volunteers, not on patients who would require mechanical ventilation on modern indications or criteria. In fact, he showed no decrease in cardiac output except in patients ventilated with positive end-expiratory pressure (PEEP) or those with a known pneumothorax, which was iatrogenically induced in all patients as part of therapy for tuberculosis.

Many previous studies (Powers *et al.*, 1973; Danek *et al.*, 1980) have shown the potential for PEEP to reduce cardiac output and thereby oxygen delivery – a typical example from one of our own patients is given in Fig. 7.6. In summary, the introduction of PEEP may increase the arterial tension of oxygen (PaO_2), as has been demonstrated repeatedly (Powers *et al.*, 1973; Danek *et al.*, 1980). However, at the same time there may be a reduction in cardiac output which reduces oxygen delivery. This effect is not a contraindication to PEEP therapy, which will reduce the need for high concentrations of inspired oxygen, but is a positive indication for the measurement of cardiac output during PEEP therapy. Indeed, determinants of PEEP therapy can be obtained by continuous measurement of mixed venous oxygen saturation or lactate, measured from samples of systemic arterial, peripheral venous or central venous blood.

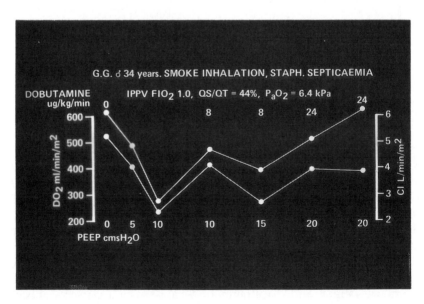

Figure 7.6   Typical example of use of PEEP to reduce cardiac output.

A more occult phenomenon is that of intrinsic PEEP or so-called 'auto-PEEP' which occurs in patients with increased airways resistance. This may be clinically evident or occult airway outflow resistance and is a sinister phenomenon as it may be difficult to recognize on some modern mechanical ventilators. The gold standard test for identification and correction of this problem is temporary occlusion of the expiratory limb of the respiratory system exactly at the end-expiratory phase. This is technically convenient with some ventilators but much more difficult with others.

All these considerations and problems should not detract from the responsible and professional use of mechanical ventilation, with or without PEEP therapy. There is accumulating evidence that manipulation and optimization of oxygen transport variables may improve outcome in severe acute respiratory failure of diverse aetiologies (Clarke *et al.*, 1991b). Primarily, this may be because of a reduced incidence of acute renal failure.

Continuous Positive Airway Pressure (CPAP)

Continuous positive airway pressure (CPAP) has been demonstrated in many studies to be an effective mode of respiratory support. In essence, a tight-fitting face mask is used to implement an adequate flow rate and concentration of inspired oxygen with some degree of limitation of the end-expiratory pressure to above the ambient atmospheric level. As with PEEP therapy this will increase the pulmonary functional residual capacity and facilitate gas exchange. This is to be regarded as a form of assisted ventilation and is most suitable for types of acute respiratory failure which may be expected to recover rapidly. The lack of airway protection in the absence of an endotracheal tube is a potential problem.

Use of Fluid and Blood Transfusion

This is extensively reviewed elsewhere in this book. It only remains to emphasize that the responses of critically ill patients are variable and unpredictable. Two studies (Haupt *et al.*, 1985; Gilbert *et al.*, 1986) using plasma and artificial colloids have shown that haemodilution without an increase in cardiac output occurs in up to one-third of patients. The same effect was demonstrated by Edwards and Wilkins (1987) using modified fluid gelatin. The biochemical composition of artificial colloids can be very variable and must be checked on the label before the fluid is infused.

The correct approach is to use volume loading and blood transfusion guided by repeated measurements of wedged pressure and cardiac output with calculations of stroke volume index and left ventricular (LV) stroke work index. When artificial colloids are used there may be haemodilution, and if the cardiac output responses are inadequate this may lead to a reduction in oxygen delivery (Edwards & Wilkins, 1987).

The oxygen transport responses of blood transfusion have been re-assessed recently by Dietricht *et al.* (1990). Once again the variability of any intervention in the critically ill patient has been emphasized.

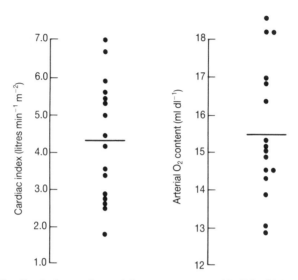

Figure 7.7 Cardiac index and arterial oxygen content (CaO_2) of 16 patients. (From Edwards *et al.*, 1988b.)

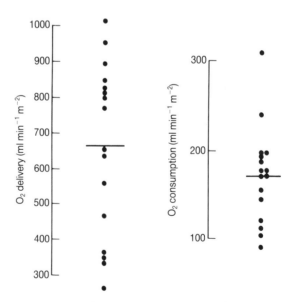

Figure 7.8 Oxygen delivery ($\dot{D}O_2$) and consumption ($\dot{V}O_2$) in 16 patients. (From Edwards *et al.*, 1988b.)

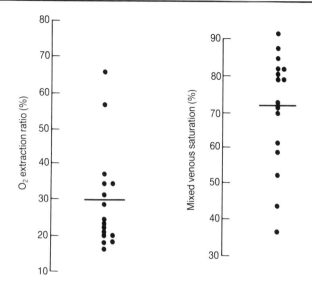

Figure 7.9   Oxygen extraction ratio (OER) and mixed venous oxygen saturation ($S\bar{v}O_2$) of 16 patients. (From Edwards *et al.*, 1988b.)

The use of fluid and blood administration has to be viewed in the light of recent investigations which have shown that even under conditions of muscle relaxation in the patient with trauma there may be an imbalance between the supply and demand of oxygen such that $S\bar{v}O_2$ values may be low (Edwards *et al.*, 1988b) (Figs. 7.7–7.9). In a separate study (Rady *et al.*, 1992) of patients with blunt thoracic trauma the patients were divided prospectively into two groups: group 1, patients with an LV stroke work index of less than 1; group 2, patients with a normal (i.e. greater than 44) LV stroke work index. There were 9 patients in group 1 with 7 deaths and in group 2 there were only 2 deaths despite the high number of patients in that

Table 7.2   Haemodynamic data for groups 1 and 2 following controlled plasma volume expansion with modified fluid gelatin and blood

	Group 1	Group 2	P^a
Heart rate (beats min^{-1})	102(23)	84(18)	n.s.
Mean arterial pressure (mm Hg)	82(9)	94(15)	n.s.
Central venous pressure (mm Hg)	11(4)	11(5)	n.s.
Wedge pressure (mm Hg)	14(7)	13(4)	n.s.
LV stroke work index (g min^{-1} m^{-2})	30(10)	62(14)	<0.001

Values are mean (S/D).
N.s. not significant.
[a] Student's paired *t*-test.

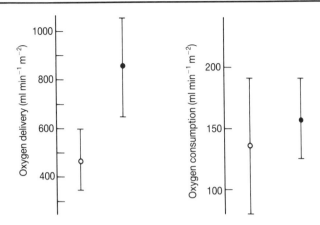

Figure 7.10   Levels of oxygen delivery ($\dot{D}O_2$) and consumption ($\dot{V}O_2$) in group 1 ($\bigcirc$) and group 2 ($\bullet$). $P < 0.001$ for oxygen delivery; there was no significant difference between the groups for oxygen consumption (Student's paired t-test). (From Rady *et al.*, 1992.)

group. The haemodynamic data are given in Table 7.2. In Fig. 7.10 it can be seen that there were major differences in the level of oxygen delivery between the two groups but no real difference between oxygen consumption. Thus the mixed venous oxygen saturation levels were significantly lower in group 2.

Conclusion

In conclusion, a variety of studies have shown that in the most critically ill patients useful information can be deduced from the measurement of oxygen transport variables.

However, at present there is only suggestive but by no means conclusive evidence of increased levels of survival. In view of repeated controversy and the importance of this issue, the next step for the future is to conduct large control studies to answer the vital question of survival rates.

Modern technology is making the use of haemodynamic measurement increasingly user-friendly. Another major requirement in terms of therapy is a new generation of critical synthetic colloids, entirely free of the risk of infection. The development of these will mean that the effects of colloids on oxygen delivery are likely to be more predictable in the future. There may be adverse effects of therapy which may not be detected by the so-called 'vital signs' and the doctor in the intensive care unit must continue to use all means at his disposal to counteract the effects of ARDS, septic shock and trauma to increase outcome. I believe oxygen therapy is one of the means whereby this can be achieved.

References

Aubier M, Trippenbach T & Roussos C (1981) Respiratory muscle fatigue during cardiogenic shock. *J. Appl. Physiol.* **51:** 499–508.

Bland RD, Shoemaker WC, Abraham E & Cobo JC (1985) Hemodynamic and oxygen transport patterns in surviving and non surviving postoperative patients. *Crit. Care Med.* **13:** 85–90.

Clarke C, Edwards JD, Nightingale P *et al.* (1991a) Persistence of supply dependency of oxygen uptake at high levels of delivery in adult respiratory distress syndrome. *Crit. Care Med.* **19:** 497–502.

Clarke C, O'Keefe N, Nightingale P & Edwards JD (1991b) Ventilatory support in ARDS and relation to outcome. *Proc. U. K. Intensive Care Soc.* (abstract).

Cournand A, Riley RL, Bradley SE *et al.* (1943) Studies of the circulation in clinical shock. *Surgery* **13:** 964.

Danek SJ, Lynch JP, Weg JG & Dantzker DR (1980) The dependece of oxygen uptake on oxygen delivery in the Adult Respiratory Distress Syndrome. *Am. Rev. Respiratory Dis.* **122:** 387–95.

Dietricht K, Conrad S, Cullen H *et al.* (1990) Cardiovascular and metabolic response to red blood cell transfusion in critically ill volume-resuscitated non-surgical patients. *Crit. Care Med.* **18:** 940–4.

Edwards JD & Wilkins RG (1987) Atrial fibrillation precipitated by acute hypovolaemia. *Br. Med. J.* **294:** 283–4.

Edwards JD, Whittaker S & Prior A (1988a) Cardiogenic shock without a critically elevated left ventricular end diastolic pressure: management and outcome in eighteen patients. *Br. Heart J.* **55:** 549–53.

Edwards JD, Redmond AD, Nightingale P & Wilkins RG (1988b) Oxygen consumption following trauma: a reappraisal in severely injured patients requiring mechanical ventilation. *Br. J. Surg.* **75:** 690–2.

Edwards JD Brown GCS, Nightingale P *et al.* (1989) Use of survivors' cardiorespiratory values as therapeutic goals in septic shock. *Crit. Care Med.* **17:** 1098–103.

Gilbert EM, Haupt MT, Mandanas RY *et al.* (1986) The effect of fluid loading, blood transfusion and catecholamine infusion on oxygen delivery and consumption in patients with sepsis. *Am. Rev. Respiratory Dis.* **134:** 873–8.

Haupt MT, Gilbert EM & Carlson RW (1985) Fluid loading increases oxygen consumption in septic patients with lactic acidosis. *Am. Rev. Respiratory Dis.* **131:** 912–6.

Nunn JF (1987) *Applied Respiratory Physiology.* London: Butterworth.

Powers SR, Mannal R, Neclerio M *et al.* (1973) Physiologic consequences of positive end-expiratory pressure (PEEP) ventilation. *Ann. Surg.* **178:** 265–72.

Rady MY, Edwards JD & Nightingale P (1992) Early cardiorespiratory findings after severe blunt thoracic trauma and their relation to outcome. *Br. J. Surg.* **79:** 65–8.

Shoemaker WC, Appel P, Waxman K *et al.* (1982) Clinical trial of survivors cardiorespiratory patterns as therapeutic goals in critically ill postoperative patients. *Crit. Care Med.* **10:** 398–403.

Shoemaker WC, Appel PL, Kram HB *et al.* (1988) Prospective trial of supranormal values of survivors as therapeutic goals in high risk surgical patients. *Chest* **94:** 1176–86.

Stoner HB (1987) Interpretation of the metabolic effects of trauma and sepsis. *J. Clin. Pathol.* **40:** 1108–17.

8 Hypovolaemic Shock

U. Kreimeier and K. Messmer

Introduction

Hypovolaemic shock is a clinical state defined as depletion of intravascular volume leading to inadequate tissue perfusion with respect to delivery of oxygen and substrates to the cells. Traumatic shock represents a subset of hypovolaemic shock, in which a critical reduction of blood volume is combined with the effects of tissue injury, eliciting the activation of inflammatory and coagulation systems. Trauma in conjunction with severe hypovolaemia and shock remains the leading cause of morbidity and mortality of patients under 45 years of age (Baker, 1986; McCabe, 1990).

Hypovolaemia triggers a sympatho-adrenergic response that results in peripheral vasoconstriction, a rise in heart rate and a decline in systolic pressure in the case of an acute reduction of circulating blood volume of more than 20% (Guyton, 1991). Blood flow to the skin and peripheral tissues is reduced in an effort to preserve perfusion of vital organs such as the brain, heart, liver and kidneys. In contrast, due to the high α-adrenergic innervation of the splanchnic vascular region, blood flow to the intestine, and to the gut mucosa in particular, is curtailed. Tachycardia and enhanced cardiac contractility elicited by the sympatho-adrenergic reaction might preserve cardiac output; however, at the same time myocardial oxygen requirement is increased. The balance between total oxygen delivery and oxygen demand is maintained as long as tissue oxygen extraction can be enhanced under conditions of reduced blood flow caused by blood loss; beyond a critical point, however, tissue perfusion becomes inadequate to the local oxygen needs, resulting in anaerobic metabolism, cellular acidosis, and reduction of specific organ functions, bringing the risk of multiple systems organ failure (MSOF) (Fig. 8.1).

Clinical Features of the Patient

The clinical presentation of the patient with established shock reflects regional perfusion deficits and is characterized by alteration of the sensorium – ranging from agitation to stupor and coma – weakness or prostration, by

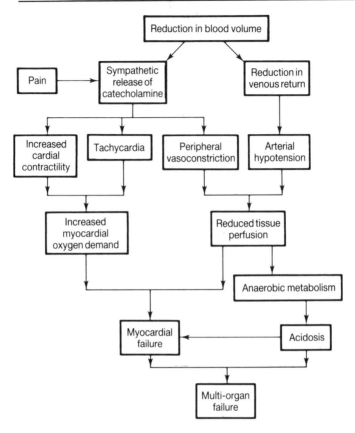

Figure 8.1 Pathophysiology of hypovolaemic shock. (From Baskett, 1990.)

cold, clammy, sometimes even cyanotic skin, tachycardia and a thready pulse, hypotension and tachypnoea. These signs are early symptoms reflecting the underlying pathophysiology, i.e. hypovolaemia, in prolonged states followed by myocardial insufficiency (leading to thirst, reduced urinary output, systemic hypotension), vasoconstriction and tachycardia due to catecholamine release (leading to skin pallor, clamminess, thready pulse), cerebral hypoxia and acidosis (leading to confusion, aggression, drowsiness, and eventually coma), and general tissue hypoxia and acidosis (leading to tachypnoea, weakness).

Shock is a dynamic process, in which the measurable haemodynamic and metabolic variables are continually changing. Table 8.1 depicts a classification of hypovolaemic shock according to blood loss (Baskett, 1990). The individual ability to maintain a normal *milieu intérieur* depends on factors such as age, pre-existing diseases, speed of blood volume reduction, and severity and duration of the shock syndrome. In previously healthy young adults, systolic blood pressure is often preserved despite a quite appreciable blood loss of up to 1.5 litres owing to the efficient compensatory response of the sympatho-adrenergic system. In children as well as in elderly patients especially with coronary heart disease, however, much smaller blood losses may provoke circulatory failure and hypotension, as myocardial stimulation and a pronounced increase in heart rate may jeopardize coronary blood flow and myocardial oxygen delivery. Also, patients under chronic medication with β-blocking drugs may not be able to respond with an appropriate sympatho-adrenergic response and may become hypotensive at moderate blood losses. In these cases myocardial ischaemia ensues as an early consequence of reduced coronary perfusion pressure.

Table 8.1   Classification of hypovolaemic shock according to blood loss

	Class I	Class II	Class III	Class IV
Blood loss:				
Volume (ml)	750	800–1500	1500–2000	>2000
Percentage	<15	15–30	30–40	>40
Blood pressure:				
Systolic	unchanged	normal	reduced	very low
Diastolic	unchanged	raised	reduced	very low or unrecordable
Pulse (beats min^{-1})	slight tachycardia	100–120	120 (thready)	>120
Capillary refill	normal	slow (>2 s)	slow (>2 s)	undetectable
Respiratory rate	normal	normal	tachypnoea (>20 min^{-1})	tachypnoea (>20 min^{-1})
Urinary flow rate ($ml\,h^{-1}$)	>30	20–30	10–20	0–10
Extremities	colour normal	pale	pale	pale and cold
Mental state	alert	anxious or aggressive	anxious, aggressive or drowsy	drowsy, confused or unconscious

From Baskett (1990).

Aetiologic Factors of Hypovolaemic Shock

The most common clinical causes of hypovolaemic shock are listed in Table 8.2. Since arterial pressure is dependent on cardiac output and peripheral vasomotor tone, marked reduction of either of these variables without a compensatory elevation of the other results in systemic hypotension. In general, reduction of cardiac output may be due to hypovolaemia, myocardial failure or obstruction of blood flow. In protracted hypovolaemic shock all three pathophysiologic features are present due to severe deterioration of nutritional blood flow at the microcirculatory level. Hypovolaemia may be caused by loss of water and electrolytes, plasma or whole blood, with the same effect on cardiovascular dynamics. Blood loss from trauma or bleeding into body cavities, muscles or the intestine can lead to shock without overt haemorrhage. Therefore, the most important clinical objectives are early recognition of hypovolaemia in the patient and detection and evaluation of occult blood or fluid loss.

Table 8.2   Aetiologic factors of hypovolaemic shock

A. *External fluid losses*
   1. Acute haemorrhage
   2. Excessive fluid loss
      a. Gastrointestinal
         I. Vomiting
         II. Severe diarrhoea
      b. Renal
      c. Cutaneous
         I. Perspiration and insensible water loss
         II. Burns
         III. Exudative lesions

B. *Internal fluid losses*
   1. Haemorrhage and trauma
   2. Ascites
   3. Intestinal obstruction

C. *Relative hypovolaemia*
   1. Vasodilatation
      a. Neurogenic
      b. Metabolic, toxic, humoral
   2. Obstructive

Hypovolaemic shock is the most common type of shock in emergency medicine as well as in major surgery. Haemorrhagic shock may be caused by external or internal bleeding, resulting from traumatic amputation of extremities or disruption of large vessels (both arteries and veins), excessive blood losses during invasive surgery, incision or rupture of large vessels (ruptured aortic aneurysm), as complication during ectopic pregnancy or of trauma to parenchymatous organs (liver, spleen, kidneys). Acute gastrointestinal or oesophageal bleeding is the most common cause of haemorrhagic shock in internal medicine. Erosive gastric or duodenal ulcera, carcinoma or intestinal polypi, but also haemorrhagic gastritis or pancreatitis, or Mallory–Weiss syndrome may result in protracted but profound loss of blood. Among the iatrogenic complications are mucosal lesions or perforation after endoscopic manoeuvres, and overdosage of antiocoagulants and thrombolytic agents with subsequent urogenital or gastrointestinal bleeding.

Cerebral, thoracic and abdominal injury are frequently found in poly-trauma patients. Lung contusion or multiple rib fractures lead to compromised breathing and thus to decreased oxygen uptake in the lungs, favouring early decompensation in previously healthy subjects despite minor blood losses. Fractures of the proximal femur or of the pelvic girdle may account for rapid (occult) blood losses of 2 litres, and call for careful clinical examination in the emergency room. Tissue trauma leads to the liberation of vasoactive mediators, involving the kallikrein–kinin, complement and coagulation system as well as activation of the arachidonic acid cascade system. The sympatho-adrenergic reaction during traumatic–haemorrhagic shock is potentiated by pain and psychologic factors such as fear and stress.

Massive loss of fluid and electrolytes may occur during profuse vomiting (pyloric or intestinal obstruction), severe diarrhoea, sweating and dehydration due to fever, heat or muscular work, as well as through fistulae and drainage tubes. Chronic pyelonephritis, the diuretic phase of acute renal failure, as well as excessive doses of diuretics are renal causes of polyuria, in contrast to extrarenal causes, e.g. diabetes mellitus and diabetes insipidus. Abdominal inflammation, e.g. peritonitis and pancreatitis, and large body surface burn injury are notoriously associated with transmembraneous loss of fluid and protein, which profoundly affects Starling forces. Common denominators in all these aetiologic factors are a rapidly developing haemo-concentration and deterioration of the rheologic properties of the blood, favouring stasis and the formation of microthrombi and thereby diminution of the capillary surface available for the exchange of oxygen and substrates (Appelgren, 1972).

Relative hypovolaemia may ensue as a consequence of vasodilatation or obstructive shock. A reduction of cardiac output in the presence of an overall normal blood volume will result in the case of compromised venous return to the heart. This is the case during compression of the *vena cava* in advanced pregnancy. Anaesthesia, ganglionic and adrenergic blockers, overdoses of barbiturates or poisons, and nervous system damage (spinal cord or brain injury) are neurogenic factors of excessive vasodilatation. These generally elicit the same pathway of sympatho-adrenergic activation as is involved in absolute hypovolaemia due to severe haemorrhage and fluid loss as described above. Among the metabolic, toxic and humoral mechanisms, anaphylactoid/anaphylactic reactions develop upon application of antigens, e.g. radiographic media. As in septic shock, hypovolaemia is not the primary cause of hypotension and shock, but develops secondary to the release of vasoactive mediators and microcirculatory alterations (*distributive shock*). The presence of bacteria and endotoxins in the bloodstream elicits an early hyperdynamic circulatory state of shock, which is also associated with profound hypovolaemia due to extravasation of fluid and macromolecules such as albumin.

Reduction of Blood Volume and the Development of Multiple Systems Organ Failure (MSOF)

As a consequence of hypovolaemia and low perfusion pressure elicited by severe blood loss and tissue trauma, nutritional blood flow is compromised and tissue hypoxia develops. The adhesion of activated polymorphonuclear leukocytes (PMNL) to the vascular endothelium and endothelial cell-swelling result in exclusion of microvessels from perfusion, which becomes highly heterogeneous at the microcirculatory level. Occlusion of microvessels either by endothelial cell-swelling or capillary plugging may completely abolish local flow. In addition, the interaction of PMNL with the venular endothelium is followed by the release of vasoactive mediators and toxic oxygen species, promoting further redistribution of tissue perfusion, macromolecular leakage, interstitial oedema, and further impediment of nutritional flow (Bihari, 1989; Messmer, 1990).

Systemic sepsis and MSOF are the most frequent and often fatal complications after trauma and major surgery (Trunkey, 1983; Carmona *et al.*, 1984; Bone *et al.*, 1989). The recognition that failure of the gut and of distant organs may be causally related has led some workers to herald the gut as the *'motor'* of MSOF (Carrico *et al.*, 1986; Border *et al.*, 1987; Cottier & Kraft, 1991). Severe trauma and shock provoke a significant reduction of splanchnic blood flow and ischaemic injury to the intestinal mucosa (Kvietys & Granger, 1989; Deitch *et al.*, 1990). Hypovolaemic shock and splanchnic hypoperfusion, by causing defects in epithelial barrier function, result in translocation of bacteria and endotoxins from the gut lumen into the liver and eventually into the systemic circulation (Billiar *et al.*, 1988; Baker *et al.*, 1988). Recently *'gut-derived infectious-toxic shock (GITS)'* has been defined as a subtype of septic shock, originating from the invasion of bacteria from the intestinal microflora (Cottier & Kraft, 1991). The generation of oxygen free radicals via the enzyme xanthine oxidase, the concentration of which is highest in the villous tip of the intestinal mucosa, has been identified as the key determinant in the process of bacterial and endotoxin translocation (Granger *et al.*, 1981; Deitch *et al.*, 1990).

Microcirculatory failure during established sepsis and endotoxaemia is caused and sustained by the direct action of endotoxin and the release of vasoactive mediators (Hack & Thijs, 1991). Cytokines such as interleukin-1 and 6 and tumour necrosis factor (TNFα) are able to elicit many of the systemic effects characteristically seen during endotoxaemia (Michie *et al.*, 1988; Natanson *et al.*, 1989; Fong *et al.*, 1990). These cytokines have recently been found to appear in the bloodstream also in response to haemorrhage and tissue trauma (Chaudry *et al.*, 1990). The ensuing activation of cascade systems and PMNL–endothelial interaction favour a significant redistribution of blood perfusion within the microvascular network resulting in a critical overall reduction of nutritional blood flow and focal ischaemia (Thijs & Groeneveld, 1987; Messmer *et al.*, 1988).

Monitoring the Patient in Hypovolaemic Shock

Patients with life-threatening injuries make up approximately 10–15% of all patients hospitalized because of injuries (Trunkey, 1991). About 50% of deaths from trauma occur at the scene of the accident, another 30% occur within a few hours of injury (Carmona *et al.*, 1984). The prognosis of patients is significantly affected by the severity and duration of shock and consequent secondary organ dysfunction, and therefore by the speed of recognition and appropriateness of medical intervention. Clinical management of the patient in hypovolaemic shock requires accurate and serial measurements of haemo-dynamic and respiratory as well as biochemical parameters, i.e. heart rate and rhythm, systemic blood pressure, respiratory rate and adequacy of gas exchange, cardiac filling pressures and eventually cardiac output (Swan–Ganz catheter), tissue perfusion indices (pulse oximetry), and organ function (mental status, urine output, liver function, etc.). The basic variables to monitor in shock are listed in Table 8.3. Careful clinical assessment allows a logical initial approach to therapy while other data are collected and considered. The objective of the management of hypovolaemic shock is to maintain tissue perfusion and oxyenation or to restore it to adequate values.

Table 8.3   Basic variables to monitor in hypovolaemic shock

Arterial pressure
Heart rate and pulse pressure
Mental state
Peripheral oxygen saturation (pulse oximetry)
Urinary output
Central venous pressure (CVP)
Alterations in the ECG
Body (core) temperature
Invasive monitoring
Central venous pressure (CVP)
Arterial pressure (A. radialis, A. femoralis)
Pulmonary arterial and pulmonary capillary wedge pressure (PAP; PCWP)
Cardiac output
Blood-gas analysis (arterial and mixed venous blood)
Biochemical analysis
(eventually) Intracranial pressure (ICP)

Haemodynamic and Respiratory Monitoring

Haemodynamic monitoring is an integral part of the diagnosis and management of hypovolaemic shock. Serial measurement of systemic arterial pressure is essential and is routinely performed non-invasively by means of a sphygmomanometer (Riva–Rocci), either manually or automatically every 3–5 min. Invasive monitoring is mandatory in cases of severe hypotension (<60 mm Hg) and shock refractory to primary resuscitation for valid quantification of systemic pressure. The arterial line, in addition, offers the advantage of frequent analyses of arterial blood gases and pH. The radial artery is the preferred site for cannulation and has the lowest complication rate. In cases of severe hypotension or the application of high doses of vasoactive drugs, which may result in peripheral vasoconstriction, larger arteries (brachial or femoral arteries) need to be cannulated.

The electrocardiogram (ECG) permits serial assessment of heart rate and prompt detection of arrhythmia. In ECG-lead II in most cases the p-wave can be analysed best, giving differentiation of a regular sinus rhythm and supraventricular and ventricular extrasystoles, respectively. In adults, the quotient of heart rate and systolic blood pressure has been referred to as the 'shock index' (Allgöwer & Burri, 1967). Although in hypovolaemic shock this quotient will increase due to tachycardia and hypotension, no definite conclusion can be drawn with regard to the amount of blood loss and severity of shock, since tachycardia may also result from the perception of pain after trauma, and, on the other hand, systolic blood pressure may be in the normal range despite considerable blood loss of up to 20% (see above).

The monitoring of central venous pressure (CVP) provides a rough index of the actual status of venous return and of the need for pushing fluids. The catheter should be inserted through the antecubital or external jugular vein; only if the physician is experienced should it be introduced through the subclavian or internal jugular vein (Trunkey et al., 1988). CVP reflects the filling pressure of the right ventricle and hence is an adequate indicator of cardiac filling pressure provided there is no underlying cardiac or pulmonary disease; it depends, however, on intrathoracic pressure, i.e. on inflation pressure in the case of mechanical ventilation, and is a poor reflection of left ventricular filling because of marked differences between right and left ventricular performance in the seriously ill (Hardaway, 1982). Central venous pressure obtained with the catheter advanced to the superior vena cava is normally between 5 and 8 mm Hg, and should be elevated to 10 mm Hg if one is to expect an adequate cardiac output in patients in shock.

Pulmonary capillary wedge pressure (PCWP) correlates well with left ventricular end-diastolic pressure and left atrial pressure. Therefore, in patients with protracted hypovolaemic shock, or with suspected cardiac or pulmonary disease, or in whom management includes the use of mechanical, particularly positive pressure ventilation, the use of a Swan–Ganz balloon-tip catheter is obligatory (Vincent, 1991). Besides monitoring body core temperature this device provides serial assessment of cardiac output and of mixed-venous blood samples to determine whole body oxygen utilization. The catheter is introduced intravenously with or without fluoroscopy, and advanced to the pulmonary artery under electrocardiographic and pressure monitoring. The refinement of fibre-optic catheters has made possible continuous monitoring of mixed-venous oxygen saturation and thus more accurate assessment of therapeutic interventions. With certain limitations, oxygen delivery to tissues can be estimated by the arteriovenous difference of oxygen content: a value of $6\,ml\,dl^{-1}$ or more in general indicates inadequate tissue perfusion.

Despite the usefulness of the Swan–Ganz catheter for determination of cardiac filling pressures and mixed-venous and pulmonary arterial blood gas monitoring, its widespread use has been questioned. The quantification of cardiac output is hardly ever needed in emergency care medicine, but is used for management of selected patients to evaluate the effects of volume therapy and of vasoactive and positive inotropic drugs, respectively, on myocardial pump function. In conjunction with blood-gas analysis, thermodilution cardiac output allows the calculation of systemic oxygen delivery ($\dot{D}O_2$) and, with certain limitations, of total body oxygen consumption ($\dot{V}O_2$).

In addition to monitoring the systemic pressure, an arterial cannula in the *A. radialis, A. brachialis* or *A. femoralis* allows the frequent determination of blood gases and pH, and therefore should be established early in cases of hypovolaemic shock and suspected respiratory dysfunction in trauma patients (lung contusion, aspiration, multiple rib fractures). Peripheral oxygenation can easily be monitored by pulse oximetry. The major advantage is its non-invasiveness, there still are, however, methodological limitations with this method in very low oxygen saturation ranges, in states of hypoperfusion and with high levels of carboxyhaemoglobin and methaemoglobin.

Blood Chemistry and Urine Analysis

The clinical laboratory plays a distinct role in the assessment of the patient with hypovolaemic shock. Initial haemoglobin and haematocrit determinations offer no clues to the magnitude of acute blood loss, since haemodilution by interstitial fluid requires time. These values, however, serve as important baseline information and therefore have to be obtained as soon as massive blood loss is suspected and volume therapy is commenced with the eventual need for blood transfusion. Serum electrolytes are of special importance in cases of excessive fluid and plasma losses (sodium, chloride) or protracted ischaemia (potassium). Severe hyponatraemia may occur during massive sweating or after fluid substitution (dilutional hyponatraemia). Hypernatraemia is seldom observed, but has recently been documented as consequences of primary resuscitation by means of small-volume hypertonic saline solutions (see below). Hyperkalaemia follows prolonged phases of (regional) ischaemia; hypokalaemia is found after profuse vomiting and therapy with diuretics (furosemide), as well as after primary resuscitation by means of hypertonic solutions. A lowered total protein content and colloid osmotic (oncotic) pressure reflect massive loss of proteins (e.g. during burn injury, septic shock).

Urinary flow should be measured in all severely traumatized patients early in the course of their resuscitation. An adequate urinary output is one of the best indices of an adequate resuscitation from hypovolaemia and shock. A volume of $50\,\text{ml}\,\text{h}^{-1}$ should be achieved in the adult patient. Since shock is a dynamic process, sequential analyses of laboratory parameters are mandatory.

General Principles of Therapy

The primary factor rendering patients at the risk of developing multiple systems organ failure after shock and trauma is the persistence of impaired microcirculation with its sequelae for cellular and organ function (Bihari, 1989; Messmer, 1990). Patients in hyopovolaemic shock should undergo evaluation and primary resuscitation simultaneously. Therapy must include control of haemorrhage (e.g. by direct pressure, medical anti-shock trousers (MAST), Sengstaken–Blakemore tube), replacing blood or fluid losses, and correcting acid–base or electrolyte disturbances (LaMuraglia & Kennedy, 1989). To ensure optimal pulmonary oxygenation, patients with hypovolaemic shock must have a clear airway, and receive assisted ventilation, if necessary, and then be adequately ventilated with oxygen at a high inspired oxygen concentration. Unconscious patients with severe shock must be intubated at once to establish and maintain an airway.

Volume Therapy by Means of Crystalloids and Colloids

The primary pathophysiological deficiency of haemorrhagic shock is the depletion of intravascular volume, resulting in inadequate venous return. Patients in shock should be placed in a horizontal position with legs slightly elevated (*autotransfusion*). In order to compensate for massive blood loss and to resolve shock, rapid infusion of large amounts of fluids is usually mandatory. Intravenous infusion of colloids and crystalloids is the mainstay of prehospital and emergency centre management of post-injury hypotension (Shoemaker & Kram, 1988; Prough, 1991) (Table 8.4). Crystalloids have a much shorter intravascular half-life compared to that of colloids (Shoemaker & Kram, 1988), and massive infusion of crystalloid solutions bears the risk of fluid overload and tissue, particularly lung, oedema.

In a prospective study on trauma patients Modig (1986) has demonstrated that stabilization of central haemodynamics (preset systolic pressure $\geq 100\,\text{mm}\,\text{Hg}$) was achieved within 2 h following primary resuscitation with the colloid 6% Dextran 70. In a second group of patients receiving as alternative regimen Ringer's acetate, almost 3 h elapsed, although volumes

Table 8.4 Main characteristics of crystalloids versus colloids for resuscitation from hypovolaemic shock

Crystalloids	Colloids
Volume effect 　small 　short	Volume effect 　large 　prolonged
Colloid osmotic 　(oncotic) pressure 　reduced	Colloid osmotic 　(oncotic) pressure 　maintained
No anaphylactic reaction	Anaphylactic reaction possible

2–3 times the infusion volume of the dextran group were administered. Within the first week following the trauma, 5 of 17 patients in the Ringer's acetate group developed pulmonary failure (ARDS), in contrast to none of the 14 patients initially treated with dextran. These authors have therefore advocated the use of dextran as a colloid for primary fluid resuscitation.

Recently, Kaweski et al. (1990) have analysed the impact of prehospital volume therapy on the survival rate of 6855 trauma patients. During the time period until arrival in a trauma centre, which averaged 36 min, either *no* volume therapy was started ('scoop and run'), or an i.v. line was inserted and 620–1550 ml of crystalloid solution were given during transport. However, even in the group of most severely injured patients (systolic blood pressure below 90 mm Hg, and injury severity score >50), as a mean not more than 1250 ± 150 ml of crystalloids were applied. The survival rate in this latter group amounted to 10%, and was not significantly different from patients with the same injury severity score without preclinical volume therapy. These results raise the question whether either patient group received adequate volume resuscitation. This study illustrates the dilemma concerning the practicability of preclinical fluid resuscitation, during which time the application of colloids or crystalloids, in adequate amounts to compensate for massive blood loss, may be limited due to difficulties in gaining intravenous access with large-bore venous cannulas.

Baker and co-workers stated that the therapeutic outcome from traumatic–haemorrhagic shock primarily depends upon the extent and duration of volume deficiency (Baker et al., 1980). New insights in the pathophysiology of shock and trauma indicate that no longer can normalization of macrocirculation alone be considered the primary goal for the prevention of organ dysfunction and MSOF; restoration of normal microcirculation must be given equal priority (Kreimeier & Messmer, 1987; Messmer & Kreimeier, 1989). Wang et al. (1990) have recently shown that fluid resuscitation from experimental haemorrhage in rats by means of 4 times the maximum bleed-out volume of Ringer's lactate increased central venous pressure to more than twice the normal value, but did not restore microvascular blood flow as determined by laser Doppler flowmetry. The authors concluded that, despite a large infusion volume of crystalloids and increased filling pressures, further pharmacological support may be needed in order to resolve the inadequacy of microvascular perfusion and capillary function.

There is no indication for routine application of sodium bicarbonate in hypovolaemic shock. In a prospective, blinded, controlled study in critically ill patients, who had metabolic acidosis and increased blood lactate, correction of acidaemia using sodium bicarbonate did not improve central haemodynamics or the cardiovascular response to catecholamines (Cooper et al., 1990). It did, however, increase $PaCO_2$ and decrease plasma ionized calcium. Possible detrimental effects of bicarbonate may be summarized as follows: venous hypercapnia, decrease in intracellular pH, cerebrospinal fluid acidosis, tissue hypoxia, circulatory congestion and hypernatraemia (Arieff, 1991).

Use of Blood and Blood Components

In order to optimize oxygen delivery to the tissues, cardiac output, blood haemoglobin content, oxygen binding to haemoglobin and arterial oxygen saturation must be normalized. Current concerns about increasingly scarce supplies, escalating costs, and the potential for transmitting severe, sometimes even fatal disease (non-A–non-B hepatitis; HIV-virus) compel us to reconsider transfusion practices (Messmer, 1987). The dynamic state of hypovolaemic shock sometimes requires infusion of a considerable amount of fluid within a short period, while bleeding is still not controlled and plasma volume is subject to changes according to the plasma half-life of crystalloids and colloids. Requirements of blood volume replacement should not be based exclusively on laboratory analysis, i.e. the haematocrit value. Furthermore, it must be remembered that large vessel haematocrit, routinely measured in clinical practice, is higher than the haematocrit in small vessels and capillaries, due to plasma skimming. Augmentation of oxygen-carrying capacity by red blood cell transfusion is a common clinical practice. However, the primary goal of hypovolaemic shock therapy should be to restore circulating volume and maintain optimum oxygen-carrying capacity with a relatively low viscosity of the blood, which can be obtained at a haematocrit of about 30% (Messmer, 1989). To optimize oxygen transport a haemoglobin level of 10–11.5 g dl^{-1} (Bryan-Brown, 1988) or a haematocrit of 30–35% (Dhainaut et al., 1990) has therefore been recommended.

Recently Dietrich and co-workers demonstrated in critically ill volume-resuscitated non-surgical patients that selective increase of global oxygen delivery (DO_2) by augmentation of red blood cell mass (increase of haemoglobin from 8.3 g dl^{-1} to 10.5 g dl^{-1} by red blood cell transfusion) and thus oxygen-carrying capacity did not improve the shock state, regardless of the aetiology of shock (Fig. 8.2) (Dietrich *et al.*, 1990). The authors concluded that, after volume and inotropic resuscitation in the critically ill anaemic patient with circulatory shock, red blood cell transfusion *per se* may fail to result in improvement in tissue oxygen metobolism. Although improvement did occur in single patients, this improvement could not be predicted on the basis of pretransfusion haemoglobin, haemodynamic status, oxygen delivery, oxygen consumption or blood lactate level.

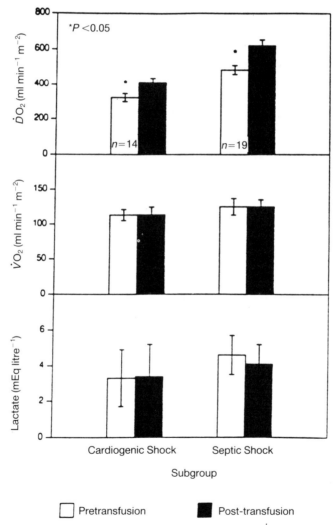

Figure 8.2   Oxygen utilization changes in oxygen delivery ($\dot{D}O_2$), oxygen consumption ($\dot{V}O_2$), and lactate after red blood cell transfusion in cardiogenic and septic shock patients. (From Dietrich *et al.*, 1990.)

Positive Inotropic and Vasoactive Drugs

The most important factor in optimizing oxygen transport is cardiac output, determined by preload, afterload, contractility and heart rate. In hypovolaemic shock, preload is primarily augmented by vigorous volume substitution. It can, however, also be increased by α-adrenoceptor agonists such as noradrenaline, adrenaline and dopamine. These agents have venoconstrictive effects. Together with the lowering of ventricular compliance this leads to increase in pulmonary capillary wedge pressure (PCWP). After haemodynamic stabilization, it is frequently possible to decrease the infusion rate of these drugs, thereby lowering the PCWP, and using additional fluid to increase the circulating volume.

A patient with a previously impaired myocardium may need inotropic support with dopamine and dobutamine. Such a support is not a substitute for adequate volume replacement but is used to enhance myocardial contraction if required. Rates of dopamine infusion should be confined to 'renal' doses (up to $5 \mu g\, kg^{-1}\, h^{-1}$) that enhance urine output. Higher doses cause vasoconstriction and tachycardia, which results in an increase in myocardial oxygen demand that may not be met adequately by myocardial blood flow. Dobutamine should then be added to improve myocardial performance. The sympathomimetic amines that are available clinically include noradrenaline, adrenaline, dopamine, isoproterenol, phenylephrine and dobutamine. The relative actions and potencies of these agents are summarized in Table 8.5 (Abboud, 1988).

Table 8.5 Relative initial haemodynamic effects of sympathomimetic amines

Amine	Heart rate	Systemic pressure	Cardiac output	Systemic resistance
Noradrenaline	↑	↑ ↑	↑ →	↑ ↑
Adrenaline	↑	↑	↑	↑ →
Dopamine	↑	↑	↑	↑ →
Isoproterenol	↑	↓ →	↑ ↑	↓
Phenylephrine	→	↑	→ ↓	↑ ↑
Dobutamine	→	→	↑	→

From Abboud (1988).
↑ = increase; ↓ = decrease; → = unchanged.

Pentoxifylline is a methylxanthine derivative which has recently been studied for its effects on microcirculatory blood flow in haemorrhagic shock. In animal models of haemorrhagic shock pentoxifylline improved tissue oxygenation and oxygen consumption post-haemorrhage, and this effect was not due to an increase in cardiac output (Waxman *et al.*, 1991). As 72-h survival rate in rats after haemorrhagic shock was found to be enhanced by pentoxifylline (Coccia *et al.*, 1989), it has been hypothetized that improvement of microcirculatory blood flow may be due to decreased polymorphonuclear leukocyte adhesiveness at the endothelium (Waxman *et al.*, 1991).

'Small-Volume Resuscitation': The New Concept for Microcirculatory Resuscitation

In 1980, Velasco and co-workers published their experimental data on resuscitation of dogs subjected to severe haemorrhagic shock, which was lethal in animals treated with isotonic saline (Velasco *et al.*, 1980). The authors demonstrated that 7.5% saline infused in a volume equivalent to only 10% of the shed blood volume rapidly increased systemic pressure, restored cardiac output, and yielded 100% long-term survival of the animals. In the same year, De Felippe *et al.* reported on 12 intensive care patients presenting with hypovolaemic shock refractory to conventional treatment (De Felippe *et al.*, 1980). These patients responded to intravenous injections of 100–400 ml of 7.5% sodium chloride – given as 50-ml portions – by a rise of arterial pressure, resumption of urine flow and recovery of consciousness, indicating reversal of the shock state. Nine of these patients could ultimately leave the hospital.

In the past years, the concept of primary resuscitation by means of hypertonic saline solution has been further elaborated and various research groups have demonstrated that, even in the presence of a 50% blood loss, a volume as small as $4\,\mathrm{ml\,kg^{-1}}$ body weight of 7.2–7.5% sodium chloride is sufficient to restore cardiac output almost instantaneously, and at the same time to significantly increase systemic pressure (Kreimeier & Messmer, 1988). During 'small-volume resuscitation' the hypertonic saline solution is applied within 2–5 min through a peripheral vein: this mode of application results in a rapid and pronounced increase of the plasma sodium concentration and thereby initiates a steep transmembraneous osmotic gradient.

The most important mechanism of action of hypertonic saline is the instantaneous mobilization of endogenous fluid along the osmotic gradient with increase of intravascular volume (Kreimeier & Messmer, 1988; Mazzoni *et al.*, 1988). In addition, direct myocardial stimulation, CNS stimulation, neurogenic reflex mechanisms, enhanced sympathetic discharge, hormone release, improvement of blood fluidity, re-establishment of spontaneous arteriolar vasomotion, and peripheral arterial vasodilatation are involved (Kreimeier & Messmer, 1988; Kreimeier *et al.*, 1992). Mazzoni *et al.* have calculated that, after a 20% blood loss, 7.5% saline solution given over 10 s in an amount equivalent to one-seventh of the actual blood loss allows re-establishment of normal blood volume within 1 min (Mazzoni *et al.*, 1988). These authors ascribe the instantaneous circulatory effect to the rapid influx of fluid, first of all from the swollen microvascular endothelium and red blood cells (Mazzoni *et al.*, 1988, 1990). Recent results from animal studies have suggested that the rapid cardiovascular response to hypertonic solutions with restoration of peripheral blood flow might in part be mediated by the release of eicosanoids (Marti-Cabrera *et al.*, 1991).

Hypertonic Saline Dextran Resuscitation

Most authors are concerned about the transience of the cardiovascular response after small-volume resuscitation using hypertonic saline. In order to preserve the intravascular volume gain, 7.2–7.5% saline solution has been combined with colloids, i.e. Dextran 60/70 or hydroxyethyl starch, to obtain a synergistic effect by increasing plasma osmolality and providing high plasma oncotic pressure. Animal studies have revealed that, compared with hypertonic sodium chloride alone, the addition of either colloid causes a sustained circulatory response and increased survival.

The concept of applying small volumes of hypertonic saline/dextran solution for primary resuscitation from severe hypovolaemia has proven effective in a prospective, randomized study of trauma patients. As compared to Ringer's lactate, the bolus infusion of 250 ml 7.5% NaCl/4.2% Dextran 70 at the site of the accident resulted in a higher systemic pressure (49 mm Hg versus 19 mm Hg) and a higher survival rate (8/10 patients versus 3/10 patients) (Holcroft *et al.*, 1987). In an extension of their first study, in 1989 Holcroft *et al.* reported on 60 trauma patients entered in a randomized, prospective double-blind trial (Holcroft *et al.*, 1989). Administration of 7.5% saline/4.2% dextran resulted in higher blood pressure when the patients reached the emergency room as compared to Ringer's lactate given in the same amount (250 ml) and followed by conventional fluid therapy. Thirty-day survival rate was significantly higher after small-volume resuscitation using hypertonic saline/dextran.

Most recently, data from the United States multicentre trial on prehospital hypertonic saline/dextran infusion for post-traumatic hypotension have been published (Mattox *et al.*, 1991). The 359 patients analysed had a mean injury severity score (ISS) of 19, and received either 250 ml of 7.5% saline in 6% Dextran 70 or Ringer's lactate, followed by conventional therapy. There was no difference in overall survival within the first 24 h, however in the subgroup of patients requiring surgery and those with penetrating injury, hypertonic saline/dextran infusion proved superior to Ringer's lactate ($P < 0.02$ and $P < 0.01$, respectively); in addition, there were fewer complications (ARDS, renal failure, coagulopathy) than in the standard treatment group. The application of hypertonic saline/dextran solutions has proven safe in patients, as Holcroft *et al.* (1989), Maningas *et al.* (1989) as well as Mattox *et al.* (1991) in the USA multicentre trial did not encounter adverse effects; in particular, no anaphylactoid reactions or dextran-related coagulo-pathies were observed.

The established effects of primary resuscitation by means of hypertonic saline either alone or in combination with dextran can be summarized on the basis of the experimental data as follow (see Table 8.6): (1) immediate increase of *systemic pressure* and *cardiac output*, while vascular resistance is reduced; (2) instantaneous increase of *nutritional blood flow* and reduction of post-ischaemic *reperfusion injury*; (3) resumption of *organ function* as seen by increase of urinary output; and (4) increased *survival rate*.

Table 8.6 Established effects of small-volume resuscitation using 7.2–7.5% saline/dextran solution

Systemic pressure	↑
Cardiac output	↑ ↑
Systemic vascular resistance	↓
Nutritional blood flow	↑ ↑
Reperfusion injury	↓
Urinary output	↑
Survival rate	(↑)

Smith and co-workers, in their studies on conscious sheep subjected to haemorrhagic shock, found an expansion of plasma volume by 8–12 ml kg^{-1} after infusion of 4 ml kg^{-1} of 2400 mOsm litre^{-1} NaCl and NaCl/6% Dextran 70, respectively (Smith *et al.*, 1985). This implicates the need for water-binding colloid molecules to conserve the fluid mobilized within the intravas-cular space, and calls for a potent colloid with high water-binding capacity. The conventional 6% Dextran 60 solution binds 20–25 ml water per 1 g dextran, i.e. 4.8–6 ml kg^{-1} body weight when applied in a dose of 4 ml kg^{-1} as with small-volume resuscitation. Therefore, we have suggested to increase the concentration of Dextran 60 to 10% and have performed our own studies with a 7.2% saline/10% Dextran 60 solution (Hyperdex; Schiwa GmbH, Glandorf, Germany). The experimental data from our group based on studies employing radioactive microspheres in protracted traumatic–haemorrhagic shock with a 50% blood loss have demonstrated that *nutri-tional blood flow* significantly increases within 5 min upon i.v. bolus infu-sion of only 4 ml kg^{-1} body weight 7.2% saline, while the peripheral shunt flow remains far below prehaemorrhage levels (Kreimeier *et al.*, 1990).

Infusion of $4\,ml\,kg^{-1}$ body weight of 10% Dextran 60 dissolved in 7.2% saline solution (hypertonic–hyperoncotic solution) in our experiments completely restored nutritional blood flow in kidney, gastric mucosa, small intestine, colon and pancreas. Despite similar changes of the central haemodynamic parameters (systemic pressure, cardiac output), blood flow to these organs remained significantly lower after hypertonic saline resuscitation without dextran (Kreimeier et al., 1990). The addition of hyperoncotic (10%) Dextran 60 therefore not only prolongs, but also significantly enhances the microcirculatory effect of 7.2% saline alone.

Summary and Conclusions

Hypovolaemic shock is a clinical state defined as depletion of intravascular volume by which tissue perfusion is rendered inadequate with respect to delivery of oxygen and substrates to the cells. It is the most common type of shock in emergency medicine as well as in major surgery. The prognosis of patients is significantly affected by the severity and the duration of shock and consecutive secondary organ dysfunction, and therefore by the speed of recognition and appropriateness of medical intervention. Management of the patient in hypovolaemic shock requires accurate and sequential measurements of haemodynamic and respiratory as well as of biochemical parameters. The objective of the management is to provide oxygen delivery adequate to tissue oxygen needs. Therapy of hypovolaemic shock must therefore include control of haemorrhage, replacement of blood or fluid losses, and correction of acid–base or electrolyte disturbances.

Fluid administration is the essential early therapy for hypovolaemic shock. Sympathicomimetic drugs are seldom needed, but may serve as transient means to ensure sufficient cardiac output. The novel concept of small-volume resuscitation using peripheral bolus infusion of hypertonic solutions has been validated in various experimental models of severe hypovolaemia and shock, and is now being investigated in clinical trials at various centres. It is attractive with regard to the small infusion volume needed to elicit an instantaneous cardiovascular effect, even in states of severe and protracted hypovolaemia, without the risk of fluid overload. By the simultaneous application of a colloid the circulatory effect is prolonged and, in the case of 10% Dextran 60, enhanced with regard to prompt normalization of tissue blood flow. Even though the optimal composition of a hypertonic–hyperoncotic solution has not yet been identified, data from our experiments have demonstrated the efficacy of 7.2% saline/10% Dextran 60 solution with regard to the instantaneous restoration of central haemodynamics and normalization of compromised microcirculation.

Besides the rapid restoration of macrohaemodynamics and prevention of early deaths, small-volume resuscitation particularly aims at the prevention of late complications, such as sepsis and MSOF, on the basis of persisting microcirculatory disturbances. The novelty of hypertonic saline/dextran resuscitation lies in its operational mechanisms at the microcirculatory level; these include the mobilization of fluid preferentially from oedematous endothelium, the reduction of post-ischaemic leukocyte adherence to the endothelium of postcapillary venules, and the restoration of spontaneous arteriolar vasomotion. Re-opening of shock-narrowed capillaries and restoration of nutritional blood flow is thus efficiently promoted.

References

Abboud FM (1988) Shock. in Wyngaarden JB & Smith LH, Jr (eds), *Cecil Textbook of Medicine* (18th edition), pp. 236–50. Philadelphia: W.B. Saunders.

Allgöwer M & Burri C (1967) Schockindex. *Dtsch. Med. Wschr.* **92:** 1947–50.

Appelgren L (1972) Perfusion and diffusion in shock. *Acta Physiol. Scand.* **Suppl. 378:** 1–72.

Arieff AI (1991) Indications for use of bicarbonate in patients with metabolic acidosis. *Br. J. Anaesth.* **67:** 165–77.

Baker CC (1986) Epidemiology of trauma: the civilian perspective. *Ann. Emerg. Med.* **15:** 1389–90.

Baker CC, Oppenheimer L, Stephens B et al. (1980) Epidemiology of trauma deaths. *Am. J. Surg.* **140:** 144–50.

Baker JW, Deitch EA, Li M et al. (1988) Hemorrhagic shock induces bacterial translocation from the gut. *J. Trauma* **28:** 896–906.

Baskett PJF (1990) Management of hypovolaemic shock. *Br. Med. J.* **300:** 1453–7.

Bihari DJ (1989) Multiple organ failure: role of tissue hypoxia. In Bihari DJ & Cerra FB (eds), *Multiple Organ Failure*, pp. 25–36. Fullerton, CA: Society of Critical Care Medicine.

Billiar TR, Maddaus MA, West MA et al. (1988) Intestinal gram-negative bacterial overgrowth in vivo augments the in vitro response of Kupffer cells to endotoxin. *Ann. Surg.* **208:** 532–40.

Bone RC, Fisher CJ, Clemmer TP et al. (1989) Sepsis syndrome: a valid clinical entity. *Crit. Care Med.* **17:** 389–93.

Border JR, Hassett J, LaDuca J et al. (1987) The gut origin septic states in blunt multiple trauma (ISS = 40) in the ICU. *Ann. Surg.* **206:** 427–48.

Bryan-Brown CW (1988) Blood flow to organs: parameters for function and survival in critical illness. *Crit. Care Med.* **16:** 170–8.

Carmona R, Catalano R & Trunkey DD (1984) Septic shock. In Shires GT (ed.), *Shock and Related Problems*, pp. 156–77. Edinburgh: Churchill Livingstone.

Carrico CJ, Meakins JL, Marshall JC et al. (1986) Multiple-organ-failure syndrome. *Arch. Surg.* **121:** 196–208.

Chaudry IH, Ayala A, Ertel W & Stephan RN (1990) Hemorrhage and resuscitation: immunological aspects (editorial review). *Am. J. Physiol.* **259:** R663–78.

Coccia MT, Waxman K, 'Soliman MH *et al.* (1989) Pentoxifylline improves survival following hemorrhagic shock. *Crit. Care Med.* **17:** 36–8.

Cooper DJ, Walley KR, Wiggs BR & Russell JA (1990) Bicarbonate does not improve hemodynamics in critically ill patients who have lactic acidosis: a prospective controlled clinical study. *Ann. Intern. Med.* **112:** 492–8.

Cottier H & Kraft R (1991) Gut-derived infectious-toxic shock (GITS). A major variant of septic shock. *Current Studies in Hematology and Blood Transfusion,* Vol. 59. Basel: Karger pp. 1–352.

De Felippe J, Jr., Timoner J, Velasco IT & Lopes OU (1980) Treatment of refractory hypovolaemic shock by 7.5% sodium chloride injections. *Lancet* **ii:** 1002–4.

Deitch EA, Bridges W, Ma L *et al.* (1990) Hemorrhagic shock-induced bacterial translocation: the role of neutrophils and hydroxyl radicals. *J. Trauma* **30:** 942–52.

Dhainaut JF, Edwards JD, Grootendorst AF *et al.* (1990) Practical aspects of oxygen transport: conclusions and recommendations of the round-table conference. *Intensive Care Med.* **16(Suppl.2):** S179–80.

Dietrich KA, Conrad SA, Hebert CA *et al.* (1990) Cardiovascular and metabolic response to red blood cell transfusion in critically ill volume-resuscitated nonsurgical patients. *Crit. Care Med.* **18:** 940–4.

Fong Y, Moldawer LL, Shires GT & Lowry SF (1990) The biologic characteristics of cytokines and their implication in surgical injury. *Surg. Gynecol. Obstet.* **170:** 363–78.

Granger DN, Rutili G & McCord JM (1981) Superoxide radicals in feline intestinal ischemia. *Gastroenterology* **81:** 22–9.

Guyton AC (1991) Circulatory shock and physiology of its treatment. In Guyton AC (ed.), *Textbook of Medical Physiology* (8th edition), pp. 263–71. Philadelphia: W.B. Saunders.

Hack CE & Thijs LG (1991) The orchestra of mediators in the pathogenesis of septic shock. In Vincent JL (ed.), *Update in Intensive Care and Emergency Medicine,* Vol. 14, Update 1991, pp. 233–41. Berlin: Springer-Verlag.

Hardaway RM (1982) Pulmonary artery pressure vs. pulmonary capillary wedge pressure and central venous pressure in shock. *Resuscitation* **10:** 47–56.

Holcroft JW, Vassar MJ, Turner JE *et al.* (1987) 3% NaCl and 7.5% NaCl/Dextran 70 in the resuscitation of severely injured patients. *Ann. Surg.* **206:** 279–86.

Holcroft JW, Vassar MJ, Perry CA *et al.* (1989) Perspectives on clinical trials for hypertonic saline/dextran solutions for the treatment of traumatic shock. *Brazilian J. Med. Biol. Res.* **22:** 291–3.

Kaweski SM, Sise MJ & Virgilio RW (1990) The effect of prehospital fluids on survival in trauma patients. *J. Trauma* **30:** 1215–19.

Kreimeier U & Messmer K (1987) New perspectives in resuscitation and prevention of multiple organ system failure. In Baethmann A & Messmer K (eds), *Surgical Research: Recent Concepts and Results,* pp. 39–50. Berlin: Springer-Verlag.

Kreimeier U & Messmer K (1988) Small-volume resuscitation. In Kox WJ & Gamble J (eds), *Fluid Resuscitation. Baillière's Clinical Anaesthesiology*, Vol. 2, pp. 545–77. London: Baillière Tindall.

Kreimeier U, Brückner UB, Niemczyk S & Messmer K (1990) Hyperosmotic saline dextran for resuscitation from traumatic–hemorrhagic hypotension: effect on regional blood flow. *Circ. Shock* **32;** 83–99.

Kreimeier U, Frey L, Pacheco A & Messmer K (1993) Hypertonic volume therapy: a feasible regimen to contribute to the prevention of multiple organ failure? In Faist E, Meakins JL and Schildberg FW (eds), *Host Defense Dysfunction in Trauma, Shock and Sepsis. Mechanisms and Therapeutic Approaches*, pp. 831–841. Berlin: Springer-Verlag.

Kvietys PR & Granger DN (1989) Hypoxia: its role in ischemic injury to the intestinal mucosa. In Marston A, Bulkley GB, Fiddian-Green RG & Haglund UH (eds), *Splanchnic Ischemia and Multiple Organ Failure*, pp. 127–34. London: E. Arnold.

LaMuraglia G & Kennedy S (1989) Shock. In Wilkins EW, Dineen JJ, Gross PL, McCabe CJ, Moncure AC & O'Malley PJ (eds), *Emergency Medicine. Scientific Foundations and Current Practice* (3rd edition), pp. 25–41. Baltimore: Williams & Wilkins.

McCabe CJ (1990) Trauma: An annotated bibliography of the recent literature. *Am. J. Emerg. Med.* **8:** 446–63.

Maningas PA, Mattox KL, Pepe PE et al. (1989) Hypertonic saline–dextran solutions for the prehospital management of traumatic hypotension. *Am. J. Surg.* **157:** 528–34.

Marti-Cabrera M, Ortiz JL, Durá JM et al. (1991) Hemodynamic effects of hyperosmotic mannitol infusion in anesthetized open-chest dogs: modification by cyclooxygenase inhibition. *Res. Surg.* **3:** 29–33.

Mattox KL, Maningas PA, Moore EE et al. (1991) Prehospital hypertonic saline/dextran infusion for post-traumatic hypotension – the U.S.A. multicenter trial. *Ann. Surg.* **213:** 482–91.

Mazzoni MC, Borgstroem P, Arfors KE & Intaglietta M (1988) Dynamic fluid redistribution in hyperosmotic resuscitation of hypovolemic hemorrhage. *Am. J. Physiol.* **255:** H629–37.

Mazzoni MC, Borgström P, Intaglietta M & Arfors KE (1990) Capillary narrowing in hemorrhagic shock is rectified by hyperosmotic saline-dextran reinfusion. *Circ. Shock* **31;** 407–18.

Messmer KFW (1987) The use of plasma substitutes with special attention to their side effects. *World J. Surg.* **11:** 69–74.

Messmer K (1989) Acute preoperative hemodilution: physiological basis and clinical application. In Tuma RF, White JV & Messmer K (eds), *The Role of Hemodilution in Optimal Patient Care*, pp. 54–74. München: W. Zuckschwerdt Verlag.

Messmer KFW (1990) Mechanisms of traumatic shock and their consequences. In Border JR, Allgöwer M, Hansen ST, Jr. & Rüedi TP (eds), *Blunt Multiple Trauma – Comprehensive Pathophysiology and Care*, pp. 39–49. New York: Marcel Dekker.

Messmer K & Kreimeier U (1989) Microcirculatory therapy in shock. *Resuscitation* **18:** S51–S61.

Messmer K, Kreimeier U & Hammersen F (1988) Multiple organ failure: clinical implications to macro- and microcirculation. In Manabe H, Zweifach BW & Messmer K (eds), *Microcirculation in Circulatory Disorders*, pp. 147–57. Berlin: Springer-Verlag.

Michie HR, Manogue KR, Spriggs DR *et al.* (1988) Detection of circulating tumor necrosis factor after endotoxin administration. *New Engl. J. Med.* **318:** 1481–6.

Modig J (1986) Effectiveness of Dextran 70 versus Ringer's acetate in traumatic shock and adult respiratory distress syndrome. *Crit. Care Med.* **14:** 454–7.

Natanson C, Eichenholz P, Danner R *et al.* (1989) Endotoxin and tumor necrosis factor challenges in dogs simulate the cardiovascular profile of human septic shock. *J. Exp. Med.* **169:** 823–32.

Prough DS (1991) Developing concepts of fluid resuscitation. *Curr. Opinion Anaesth.* **4:** 212–17.

Shoemaker WC & Kram HB (1988) Crystalloid and colloid fluid therapy in resuscitation and subsequent ICU management. In Kox WJ & Gamble J (eds), *Fluid Resuscitation*, pp. 509–44. London: Baillière Tindall.

Smith GJ, Kramer GC, Perron P *et al.* (1985) A comparison of several hypertonic solutions for resuscitation of bled sheep. *J. Surg. Res.* **39:** 517–28.

Thijs LG & Groeneveld ABJ (1987) The circulatory defect of septic shock. In Vincent JL & Thijs LG (eds), *Septic Shock. Update in Intensive Care and Emergency Medicine*, Vol. 6, pp. 161–78. Berlin: Springer-Verlag.

Trunkey DD (1983) Trauma. *Sci. Am.* **249:** 20–7.

Trunkey D (1991) Initial treatment of patients with extensive trauma. *New Engl. J. Med.* **324:** 1259–63.

Trunkey DD, Catalano R & Carmona RH (1988) Hypovolemic and traumatic shock. In Hardaway RM (ed.), *Shock: the Reversible Stage of Dying*, pp. 158–77. Littleton, MA: PSG Publishing Company.

Velasco IT, Pontieri V, Rocha e Silva M, Jr. & Lopes OU (1980) Hyperosmotic NaCl and severe hemorrhagic shock. *Am. J. Physiol.* **239:** 664–73.

Vincent JL (1991) Expert panel: the use of the pulmonary artery catheter. *Intensive Care Med.* **17:** I–VIII.

Wang P, Hauptman JG & Chaudry IH (1990) Hemorrhage produces depression in microvascular blood flow which persists despite fluid resuscitation. *Circ. Shock* **32:** 307–18.

Waxman K, Clark L, Soliman MH & Parazin S (1991) Pentoxifylline in resuscitation of experimental hemorrhagic shock. *Crit. Care Med.* **19:** 728–31.

9 Therapy: Effects of Fluid Resuscitation

Marilyn T. Haupt

Introduction

Fluid loading is widely recognized to be an effective and safe intervention in the treatment of critically ill patients with signs of decreased blood volume and circulatory failure. During the past century, the ability of fluids to reverse hypotension and oliguria, increase cardiac output and increase survival has been repeatedly documented in laboratory and clinical studies of shock. In addition, these goals are usually accomplished by fluids without adverse effects on heart rate, metabolic demands and distribution of perfusion attributed to inotropic and vasopressor drugs which are also used to treat circulatory shock. Because of these favourable effects, fluid loading with asanguinous colloidal and crystalloidal solutions, and blood and blood products has been recommended as initial therapy for numerous and diverse conditions associated with hypovolaemia including sepsis, burns, trauma, haemorrhage, drug overdose, and many others (Thompson, 1975; Weil & Nishijima, 1978; Falk *et al.*, 1989; Carcillo *et al.*, 1991).

Blood transfusion may be considered a special type of fluid loading since blood carries significantly more oxygen than asanguinous fluids. Blood transfusion, often with supplemental colloidal or crystalloidal fluids, is frequently employed in patients with severe haemorrhage or patients undergoing surgical procedures associated with significant blood loss (Skillman *et al.*, 1975; Virgilio *et al.*, 1979). In addition, blood may be given to patients who may not be actively bleeding but who are anaemic and have critical reductions in haemoglobin levels.

In recent years, clinical and laboratory studies of fluid resuscitation have been influenced by an emerging understanding of critical illness and circulatory shock at the microvascular, cellular and subcellar level. Because of the established importance of oxygen in the energy metabolism of the cell, a variety of clinical investigations of critically ill patients have examined the effects of fluid loading on the systemic and regional utilization of oxygen.

The importance of defining the effects of therapeutic interventions on oxygen utilization has been highlighted by several recent prospective investigations of high-risk surgical patients, patients with cardiogenic shock, and septic patients. In these studies, patients who were treated with therapeutic interventions designed to achieve the goal of supranormal systemic oxygen delivery and/or consumption exhibited significantly improved survival when compared to controls who were treated conventionally (Shoemaker *et al.*, 1988; Tuchschmidt *et al.*, 1991). Indirect support for therapeutically optimizing oxygen utilization has been provided by several prospective (Hankeln *et al.*, 1987; Edwards *et al.*, 1989; Creamer *et al.*, 1990) and retrospective studies (Tuchschmidt *et al.*, 1989; Russell *et al.*, 1990; Kruse *et al.*, 1990; Bakker *et al.*, 1991) which demonstrated improved outcome in patients meeting criteria for optimal oxygen utilization. The contribution of fluid therapy to oxygen utilization thus warrants critical analysis because of its widespread use as an intervention, frequently the first intervention, to correct haemodynamic abnormalities, and systemic and regional hypoperfusion in critically ill patients.

Effects of Fluids on Systemic Oxygen Delivery

Systemic oxygen delivery or transport ($\dot{D}O_2$) is defined as the product of the cardiac output or systemic blood flow (cardiac output) and the arterial oxygen content (CaO_2). Both may be significantly influenced by fluid loading. CaO_2 includes oxygen bound to haemoglobin plus oxygen dissolved in plasma. Because CaO_2 is a function of blood haemoglobin levels (Hb), arterial haemoglobin oxygen saturation (SaO_2), and arterial oxygen pressure (PaO_2), $\dot{D}O_2$ is defined by the following equation: $\dot{D}O_2 =$ cardiac output $\times CaO_2 =$ cardiac output $\times [(1.36 \times SaO_2 \times Hb + 0.003 \times PaO_2)]$ where 1.36 is the oxygen-carrying capacity of haemoglobin (ml $O_2 \, g^{-1}$), and 0.003 is the solubility of oxygen in blood (ml $O_2 \, dl^{-1} \, mm \, Hg$). In this equation, cardiac output is expressed in litres per minute, SaO_2 as a fraction, Hb in grammes per decilitre, and PaO_2 in millimetres of mercury. $\dot{D}O_2$ may be divided by body surface area (BSA) or body weight to account for differences in size. The intravenous infusion of clinically available colloidal and crystalloidal fluids, blood, and blood products may influence one or more components of this equation. In order to predict changes in $\dot{D}O_2$ after fluid infusion, it is useful to understand the effects of fluid infusion on each component of the $\dot{D}O_2$ equation.

Cardiac Output

The main determinants of cardiac output are preload, afterload, contractility and heart rate (HR). Fluid loading with asanguinous fluids or blood increases cardiac output primarily by increasing venous return and preload. Right and left ventricular end-diastolic volumes and stroke volume are therefore augmented by fluids. (Braunwald & Ross, 1964). Because fluid loading increases LV end-diastolic volume, the Frank–Starling curve is useful in describing the effects of this intervention on cardiac output (Fig. 9.1). Accordingly, this relationship predicts that as ventricular end-diastolic volume increases from low values, stroke volume and thus cardiac output will increase until plateau levels are reached.

With continued increases in ventricular end-diastolic volume, a decrease in cardiac output may be observed (Fig. 9.1, descending limb). The mechanism for the descending limb is unclear, however. Laboratory studies suggest that the decline in cardiac output with continued increases in ventricular end-diastolic volume is not due to overstretched sarcomeres leading to reduced tension development from decreased overlap of actin and myosin filaments. Rather, it is thought from the results of clinical and laboratory studies that an 'apparent descending limb' may be a response to volume induced increases in aortic pressure and afterload in the absence of adequate preload reserve. (Monroe *et al.*, 1971; MacGregor *et al.*, 1974; Braunwald *et al.*, 1984).

Clinical studies also validate the Frank–Starling mechanism in patients when left ventricular preload, usually estimated by the pulmonary artery wedge pressure (PAWP), is increased by fluid loading. Although the PAWP may not accurately reflect preload in conditions associated with dynamic changes in cardiac compliance (Calvin *et al.*, 1986), an increase in both PAWP and cardiac output is a predictable response to fluid loading in most clinical studies of fluid resuscitation in circulatory shock. In a large clinical study of colloid and crystalloid fluid resuscitation reported by Rackow, for example, large volumes of fluid given as initial therapy in circulatory shock were associated with 40–50% increases in cardiac output (Rackow *et al.*, 1983). Severe additional studies have described plateau cardiac output values with continued fluid loading in critically ill patients (Calvin *et al.*, 1981b; Packman & Rackow, 1983). In the study reported by Packman, for example, plateau values for cardiac output were attained in

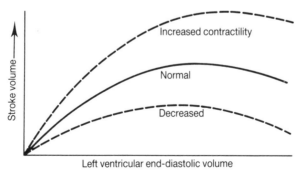

Figure 9.1   The Frank–Starling curve illustrates the relationship between left ventricular end-diastolic volume (preload) and stroke volume. The position and shape of the curve is influenced by changes in cardiac contractility. Fluid loading increases end-diastolic volume and stroke volume according to this relationship.

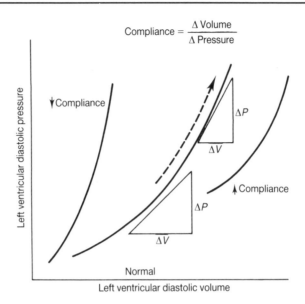

$$\text{Compliance} = \frac{\Delta \text{ Volume}}{\Delta \text{ Pressure}}$$

Figure 9.2 The compliance characteristics of the left ventricle, when applied to fluid loading, predicts that continued loading will result in precipitous increases in pressure, a signal that the limits of myocardial stretch have been reached. A similar relationship applies to the right ventricle.

patients with septic and hypovolaemic shock as fluid increased the PAWP beyond 15 mm Hg (Packman & Rackow, 1983). The PAWP associated with optimal cardiac output is higher for patients with cardiac failure. Because of the reduced cardiac compliance in these patients, higher LV end-diastolic pressures are required to achieve end-diastolic volumes comparable to those in patients with normal cardiac compliance (Fig. 9.2). For patients with cardiogenic shock with associated hypovolaemia, cautious fluid administration to PAWPs of approximately 20 mm Hg have been recommended to achieve optimal cardiac outputs (Rackley *et al.*, 1975; Rackow *et al.*, 1987). A descending limb in the cardiac function curve has been described in several clinical studies. Fifty per cent of patients with sepsis, for example, exhibited downslopes in their cardiac function curves in a study reported by Weisel (1977). Crexells (1973) reported cardiac function curve downslopes in 22% of patients with acute myocardial infarctions.

Because the shape and position of the Frank–Starling curve is dependent on left ventricular contractility, compliance and afterload, it may be difficult to predict when cardiac output is optimal or at plateau levels during a fluid challenge without direct sequential measurements. The list of conditions and drugs which alter these haemodynamic characteristics is exhaustive and includes myocardial and pericardial disease, vasoactive and inotropic medications, and positive pressure mechanical ventilation. Although 'optimal

PAWPs' have been defined using pooled values from subsets of patients with critical illness, these values may not be optimal for an individual patient. Frequent measurements of cardiac output during fluid loading may thus be necessary to determine optimal cardiac outputs for individual patients. Because it may be difficult to obtain frequent determinations of cardiac output in some clinical settings, fluid challenge techniques may be used to estimate when cardiac output is optimal. These techniques employ the principle that a decrease in cardiac compliance reflected in a precipitous increase in PAWP or CVP during fluid loading signals that the limit of stretch of the myocardium has been reached and thus signals optimal cardiac filling. Precipitous increases in PAWP or CVP therefore caution the clinician to stop the fluid challenge and observe the patients for signs of clinical improvement (Weil & Shubin, 1969; Rackley *et al.*, 1975; Starchuck *et al.*, 1975; Weil & Henning, 1979). A technique described by Weil & Henning to optimally guide fluid therapy is described in Tables 9.1 and 9.2.

Table 9.1 Guidelines for fluid challenge utilizing central venous pressure (CVP) monitoring

Fluid challenge: CVP cm H_2O (5–2 rule)		
Observe CVP for 10 min	< 8 cm H_2O	200 ml × 10 min
	< 14 cm H_2O	100 ml × 10 min
	≥ 14 cm H_2O	50 ml × 10 min
During infusion 0–9 min	> 5 cm	STOP
Following infusion	> 2 cm < 5 cm	Wait 10 min
	> 5 cm	Wait STOP
	≤ 3 cm	Continue infusion

Adapted from Weil and Henning (1979).

Table 9.2 Guidelines for fluid challenge utilizing pulmonary artery diastolic or pulmonary artery wedge pressure monitoring

Fluid challenge: PAWP, PADP mm Hg (7–3 rule)		
Observe PADP/PAWP for 10 min	< 12 mm Hg	200 ml × 10 min
	< 16 cm Hg	100 ml × 10 min
	≥ 16 mm Hg	50 ml × 10 min
During infusion 0–9 min	> 7 mm Hg	STOP
Immediately following 10 min infusion	> 3 < 7 mm Hg	Wait 10 min
	> 7 mm Hg	Wait STOP
	≤ 3 mm Hg	Continue infusion

PAWP, pulmonary artery wedge pressure; PADP, pulmonary artery diastolic pressure.
Adapted from Weil and Henning (1979).

One would expect blood transfusions, like asanguinous fluids, to also increase venous return, ventricular end-diastolic volumes, and cardiac output according to the Frank–Starling relationship. Although an increase in cardiac output has been documented with the rapid infusion of blood for volume expansion (Czer & Shoemaker, 1980), significant increases in cardiac output after blood transfusion have not been observed in critically ill patients in several recent studies (Dennis *et al.*, 1978; Rice *et al.*, 1978; Gilbert *et al.*, 1986; Conrad *et al.*, 1990; Dietrich *et al.*, 1990; Mink & Pollack, 1990; Lucking *et al.*, 1990; Ronco *et al.*, 1991). Several factors may account for these negative results: (1) Blood is typically administered to critically ill patients after fluid resuscitation and stabilization with asanguinous fluids. At this period, cardiac preload and output may already be at optimal levels. In studies in which the pretransfusion PAWP was documented, values of 12 mm Hg or greater were recorded. These PAWP values correspond to those associated with optimal cardiac outputs in studies of critically ill patients (Packman & Rackow, 1983). (2) Blood is usually administered more slowly than asanguinous fluids, especially in patients who are not actively bleeding. The slow administration of blood may permit a compensatory return of the cardiac output to baseline levels. These changes may include decreases in vascular tone and heart rate, and increase in urine output. (3) Blood transfusion, especially with packed red cells, increases blood viscosity, a change which may prevent increases in cardiac output by increasing afterload (Guyton & Richardson, 1961; Murray *et al.*, 1969).

It is important to note, however, that equivalent volumes of clinically available asanguinous fluids and blood expand intravascular volume, augment LV end-diastolic volume, and increase cardiac output to different extents. In general, packed red cells and whole blood expand intravascular volume to a greater extent than equivalent volumes of clinically available colloidal and crystalloidal fluids. Colloidal fluids are better intravascular volume expanders than crystalloidal fluids. In a study of fluid resuscitation of critically ill patients reported by Rackow, 1.5 to 4 times as much crystalloid (normal saline) was required to achieve comparable volume expansion to colloids (5% albumin or 6% hydroxyethylstarch (Rackow *et al.*, 1983). Even more crystalloids compared to colloids may be needed to achieve comparable volume expansion in conditions associated with severe increases in microvascular permeability. In a laboratory study of intravenous rattlesnake venom shock, for example, six times as much crystalloid was required to achieve volume expansion similar to colloids (Haupt *et al.*, 1984). A summary of the intravascular volume-expanding effects of clinically available fluids is provided in Table 9.3 (Lamke & Liijedahl, 1976; Carlson *et al.*, 1990). The volumes used in this table have been estimated in patients without significant permeability problems. In general, when permeability is increased, greater volumes of both colloids or crystalloids are required since both fluid and colloidal particles escape into the interstitium. Haemodynamic monitoring to assess cardiac output and PAWP is especially

Table 9.3   Representative effects (ml) of the intravenous infusion of 1 litre of fluids on body compartments of normal subjects

Fluid	Intracellular volume	Extracellular volume	Interstitial volume	Plasma volume
0.9% NaCl	−100	1100	825	275
5% Dextrose in water	660	340	255	85
5% NaCl	−2950	3950	2690	990
5% Albumin	0	1000	≥500	≥500
Whole blood	0	1000	0	1000

Adapted from Lamke and Liljedahl (1976) and Carlson *et al.* (1990).
   In patients with increases in vascular permeability, the plasma volume-expanding properties of all fluids is decreased.

important in patients with increased vascular permeability since it is difficult to predict the extent to which fluids will remain in the vascular space.

Crystalloid fluid loading may expand intravascular volume and increase cardiac output more transiently than colloidal fluids. This was first demonstrated by André Cournand in patients with cardiogenic shock utilizing the cardiac catheterization techniques that he developed (Cournand *et al.*, 1944). A more recent study has also confirmed the transient effects of crystalloids when compared to colloids in patients after cardiac surgery (Ley *et al.*, 1990). Similar findings came from a large prospective study of hypotensive emergency patients (Shoemaker *et al.*, 1981) where resuscitation times were significantly longer in the patients treated with cystalloids.

Haemoglobin

Blood haemoglobin levels as well as haematocrit are predictably decreased by fluid loading with asanguinous fluids. This effect of asanguinous fluids contrasts with the reliable increases in haemoglobin and haematocrit associated with the transfusion of packed red cells and whole blood. The degree of haemodilution caused by an asanguinous resuscitative fluid will depend on the extent to which the fluid increases intravascular volume. Table 9.3 provides estimates of the plasma volume-expanding effects for the most commonly used asanguinous fluids in patients without permeability disorders. In general, because of the oncotic effects of colloids, these fluids produce more haemodilution from plasma volume expansion when compared to equivalent volumes of crystalloidal fluids. The ability of colloids to produce more haemodilution than crystalloids also applies to conditions associated with increased permeability, in spite of the predicted loss of colloid into the interstitium (Hauser *et al.*, 1980; Appel & Shoemaker, 1981).

The haemodilution associated with asanguinous fluid loading will decrease $\dot{D}O_2$ when the decrease in haemoglobin outweighs the increase in cardiac output in the oxygen delivery equation. Thus decreases in $\dot{D}O_2$

predictably occur when the effects of fluids produce minimal or no increases in cardiac output. In one study of sepsis, initial resuscitation with colloidal fluids produced a decrease in $\dot{D}O_2$ in 30% of patients in spite of increases in arterial pressure and cardiac output (Haupt *et al.*, 1985).

Arterial Oxygen Saturation of Haemoglobin and Arterial Oxygen Pressure

The effect of fluid therapy on arterial haemoglobin oxygen saturation (SaO_2) and arterial oxygen pressure (PaO_2) may be due to effects on the gas exchanging properties of the lung, changes in cardiac output, and changes in P_{50}. The balance of these changes may also influence $\dot{D}O_2$.

The effects of fluid loading on the gas exchanging properties of the lung may be predicted from knowledge of the effects of both colloids and crystalloids on the relationship between microvascular (capillary) and perimicrovascular (interstitium) hydrostatic and oncotic forces. When applied to the lung, the balance of these forces, initially described by Earnest Starling (1896, 1898), influences the accumulation of interstitial oedema. In turn, the accumulation of oedema in the pulmonary interstitium will impair the diffusion of oxygen from the airways to the microvasculature. This relationship, which was subsequently modified to account for changes in microvascular permeability (Pappenheimer & Soto Rivera, 1948; Staverman, 1951; Kedem & Katchalsky, 1958) is expressed in terms of the following formula:

$$\dot{Q}c = K_f [(Pmv - Ppmv) - \sigma (\pi mv - \pi pmv)]$$

where $\dot{Q}c$ = volume flow across the capillary wall, K_f = the filtration coefficient representing volume flow per unit time per unit pressure per 100 g tissue; Pmv, $Ppmv$ = hydrostatic pressure of the microvascular and perimicrovascular spaces, πmv, πpmv = colloid osmotic pressure of the microvascular and perimicrovascular space; σ = the osmotic reflection coefficient, a value that reflects the degree of permeability of the membrane to plasma proteins relative to water. A positive value for $\dot{Q}c$ represents the movements of fluid from the capillary to the interstitium.

The modified Starling equation has been used to predict changes in pulmonary interstitial oedema during fluid challenges in critically ill patients with and without permeability disorders. The Starling equation, for example, predicts that volume resuscitation with clinically available colloidal and crystalloidal fluids will increase $\dot{Q}c$ through increases in Pmv. In addition, it is also predicted that crystalloidal fluids, which have no oncotically active particles, will also increase $\dot{Q}c$ as πmv is decreased through the dilution of oncotically active plasma proteins (Haupt & Rackow, 1982). Clinically available colloidal fluids, diluted in normal saline, have oncotic pressures that are close to normal values in healthy adults (e.g. 25 mm Hg for 5% albumin and 30 mm Hg for 6% hydroxyethylstarch) (Haupt &

Rackow, 1982). Because critically ill patients tend to have reduced plasma colloid osmotic pressures (COP) from poor nutrition, reduced albumin synthetic capacity of the liver and hypercatabolism (Rackow *et al.*, 1977; Weil *et al.*, 1981), colloids tend to increase πmv as assessed by measurements of COP (Haupt & Rackow, 1982). This change may favourably influence pulmonary oedema accumulation. However, the theoretical benefit of colloids in promoting intravascular fluid retention is diminished when microvascular permeability is increased. As predicted by the Starling equation, the osmotic reflection coefficient, σ, approaches zero in these conditions and hydrostatic pressures becomes the main determinant of $\dot{Q}$c.

In spite of evidence to suggest that the Starling equation represents an oversimplification (Altschule, 1986), clinical studies support the predictive value of the modified equation in determining transcapillary fluid flux (Falk *et al.*, 1989; Haupt, 1989; Haupt *et al.*, 1993). For example, increases in PAWP, an estimate of Pmv, from fluid loading positively correlates with pulmonary oedema formation (Sibbald *et al.*, 1981, 1985). The combination of the PAWP and plasma COP also appears to predict pulmonary oedema better than either value alone (Rackow *et al.*, 1977). Several studies of criticallly ill patients, which used physiologic end-points such as an optimal PAWP as a guide to fluid resuscitation, have demonstrated a deterioration in pulmonary function reflected in an increase in radiographically determined lung water accumulation or increased intrapulmonary shunt fraction ($\dot{Q}$s/$\dot{Q}$T) associated with crystalloid resuscitation. These pulmonary changes were not observed in patients similarly resuscitated with colloidal fluids (Rackow *et al.*, 1983; Metildi *et al.*, 1984). An increase in $\dot{Q}$c from crystalloid was implied by the results of a study reported by Metildi. This study revealed a crystalloid-associated increase in $\dot{Q}$s/$\dot{Q}$T in patients with ARDS, a condition associated with increased permeability of the pulmonary microcirculation (Metildi *et al.*, 1984). Failure to observe an increase in $\dot{Q}$s/$\dot{Q}$T in colloid-resuscitated ARDS patients suggests that the pulmonary microvasculature in ARDS was, at least to some extent, a barrier to colloidal particles. Although crystalloidal fluids increase $\dot{Q}$s/$\dot{Q}$T and radiographic oedema in these clinical studies, their effect on PaO_2 and SaO_2, factors contributing to the determination of $\dot{D}O_2$, nevertheless appears to be minimal. Both studies reported by Metildi and Rackow failed to show statistically significant decreases in PaO_2 and SaO_2 after crystalloidal fluid loading, although a downward trend in PaO_2 was observed in Rackow's study (Rackow *et al.*, 1983; Metildi *et al.*, 1984).

Failure to observe major declines in PaO_2 and SaO_2 after fluid loading may, in part, be due to the effects of increased cardiac output to increase SaO_2 in the presence of a fixed intrapulmonary shunt and in the absence of increases in oxygen demand or oxygen debt. The effects of cardiac ouput on CaO_2 may be especially significant in patients with pulmonary disease who have increased intrapulmonary shunting and has been observed in several studies of fluid loading (Gilbert *et al.*, 1986; Haupt *et al.*, 1985). In addition, compensatory mechanisms in the lung may also minimize the effects of a fluid induced increase in $\dot{Q}c$ on the gas exchanging properties of the lung. These mechanisms include a compensatory decrease in πpmv, increase in πmv, and increase in Ppmv as fluid or plasma filtrate moves into the normally non-compliant interstitial space (Guyton, 1986). Compensatory mechanisms not predicted by the modified Starling equation may also be operative. These include the removal of interstitial fluid and protein by actively contracting lymphatic vessels as well as by smaller passive lymphatics with unidirectional valves (Smith, 1948; Guyton & Coleman, 1968; Staub, 1974).

Changes in P_{50} are associated with changes in the relationship between SaO_2 and PaO_2 and may thus affect CaO_2 and $\dot{D}O_2$. Large volumes of crystalloidal fluid loading, for example, may influence P_{50} through changes produced in acid–base status. Large volumes of infused normal saline are associated with the production of a hyperchloraemic metabolic acidosis, a change which may increase P_{50} and decrease SaO_2 in the pulmonary capillary. Opposite effects on P_{50} may be observed after volume loading with Ringer's lactate. Clinical studies that describe changes in P_{50} associated with fluid loading are rare, however. Changes in both *in vivo* and *in vivo* P_{50} could not be demonstrated in a study of fluid loading with the colloids 5% albumin and 6% hydroxyethylstarch (both in normal saline). Transfusions employing modern blood banking techniques also rarely produce changes in P_{50}. However, if blood is stored for prolonged periods, intracellular 2,3-diphosphoglyceric acid (2,3-DPG) will become depleted and will decrease P_{50} (Collins, 1974).

The results of these clinical investigations reveal that fluid loading in the clinical setting appears to be associated with minimal effects on the gas exchanging properties of the lung when given cautiously in a monitored setting to achieve accepted physiologic end-points. Although crystalloidal fluids have been associated with increased radiographic oedema and increased pulmonary shunt fractions in some studies, associated decreases in PaO_2 and SaO_2 are usually absent or minimal. However, the Starling equation which predicts fluid movement into the lung, when pmv increases or πmv decreases, cautions the physician to avoid extreme increases in PAWP or decreases in plasma COP during fluid loading.

In summary, the effects of fluid loading on $\dot{D}O_2$ of critically ill patients are influenced by multiple factors. These factors include changes in haemoglobin levels and cardiac output. When both colloidal and crystalloidal fluids are administered under the guidance of haemodynamic monitoring, changes in the gas exchanging properties of the lung and P_{50} appear to be minimal. It thus remains difficult in the clinical setting to predict changes in $\dot{D}O_2$ in response to fluid loading without repeated assessment of haemoglobin levels, cardiac output and arterial oxygen tension and saturation, values required for the calculation of this value. This difficulty is augmented in the unstable patient with circulatory shock who may have independent changes in volume status and cardiac function during fluid resuscitation.

Effects of Fluids on Systemic Oxygen Consumption

Oxygen consumption ($\dot{V}O_2$) is also influenced by fluid loading. This value may be calculated with the following equation: $\dot{V}O_2 =$ cardiac output $\times (CaO_2 - C\bar{v}O_2)$, where $C\bar{v}O_2 = (1.36 \times S\bar{v}O_2 \times Hb) + (0.003 \times P\bar{v}O_2)$. $S\bar{v}O_2$ and $P\bar{v}O_2$ are mixed venous oxygen saturations and pressures respectively. Alternatively, oxygen consumption may be directly determined using a variety of techniques (Houtchens & Westenkow, 1984; Buran, 1987).

Changes in $\dot{V}O_2$ are also difficult to predict during fluid loading. Both increases and decreases may be observed. This is partly due to the unpredictability of $\dot{D}O_2$ in response to fluids. Both increases and decreases in $\dot{V}O_2$ may be observed after fluid loading and may depend on the direction of change of $\dot{D}O_2$. In one clinical study, when fluid loading was associated with decreases in $\dot{D}O_2$, for example, a downward trend in $\dot{V}O_2$ was observed, although statistical significance was not reached (Haupt et al., 1985).

When $\dot{D}O_2$ is increased by fluid loading or blood transfusion, subsets of patients exhibiting an increase in $\dot{V}O_2$ (Lazrove et al., 1980; Kaufman et al., 1984; Haupt et al., 1985; Gilbert et al., 1986; Fenwick et al., 1990) and subsets with a decrease or no change in $\dot{V}O_2$ have been identified in others (Haupt et al., 1985; Gilbert et al., 1986). These subsets (see Figs. 9.3 and 9.4) thus exhibit supply-dependent and supply-independent oxygen uptake respectively. A biphasic pattern of oxygen utilization is suggested and is consistent with patterns of oxygen utilization observed in the laboratory (Cain, 1984) below and above a critical level of $\dot{D}O_2$.

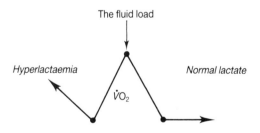

Figure 9.3   A summary of the effects of fluid loading in hypovolaemic shock.

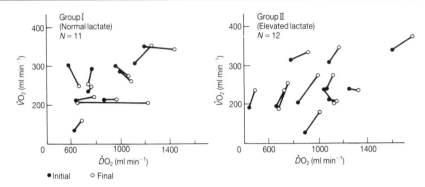

Figure 9.4 Patterns of oxygen utilization before and after fluid loading are illustrated for patient with sepsis with and without lactic acidosis. Patients with lactic acidosis (lactate ≥ 2.2 mmol litre^{-1}) tend to exhibit increased oxygen uptake, a pattern not observed in patients without lactic acidosis. (Adapted from Gilbert et al., 1986.)

In several clinical studies of fluid loading, an association between supply-dependent oxygen utilization and lactic acidosis has been described (Kaufman et al., 1984; Haupt et al., 1985, Gilbert et al., 1986). These studies showed that subsets of patients with lactic acidosis exhibited an increase in $\dot{V}O_2$ in response to an increase in $\dot{D}O_2$. Because lactic acidosis is a consequence of anaerobic metabolism, it has been postulated that the increase in $\dot{V}O_2$ from fluid-induced increases in $\dot{D}O_2$ represents a reduction in the imbalance between oxygen supply and demands. In contrast, subsets of patients without lactic acidosis do not exhibit an increase in $\dot{V}O_2$ in response to an increase in $\dot{D}O_2$ (Haupt et al., 1985; Gilbert et al., 1986) (Fig. 9.5). Thus, these clinical studies of critically ill patients support the presence of a biphasic pattern of oxygen utilization. Accordingly, supply-dependent $\dot{V}O_2$ characterizes patients with lactate acidosis but is not characteristic of patients without lactic acidosis (Table 9.4). These findings are consistent with laboratory models of critical illness which demonstrate an increase in blood lactate levels as $\dot{D}O_2$ is decreased below a critical value which represents a transition from supply-independent to supply-dependent oxygen utilization (Fahey & Lister, 1987; Heusser et al., 1989).

Table 9.4 Oxygen delivery, consumption, and lactate levels in patients with sepsis

	Normal lactate ($n = 6$)		Elevated lactate ($n = 14$)	
	Initial	Final	Initial	Final
$\dot{D}O_2$ (ml min^{-1} m^{-2})	448 ± 111**	499 ± 115	494 ± 165*	575 ± 206
$\dot{V}O_2$ (ml min^{-1} m^{-2})	147 ± 31	137 ± 38	132 ± 33*	163 ± 70
Lactate (mmol litre^{-1})	1.5 ± 0.6	1.6 ± 0.5	5.8 ± 3.4	4.8 ± 2.9

Adapted from Gilbert et al. (1986).
* $P < 0.05$; ** $P < 0.01$.

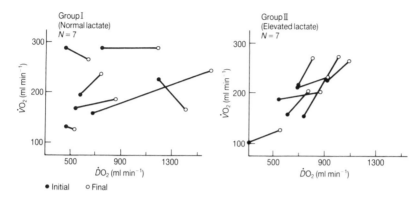

Figure 9.5 Patterns of oxygen utilization before and after blood transfusion are illustrated for patients with sepsis with and without lactic acidosis (lactate $\geq$ mmol litre^{-1}). (Adapted from Gilbert *et al.*, 1986.)

However, conflicting data from several clinical studies has been reported. These studies do not support an association of supply-dependent oxygen uptake with lactic acidosis when applied to the critically ill patient receiving fluids. Failure to observe supply dependence in patients transfused with blood, for example, has been described in several studies of patients with lactic acidosis (Conrad *et al.*, 1990; Dietrich *et al.*, 1990; Steffes *et al.*, 1991). The reasons for these negative results are unclear. These studies vary with respect to experimental design, duration of fluid challenge, age of patients, and patient diagnoses. Factors such as prolonged time between assessments of $\dot{D}O_2$ and $\dot{V}O_2$ post-operative pain, fluctuating levels of analgesia and anaesthesia, may have contributed to the negative results of these studies by leading to highly variable levels of $\dot{V}O_2$ from changes in oxygen demands (Villar *et al.*, 1990; Weissman & Kemper, 1991).

Some have postulated that supply-dependent $\dot{V}O_2$ is artifactual in studies which use indirect, calculated methods to assess $\dot{V}O_2$. Thus, supply dependency in these studies may be secondary to the mathematical coupling of variables shared in the equations for $\dot{D}O_2$ and $\dot{V}O_2$ described in reviews by Archie (1981) and Stratton *et al.* (1987). Others have postulated that increases in $\dot{V}O_2$ may be secondary to spontaneous change in oxygen demands that also result in corresponding changes in $\dot{D}O_2$ (Dantzker, 1987; Villar *et al.*, 1990). One would anticipate these mechanisms for supply-dependent oxygen utilization should be applicable to all critically ill patients and for all studies using calculated assessments of $\dot{D}O_2$ and $\dot{V}O_2$. However, several studies of fluid loading and blood transfusion, as well as a study utilizing positive end-expiratory pressure and a study using dobutamine reveal identically studied subsets of patients exhibiting supply-dependent and supply-independent oxygen uptake (Haupt *et al.*, 1985; Gilbert *et al.*, 1986; Fenwick *et al.*, 1990; Kruse *et al.*, 1990; Vincent *et al.*, 1990). Furthermore, these subsets are associated with elevated and normal lactate levels respectively. These studies refute the possibility that supply dependency is due solely to fluctuations in oxygen demands and mathematical coupling. Rather, the association of supply-dependent oxygen uptake with lactic acidosis supports the hypothesis that an imbalance between oxygen supply and demand and anaerobic metabolism is characteristic of critically ill patients.

In summary, fluids and blood increase $\dot{V}O_2$ in many critically ill patients, especially when $\dot{D}O_2$ increases and lactic acidosis is present. The association of supply-dependent oxygen uptake with lactic acidosis supports the hypothesis that critically ill patients have an imbalance between oxygen supply and demand. It is logical therefore to give fluid therapy to critically ill patients, especially those with lactic acidosis under the guidance of monitoring sufficient to achieve levels of $\dot{D}O_2$ that result in plateau levels of $\dot{V}O_2$.

References

Altschule M, (1986) Vagaries of transcapillary albumin flux. *Chest* **90**: 280.

Appel PI & Shoemaker WC (1981) Evaluation of fluid therapy in adult respiratory failure. *Crit. Care Med.* **9**: 862.

Archie JP (1981) Mathematic coupling of data. A common source of error. *Ann. Surg.* **193**: 296.

Bakker J, Caffernils M, Leon M *et al.* (1991). Blood lactate levels are superior to oxygen-derived variables in predicting outcome in human septic shock. *Chest* **99**: 956–62.

Braunwald E & Ross J (1964) Applicability of Starling's law of the heart to man. *Circ. Res.* (suppl. II) 14 and 15: II–169.

Braunwald E, Sonnenblick EH & Ross J (1984) Contraction of the normal heart. In Brunwald E. (ed.) *Heart Disease, A Textbook of Cardiovascular Medicine*, Philadelphia: W.B. Saunders Co. pp 409–46.

Buran MJ (1987) Oxygen consumption. In Snyder JV & Pinsky MR (eds), *Oxygen Transport in the Critically Ill.* Year Book Medical Publishers.

Cain SM (1984) Review: Supply dependency of oxygen uptake in ARDS: Myth or reality? *Am. J. Med. Sci.* **288**: 119.

Calvin JE, Driedger AA & Sibbald WJ (1981a) Does the pulmonary capillary wedge pressure predict left ventricular preload in critically ill patients? *Crit. Care Med.* **9**: 437.

Calvin JE, Driedgar AA & Sibbald WJ (1981b) The hemodynamic effect of rapid fluid infusion in critically ill patients. *Surgery* **90**: 61.

Carcillo JA, Davis AL & Zaritsky A (1991) Role of early fluid resuscitation in pediatric septic shock. *J. Am. Med. Assoc.* **266**: 1242.

Carlson RW, Rattan S & Haupt MT (1990) Fluid resuscitation in conditions of increased permeability. *Anesth. Rev.* **17**: 14.

Collins JA (1974) Problems associated with the massive transfusion of stored blood. *Surgery* **75**: 274.

Conrad SA, Dietrich KA, Herbert CA & Romero MD (1990) Effect of red cell transfusion on oxygen consumption following fluid resuscitation in septic shock. *Circ. Shock* **31:** 3419.

Cournand A, Nobel RP, Brud ES *et al*. (1944) Chemical, clinical and immunologic studies on the product of human plasma fractionation. VIII. Clinical use of concentrated human serum albumin in shock and comparison with whole blood and with rapid saline infusion. *J. Clin. Invest.* **23:** 491.

Creamer J, Edwards JD & Nightingale P (1990) Hemodynamic and oxygen transport variables in cardiogenic shock following acute myocardial infarction and their response to treatment. *Am. J. Cardiol.* **65:** 1297.

Crexells C, Chatterjee, Forrester JS *et al*. (1973) Optimal level of filling pressure in the left side of the heart in acute myocardial infarction. *New Engl. J. Med.* **289:** 1263.

Czer LSC & Shoemaker WC (1980) Myocardial performance in acutely ill patients: response to whole blood transfusion and catecholamine infusion in patients with sepsis. *Am. Rev. Respir. Dis.* **134:** 878.

Dantzker DR (1987) Interpretation of data in the hypoxic patient. In Bryan-Brown CW & Ayres SM (eds), *New Horizons,* pp. 93–108. Society of Critical Care Medicine.

Dennis RC, Hechtman HB, Berger RH *et al*. (1978) Transfusion of 2, 3 DPG-enriched red blood cells to improve cardiac function. *Ann. Thoracic Surg.* **26:** 18.

Dietrich KA, Conrad SA, Herbert CA *et al*. (1990) Cardiovascular and metabolic response to red blood cell transfusion in critically ill volume – resuscitated non-surgical patients. *Crit. Care Med.* **18:** 940.

Edwards JD, Brown GCS, Nightingale P *et al*. (1989) Use of survivors cardiorespiratory values as therapeutic goals in septic shock. *Crit. Care Med.* **17:** 1098.

Fahey JT & Lister G (1987) Postnatal changes in critical cardiac output and oxygen transport in conscious lambs. *Am. J. Physiol.* **253:** H100.

Falk JL, Rackow EC & Weil MH (1989) Colloid and crystalloid fluid resuscitation. In Shoemaker, Ayers, Grenvik, Holbrook, Thompson (eds), *Textbook of Critical Care* (2nd edition), pp. 1055–73. Philadelphia: W.B. Saunders Co.

Fenwick JC, Dodek PM, Ronco JJ *et al*. (1990) Increased concentrations of plasma lactate predict pathological supply dependence of O_2 consumption on O_2 delivery in patients with the adult respiratory distress syndrome. *J. Crit. Care.* **5:** 81.

Gilbert EM, Haupt MT, Mandanas RY *et al*. (1986) The effect of fluid loading, blood transfusion, and catecholamine infusion patients with sepsis. *Am. Rev. Respiratory Dis.* **134:** 878.

Guyton AC (1986) The lymphatic system, interstitial fluid dynamics, edema, and pulmonary fluid. In Guyton AC (ed.), *Textbook of Medical Physiology,* p. 361. Philadelphia: W.B. Saunders.

Guyton AC & Coleman TG (1968) Regulation of interstitial volume and pressure. *Ann. NY Acad. Sci.* **150:** 537.

Guyton AC & Richardson TW (1961) Effect of the hemotocrit on venous return. *Circ. Res.* **9:** 157.

Hankeln KB, Senker R, Schwarten JU et al. (1987) Evaluation of prognostic indices based on hemodynamic and oxygen transport variables in shock patients with adult respiratory distress syndrome. *Crit. Care Med.* **15**: 1.

Haupt MT (1989) The use of crystalloidal and colloidal solutions for volume replacement in hypovolemic shock. *CRC Crit. Rev. Clin. Lab. Sci* **27**: 1.

Haupt MT & Rackow EC (1982) Colloid osmotic pressure and fluid resuscitation with hetastarch, albumin, and saline solutions. *Crit. Care Med.* **10**: 159.

Haupt MT, Teerapong P, Green D et al. (1984) Increased pulmonary edema with crystalloid compared to colloid resuscitation of shock associated with increased vascular permeability. *Circ. Shock* **12**: 213.

Haupt MT, Gilbert EM & Carlson RW (1985) Fluid loading increases oxygen consumption in septic patients with lactic acidosis. *Am. Rev. Respiratory Dis.* **131**: 412.

Haupt MT, Kaufman BF & Carlson RW (1993) Fluid resuscitation in patients with increased vascular permeability. In Kaufman B. (ed.), *Critical Care Clinics.* Philadelphia: W.B. Saunders Co (in press).

Hauser CJ, Shoemaker WC, Turpin I & Goldberg SJ (1980) Oxygen transport responses to colloids and crystalloids in critically ill surgical patients. *Surg. Gynecol. Obstet.* **150**: 811.

Heusser F, Fahey JT & Lister G (1989) Effect of hemoglobin concentration on critical cardiac output and oxygen transport. *Am. J. Physiol.* **256**: H527.

Houtchens BA & Westenkow DR (1984) Oxygen consumption in septic shock. *Circ. Shock* **13**: 361.

Kaufman BS, Rackow EC & Falk JL (1984) The relationship between oxygen delivery and consumption during fluid resuscitation of hypovolemic and septic shock. *Chest* **85**: 336.

Kedem O & Katchalsky A (1958) Thermodynamic analysis of the permeability of biological membranes to non-electrolytes. *Biochim. Biophys. Acta* **27**: 229.

Kruse JA, Haupt MT, Puri VK et al. (1990) Lactate levels as predictors of the relationship between oxygen delivery and consumption in ARDS. **98**: 959.

Lamke LO & Liijedahl GSO (1976) Plasma volume changes after infusion of various plasma expanders. *Resuscitation* **5**: 93.

Lazrove S, Waxman K, Shippy C & Shoemaker WC (1980) Hemodynamic, blood volume, and oxygen transport responses to albumin and hydroxyethyl starch infusions in critically ill postoperative patients. *Crit. Care Med.* **8**: 302.

Ley SJ, Miller K, Skov P & Preisig P (1990) Crystalloid versus colloid fluid therapy after cardiac surgery. *Heart and Lung* **19**: 31.

Lucking SE, Williams TM, Chaten FC et al. (1990) Dependence of oxygen consumption on oxygen delivery in children with hyperdynamic septic shock and low oxygen extraction. *Crit. Care Med.* **18**: 1316.

MacGregor DC, Cavell JW, Mahler F et al. (1974) Relations between afterload, stroke volume, and the descending limb of the Starling curve. *Am. J. Physiol.* **227**: 884.

Metildi LA, Shackford SR, Virgilio RW et al. (1984) Crystalloid versus colloid in fluid resuscitation of patients with severe pulmonary insufficiency. *Surg. Gynecol. Obstet.* **58**: 207.

Mink RB & Pollack MM (1990) Effect of blood transfusion on oxygen consumption in pediatric septic shock. *Crit. Care Med.* **18:** 1087.

Monroe RG, Gamble WJ, LaFarge CG *et al.* (1971) Left ventricular performance at high end-diastolic pressures in isolated, perfused dog hearts. *Circ. Res.* **28:** 49.

Murray JF, Escober E & Rapaport E (1969) Effects of blood viscosity on hemodynamic responses in acute experimental anemia. *Am. J. Physiol.* **216:** 638.

Packman MI & Rackow EC (1983) Optimal left heart filling pressure during fluid resuscitation of patients with hypovolemia and septic shock. *Crit. Care Med.* **11:** 165.

Pappenheimer J & Soto Rivera A (1948) Effective osmotic pressure of the plasma proteins and other quantities associated with the capillary circulation of the hind limbs of cats and dogs. *Am. J. Physiol.* **152:** 471.

Rackley CE, Russell RO Jr, Mantle JA & Maraski RE (1975) Cardiogenic shock: Recognition and management. *Cardiovasc. Clin.* **7:** 251.

Rackow EC, Kaufman BS, Falk JL *et al.* (1987) Hemodynamic response to fluid repletion in patients with septic shock: evidence for early depression of cardiac performance. *Circ. Shock* **22:** 11.

Rackow EC, Fein LA & Leppo J (1977) Colloid osmotic pressure as a prognostic indicator of pulmonary edema and mortality in the critically ill. *Chest* **72:** 709.

Rackow EC, Falk JL, Fein IA *et al.* (1983) Fluid resuscitation in circulatory shock: a comparison of the cardiorespiratory effects of albumin, hetastarch, and saline solutions in patients with hypovolemic and septic shock. *Crit. Care Med.* **11:** 835.

Rice CH, Herman CM, Kiesow LA *et al.* (1978) Benefits from improved oxygen delivery of blood in shock therapy. *J. Surg. Res.* **19:** 193.

Ronco JJ, Phang PT, Walley KR *et al.* (1991) Oxygen consumption is independent of changes in oxygen delivery in severe adult respiratory distress syndrome. *Am. Rev. Respiratory Dis.* **143:** 1267.

Russell JA, Ronco JJ, Lockhart D *et al.* (1990) Oxygen delivery and consumption and ventricular preload are greater in survivors than in nonsurvivors of the adult respiratory distress syndrome. *Am. Rev. Respiratory Dis.* **141:** 659.

Shoemaker WC, Schluchter M, Hopkins JA *et al.* (1981) Comparison of the relative effectiveness of colloids and crystalloids in emergency resuscitation. *Am. J. Surg.* **142:** 73.

Shoemaker WC, Appel PL, Kram HB *et al.* (1988) Prospective trial of supernormal values of survivors as therapeutic goals in high-risk surgical patients. *Chest* **94:** 1176.

Shimoda V, Yoshiya I & Hirata TP (1984) Evaluation of a system for on-line analysis of $\dot{V}O_2$ and $\dot{V}CO_2$ for clinical applicability. *Anesthesiology* **61:** 311.

Sibbald WJ, Driedger AA, Moffat JD *et al.* (1981) Pulmonary microvascular clearance of radiotracers in human cardiac and non-cardiac pulmonary edema. *J. Appl. Physiol.* **50:** 1337.

Sibbald WJ, Short AK, Warshawski FJ *et al.* (1985) Thermal dye measurements of extravascular lung water in critically ill patients: Intravascular Starling forces and extravascular lung water in the adult respiratory distress syndrome. *Chest* **87**: 585.

Skillman JJ, Restall DS & Salzman EW (1975) Randomized trial of albumin vs electrolyte solutions during abdominal aortic operations. *Surgery* **78**: 291.

Smith RO (1948) Lymphatic contractility. A possible intrinsic mechanism of lymphatic vessels on the transport of lymph. *J. Exp. Med.* **90**: 497.

Starchuck E, Weil MH & Shubin H (1975) Fluid challenge. In Weil MH & Shubin H (eds), *Critical Care Medicine Handbook*. New York: John N. Kolen.

Starling EH (1896) On the absorption of fluids from the connective tissue spaces. *J. Physiol. (Lond.)* **4**: 55.

Starling EH (1898) Production and absorption of lymph. Shaefer EA (ed.), *Textbook of Physiology*. Vol. 1, p. 285. London: Caxton.

Staub NC (1974) Pathogenesis of pulmonary edema. *Am. Rev. Respiratory Dis.* **109**: 358.

Staverman AJ (1951) The theory of measurement of osmotic pressure. *Recl. Trav. Chi Pays Bas.* **70**: 344.

Steffes CP, Bender JS & Levison MA (1991) Blood transfusion and oxygen consumption in surgical sepsis. *Crit. Care Med.* **19**: 512.

Strattan HH, Feustel PJ & Newell JC (1987) Regression of calculated variables in the presence of shared measurement error. *J. App. Physiol.* **62**: 2083.

Thompson WL (1975) Rational use of albumin and plasma substitutes. *Johns Hopkins Med. J.* **136**: 220.

Tuchschmidt J, Fried J, Swinney R & Sharma OP (1989) Early hemodynamic correlates of survival in patients with septic shock. *Crit. Care Med.* **17**: 719–23.

Tuchschmidt J, Fried J, Astiz M, *et al.* (1991) Supranormal oxygen delivery in septic shock patients. *Crit. Care Med.* **19**: S66 (abstract).

Villar J, Slutsky AS, Hew E & Aberman A (1990) Oxygen transport and oxygen consumption in critically ill patients. *Chest* **98**: 687.

Vincent JL, Roman A, DeBacker D & Kahn RJ (1990) Oxygen uptake/supply dependency. Effects of a short-term dobutamine infusion. *Am. Rev. Respiratory Dis.* **142**: 2.

Virgilio RW, Rice CH, Smith DE *et al.* (1979) Crystalloid vs colloid resuscitation: Is one better? *Surgery* **85**: 129.

Weil MH & Henning RJ (1979) New concepts in the diagnosis and fluid treatment of circulatory shock. *Anesthesia Analgesia* **58**: 124.

Weil MH & Nishijima H (1978) Cardiac output in bacterial shock. *Am. J. Med.* **64**: 920.

Weil MH & Shubin H (1969) The 'VIP' approach to the bedside management of shock. *J. Am. Med. Assoc.* **107**: 337.

Weil MH, Michael S, Puri VK & Carlson RW (1981) The stat laboratory. Facilitating blood gas and biochemical measurements for the critically ill and injured. *Am. J. Clin. Pathol.* **76**: 34.

Weisel RD, Vito L, Dennis RC *et al.* (1977). Myocardial depression in sepsis. *Am. J. Surgery* **133**: 512.

Weissman C & Kemper M (1991) The oxygen uptake–oxygen delivery relationship during ICU interventions. *Chest* **99**: 430.

10 Therapy: The Effects of Vasoactive Drugs

Jean-Louis Teboul

Rationale For the Use of Vasoactive Drugs in Critically Ill Patients

Transport of oxygen from the external environment into the mitochondria involves a sequence of convective and diffuse steps. In this chapter we focus on the manipulation of the convective step of oxygen transport by vasoactive drugs. Oxygen delivery (DO_2) is defined as the product of the cardiac output (and arterial oxygen content (CaO_2). There are many arguments suggesting that optimization of DO_2 must be considered as a major goal for the management of critically ill patients.

A pathological oxygen consumption (VO_2) supply dependency has been reported in various critical illnesses including sepsis (Haupt *et al.*, 1985; Gilbert *et al.*, 1986; Vincent *et al.*, 1990a), adult respiratory distress syndrome (ARDS) (Danek *et al.*, 1980), congestive heart failure (CHF) (Moshenifar *et al.*, 1987). The relevance of VO_2/DO_2 dependency in indicating oxygen debt has been supported in several studies by its correlation with hyperlactaemia, another marker of tissue hypoxia (Haupt *et al.*, 1985; Gilbert *et al.*, 1986; Fenwick *et al.*, 1990; Vincent *et al.*, 1990a). However, some investigators have questioned the reality of a supply dependency observed when VO_2 and DO_2 that share common variables (cadiac output, CaO_2), are not measured independently. Indeed, in recent studies where VO_2 and DO_2 were assessed independently, VO_2 supply dependency was not observed in patients with ARDS (Ronco *et al.*, 1991) or in septic (Ronco *et al.*, 1993) or post-operative patients (Vermeij *et al.*, 1990), even in the presence of hyperlactaemia. Despite these latter disconcerting findings, which need further confirmation, a prognostic value of supply dependency in critically ill patients has been suggested by some studies, in which patients who exhibited supply dependency had a mortality rate higher than those who did not (Gutierrez & Pohil, 1986; Bihari *et al.*, 1987; Ranieri *et al.*, 1992). Supply dependency would thus indicate a significant tissue oxygen deprivation which finally resulted in organ failure and death.

Other types of prognostic studies have supported the concept of optimization of DO_2 to reduce oxygen debt in acute illnesses. Shoemaker and co-workers showed that critically ill surgical patients are more likely to survive if they have a $\dot{D}O_2$ >600 ml min^{-1} m^{-2} and a $\dot{V}O_2$ >170 ml min^{-1} m^{-2} (Shoemaker *et al.*, 1973). Furthermore, the use of these supranormal haemodynamic values as therapeutic goals in controlled clinical trials resulted in a significant reduction in mortality (Shoemaker *et al.*, 1988). Similar conclusions could be drawn from reports in patients with ARDS (Russell *et al.*, 1990) or septic shock (Tuchschmidt *et al.*, 1989, 1992). Yet, in prospective studies in septic patients, others failed to find any difference in $\dot{D}O_2$ between survivors and non-survivors (Reinhart *et al.*, 1990; Bakker *et al.*, 1991). Although it is difficult to draw definitive conclusions from such conflicting findings, it must be remembered that there is probably a great heterogeneity in optimal levels of $\dot{D}O_2$ among critically ill patients. Therefore, in any individual acutely ill patient, it seems logical to try to increase $\dot{D}O_2$ until no further increase in $\dot{V}O_2$ is realized.

Although optimizing haemoglobin and arterial oxygen saturation (SaO_2) are first therapeutic options, the most effective means to increase $\dot{D}O_2$ is to increase cardiac output. This is first, because large increases in cardiac output can often be obtained with fluid or drugs, whereas increasing SaO_2 by more than 10% is rarely possible; and second, because hypovolaemia or cardiac dysfunction are common in critically ill patients. Clearly, optimizing cardiac preload by fluid loading must be the first step for increasing cardiac output. If cardiac output remains low or inadequate despite adjusted volume loading, vasoactive drugs should be used.

In the following sections we analyse the main effects of the vasoactive drugs commonly used in critical care situations on $\dot{D}O_2$ and on tissue oxygen utilization.

Effects of Vasoactive Drugs on Oxygen Delivery

Effects on Cardiac Output

Catecholamines

Dopamine and Dobutamine: These are the most widely used β-adrenergic positive inotropic agents. Stimulation of myocardial β-adrenergic receptors activates adenylate cyclase and causes accumulation of cyclic adenosine monophosphate (cAMP) which enhances myocardial contractility by increasing the influx of calcium through voltage-dependent channels.

Dopamine is the naturally occurring immediate precursor of noradrenaline. In doses of less than $4 \mu g \, kg^{-1} \, min^{-1}$, dopamine stimulates dopaminergic receptors in the renal, splanchnic, cerebral and coronary vascular beds. This results in vasodilation of these regional circulations. At intermediate doses (4–$8 \mu g \, kg^{-1} \, min^{-1}$) dopamine also stimulates α- and β-adrenergic receptors in the vasculature and the myocardium. β-Adrenergic stimulation results in increased stroke volume, and heart rate (HR) and hence cardiac output.

α-Adrenergic stimulation results in arterial and venous constriction, leading to increases in blood pressure, systemic venous return and cardiac filling pressures. At higher doses, the predominant α-adrenergic effect leads to a marked vasoconstriction able to counteract the dopaminergic renal effect.

Dobutamine is a sympathomimetic amine that acts primarily to increase myocardial contractility through β-adrenergic stimulation. In fact, dobutamine is a racemic mixture of two stereoisomers: an α_1-adrenorecep-tor agonist activity resides in the $(-)$ isomer while β_1- and β_2-adrenoreceptor agonist activities reside in the $(+)$ isomer. The inotropic activity of dobutamine appears related to its combined β_1 and α_1 activities. By contrast, the activation of the opposing α_1 and β_2 vascular adrenoreceptors results in little direct effect on systemic vasculature. Tachycardia and arrythmias are the major dose-limiting side-effects of dobutamine.

In a cross-over trial of dopamine and dobutamine in patients with CHF (Leier et al., 1978), dobutamine ($2.5-10\ \mu g\ kg^{-1}\ mm^{-1}$) increased cardiac output by increasing SV in a dose–response fashion. In contrast, dopamine increased SV and cardiac output at $4\ \mu g\ kg^{-1}\ mm^{-1}$ but not at higher doses, presumably because of an increase in left ventricular afterload. It was also noted that pulmonary artery occlusion pressure (PAOP) decreased with dobutamine, but increased with incremental doses of dopamine. Similar findings were reported in patients with acute respiratory failure (Molloy et al., 1986). In this report dopamine also increased left ventricular end-diastolic volume (measured by scintigraphic technique) while dobutamine did not; presumably dopamine increases systemic venous tone (Lang et al., 1988) and thereby preload. However, dopamine could be recommended in combination with dobutamine for the management of patients with cardiogenic shock (Richard et al., 1983): indeed, the additional inotropic effect of dobutamine, which alone failed to rise BP, allowed a lower dose of dopamine to be effective in increasing BP while avoiding the harmful effects of higher doses of dopamine on PAOP and arterial oxygen tension (PaO_2).

In septic shock, among vasoactive drugs, dopamine is probably the most widely used. Comparison of dopamine with dobutamine has shown a similar increase in cardiac output and SV with the two agents, but only dopamine increased blood pressure (Regnier et al., 1979). However, it was observed that even at low dosage, dopamine sometimes caused peripheral vasoconstriction, resulting in unaltered or even decreased cardiac output (Edwards, 1990). For this author, since improving DO_2 rather than blood pressure is recognized as a major therapeutic goal in septic shock, dopamine alone may not be an ideal agent. As an early myocardial depression commonly occurs in septic shock (Parker et al., 1984), the use of dobutamine, a potent inotropic agent should be licit. Moreover, in lowering PAOP more than dopamine, dobutamine could allow an additional fluid volume infusion and hence a further increase in cardiac output. This hypothesis was verified in study using a canine endotoxinic shock (Vincent et al., 1987). In human septic shock dobutamine could produce substantial increases in cardiac output while decreasing PAOP (Jardin et al., 1981). More recently, Vincent et al. demonstrated that the addition of $5\,\mu g\,kg^{-1}\,min^{-1}$ to a standard treatment of septic shock allowed an increase in cardiac output, DO_2 and $\dot{V}O_2$ without altering BP (Vincent et al., 1990b).

In summary, dobutamine seems to be a drug of choice in critical care settings because of its efficiency in increasing cardiac output in patients with CHF (Richard et al., 1983), septic shock (Vincent et al., 1990b), acute respiratory failure (Molloy et al., 1986), massive pulmonary embolism (Jardin et al., 1985) and in the post-operative period (Shoemaker et al., 1986). However, intravascular volume replacement is required before institution of dobutamine to avoid hypotension and tachycardia (Shoemaker et al., 1986).

Noradrenaline and Adrenaline: Noradrenaline is a natural catecholamine. As a β_1-agonist noradrenaline increases myocardial contractility. However, its α-agonist effects lead to a marked peripheral vasoconstriction resulting in increased blood pressure and left ventricular afterload. HR usually remains constant due to a baroreceptor stimulation. In recent years there has been a renewed interest in this agent in hyperdynamic septic shock (Desjars et al., 1987). In this setting, noradrenaline can restore adequate organ perfusion pressure, thereby preventing myocardial or renal ischaemia. Recent clinical studies in septic shock have reported its efficiency in reversing hypotension refractory to fluids and other catecholamines (Desjars et al., 1987; Meadows et al., 1988). In reversing classical signs of shock (hypotension and oliguria) noradrenaline would have been judged effective. However, although cardiac output increased in some patients, it was unchanged or decreased in others, so that changes in DO_2 and $\dot{V}O_2$ induced by noradrenaline were highly variable (Meadows et al., 1988). This re-emphasizes the unpredictability of the effects of catecholamines (except dobutamine) in septic shock. Nevertheless, noradrenaline could be a useful adjuvant therapy to maintain sufficient vital organ perfusion pressures provided that a powerful inotropic agent like dobutamine is used concomitantly to increase cardiac output and DO_2. Edwards et al. (1989) proposed this option for the management of septic shock. However, further controlled trials are needed.

Adrenaline is an endogenous adrenal hormone. At low doses, its potent β_1- and moderate β_2-agonist effects result in increased SV, HR and cardiac output. At doses higher than $1\,\mu g\,kg^{-1}\,min^{-1}$, α-adrenergic effects predominate, resulting in peripheral vasoconstriction. The use of adrenaline in shock – except for anaphylactic shock – is not currently recommended. Nevertheless, two studies provide promising haemodynamic data in septic shock: in patients who remained hypotensive despite adequate fluid loading, adrenaline infusion produced significant increases in blood pressure, cardiac output and DO_2 (Bollaert et al., 1990; Mackenzie et al., 1991), of note in one study a slight but significant increase in $\dot{V}O_2$ (Bollaert et al., 1990).

Dopexamine: This new synthetic catecholamine has β_2-agonist and dopaminergic receptor activities, but only weak β_1-agonist and no α-agonist activities. It also inhibits neuronal re-uptake of noradrenaline. This results in a combination of inotropic, afterload-reducing and renal vasodilating effects which could be useful for the management of CHF. In patients with low output CHF, dopexamine substantially increased cardiac output without altering blood pressure: at doses up to $4\,\mu g\,kg^{-1}\,min^{-1}$, the majority of the effects resulted from increased SV; at higher doses the increase in HR makes a greater contribution (Smith & Filcek, 1989). In patients with acute respiratory failure and previous cardiomyopathy, dopexamine produced significant increases in cardiac output: below $3\,\mu g\,kg^{-1}\,min^{-1}$ HR was unchanged, whereas above $3\,\mu g\,kg^{-1}\,min^{-1}$ only increased HR accounted for the further increase in cardiac output (Vincent *et al.*, 1989). In human septic shock, dopexamine produced dose-dependent increases in cardiac output, SV and HR, but blood pressure and urine output did not change significantly (Colardyn *et al.*, 1989). Further studies in critical care settings are needed (1) to assess the usefulness of dopexamine alone or combined with other drugs, and (2) to identify the characteristics of patients in whom beneficial effects could be expected.

Phosphodiesterase (PDE) Inhibitors
Despite the major role of catecholamines in the management of critically ill patients with inadequate cardiac output, problems such as tachycardia, arrythmias, increased myocardial oxygen consumption or excessive vaso-constriction may occur. In addition, loss of effectiveness with prolonged exposure to β-agonist agents (Bristow *et al.*, 1982) may result in recurrence of clinical symptoms. Thus, other inotropic drugs like PDE inhibitors have been investigated for the acute management of cardiac dysfunction. PDE inhibitors (amrinone, milrinone, enoximone) inhibit the degradation of cAMP by peak-III phosphodiesterase, in both myocardium and vascular smooth muscle. In the myocardium, cAMP improves the calcium influx through voltage-dependent channels, and promotes calcium uptake by the sarcoplastic reticulum; thus both myocardial contractility and relaxation are improved. In the vascular smooth muscle, cAMP induces vasodilation. In CHF patients, PDE inhibitors significantly increased cardiac output and decreased cardiac filling pressures, while blood pressure did not change or slightly decreased (Benotti *et al.*, 1978; Ludmer *et al.*, 1986). Both inotropic and vasodilating properties contribute to the overall haemodynamic effect (Ludmer *et al.*, 1986). Because of the ability of β-agonist agents to increase cAMP levels, thereby providing increased substrate for PDE inhibitors, the combination of these two types of drugs should be attractive. Thus, coadministration of amrinone and dobutamine resulted in a higher left ventricular dP/dt and SV than did the infusion of either agent alone (Gage *et al.*, 1986). Synergic effect on CO of dobutamine and enoximone was observed in

patients with CHF (Thuillez *et al.*, 1993). Addition of low doses of enoximone to adrenergic agents was demonstrated to improve cardiac output without decreased blood pressure in patients wih cardiogenic shock (Vincent *et al.*, 1988). In septic shock, enoximone increased cardiac output and DO_2 substantially without altering blood pressure because of the concomitant fluid infusion allowed by the lowered PAOP induced by this agent (Kox & Brydon, 1991). Further investigational studies are obviously required to assess the usefulness of these agents in this setting.

Vasodilators

If vasodilators, which act on both arterial and venous tone, are administered in subjects with normal heart, cardiac output decreases because of a predominant effect of preload (Pouleur *et al.*, 1980). By contrast, in patients with reduced myocardial contractility vasodilators increase SV and cardiac output, because a failing heart is more responsive to changes in afterload than those in preload (Pouleur *et al.*, 1980). A consistent advantage of vasodilators over inotropic drugs is their potential to reduce myocardial oxygen demand by reducing myocardial wall stress. However, in patients with low blood pressure there is some limitation to the use of vasodilators alone since the improved SV does not always sufficiently compensate for the lowered vascular resistance and so further reduction in blood pressure may occur.

Nitrates: These act directly on vascular smooth muscle to cause arteriolar and venous dilation. After generating nitric oxide they activate guanylate cyclase, which stimulates the synthesis of cyclic GMP (guanosine monophosphate), resulting in activation of muscle relaxation.

Nitroprusside is of particular benefit in patients with low cardiac output, pulmonary oedema and normal or increased blood pressure, because it quickly and markedly reduces PAOP while increasing forward flow without myocardial metabolic cost (Installé *et al.*, 1987). It is also helpful in shock due to mitral regurgitation, ventricular septal defect or acute aortic regurgitation because it reduces volume regurgitation and improves forward flow. Nitroprusside may be combined either with dobutamine to further increase cardiac output or with dopamine to maintain blood pressure.

At low doses, nitroglycerine is predominantly a venodilator indicated to reduce pulmonary oedema, but at high doses it produces similar haemodynamic effects to those of nitroprusside.

Prostaglandins: Prostacyclin is a potent microvascular vasodilator, antagonizing the effects of excessive thromboxane-A_2 release. Its use is investigational in septic shock, because of its anti-inflammatory properties. It was reported to increase substantially cardiac output, DO_2 (and VO_2) with no (Pittet *et al.*, 1990) or small decrease in blood pressure (Bihari *et al.*, 1987).

PGE_1 is a pulmonary and systemic vasodilator. Its use is investigational in ARDS where it could substantially increase cardiac output and $\dot{D}O_2$ (Radermacher et al., 1989; Silverman et al., 1990) with variable effects on $\dot{V}O_2$.

Effects on Arterial Oxygen Content

Effects Related to Drug-induced Changes in Cardiac Patterns

A decrease in PAOP may reduce pulmonary fluid filtration rate, pulmonary oedema and intrapulmonary shunt fraction ($\dot{Q}s/\dot{Q}T$), resulting in improved PaO_2.

The increase in cardiac output may affect PaO_2 by two means:

(1) The increase in cardiac output was demonstrated to be responsible for an increase in $\dot{Q}s/\dot{Q}T$ (Lemaire et al., 1976; Lynch et al., 1979). One part of this effect was ascribed to the increased mixed venous oxygen tension ($P\bar{v}O_2$) induced by increased cardiac output. Indeed, increased $P\bar{v}O_2$ decreases hypoxic pulmonary vasoconstriction (Pease et al., 1982). However, at least partly, $P\bar{v}O_2$ and cardiac output affect $\dot{Q}s/\dot{Q}T$ independently.

(2) The increase in cardiac output may result in increased $P\bar{v}O_2$ which may improve PaO_2 in the presence of ventilation/perfusion ($\dot{V}A/\dot{Q}$) mismatching, and independently of its aggravating effect on $\dot{Q}s/\dot{Q}T$ (Dantzker & Gutierrez, 1989). Thus, the beneficial effect of increased $P\bar{v}O_2$ on PaO_2 may compensate for the deleterious effect of increased cardiac output on $\dot{Q}s/\dot{Q}T$.

However, it must be remembered that $P\bar{v}O_2$ changes do not parallel changes in cardiac output in patients with $\dot{V}O_2$ supply dependency. Yet, it is particularly in this setting that a substantial increase in cardiac output could be required to reduce oxygen debt.

Direct Effects on Pulmonary Vasculature

In animal and clinical studies most vasodilators have been demonstrated to decrease or inhibit hypoxic pulmonary vasoconstriction (Voelkel, 1986). In ARDS, multiple inert gas analysis showed that nitroprusside (Radermacher et al., 1988) and nitroglycerin (Radermacher et al., 1989) induced profound hypoxaemia by increasing $\dot{Q}s/\dot{Q}T$ without altering cardiac output or $P\bar{v}O_2$. A direct effect of nitrates on pulmonary vasculature (inhibition of hypoxic pulmonary vasoconstriction) is likely. Indirect evidence of detrimental redistribution of pulmonary blood flow with drugs was given by the compared effects of dobutamine, nitroprusside and enoximone in the same patients with CHF (Installé et al., 1987). Despite similar increases in cardiac output and $P\bar{v}O_2$ with the three drugs, PaO_2 decreased with nitroprusside and enoximone, while it remained constant with dobutamine.

In summary, the effects of vasoactive drugs on gas exchange are complex (Fig. 10.1) and vary according to the patient's cardiopulmonary conditions: integrity of hypoxic pulmonary vasoconstriction, degree of alveolar hypoxia, degree of $\dot{V}A/\dot{Q}$ mismaching, level of basal $P\bar{v}O_2$, level of filling pressures, existence of $\dot{V}O_2$ supply dependency, etc. Therefore, in a given patient, it is impossible to predict accurately the resultant effect on PaO_2 of any vasoactive drug. However, from available clinical data, changes in PaO_2 induced by vasoactive drugs are relatively limited (Regnier *et al.*, 1979, Richard *et al.*, 1983; Molloy *et al.*, 1986) except for nitrates in ARDS (Radermacher *et al.*, 1988, 1989). Furthermore, even when PaO_2 slightly decreases, this rarely results in falls in SaO_2 (Vincent *et al.*, 1990a) and CaO_2 (Installé *et al.*, 1987) because of the sigmoid-shaped oxyhaemoglobin dissociation curve. Therefore, in most cases, increased $\dot{D}O_2$ parallels increased cardiac ouput.

Effects of Vasoactive Drugs on Tissue Oxygen Utilization

Even though a vasoactive drug produces a large increase in $\dot{D}O_2$, its effectiveness in reducing oxygen debt in the most severely ill patients depends upon its capacity to provide oxygen to the most hypoxic tissues. This concern is particularly crucial since first redistribution of blood flow is a characteristic pattern of shock states, and second, vasoactive drugs have their own influence on blood flow distribution. In cardiogenic shock redistribution of flow is recognized as a potent adaptative mechanism, which, in

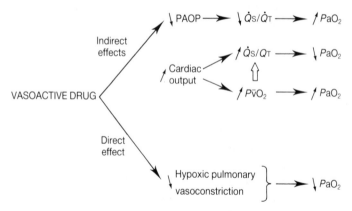

Figure 10.1   Potential effects of vasoactive drugs on PaO_2. PaO_2, Arterial oxygen tension; $P\bar{v}O_2$, mixed venous oxygen tension; PAOP, pulmonary arterial occlusion pressure; $\dot{Q}s/\dot{Q}T$, intrapulmonary shunt fraction.

response to reduced global $\dot{D}O_2$, attempts to deviate flow from non-vital organs with low oxygen extraction ratio toward vital organs with high oxygen extraction ratio. Clinicians must be aware that administration of vasoactive drugs in this setting may interfere with vasoregulation of regional flow in either a beneficial or a deleterious manner.

Studies in patients with CHF (Leier et al., 1988) demonstrated that for a global increased CO, limb blood flow increased markedly with dobutamine, nitroprusside, nitroglycerin and enoximone, hepatosplanchnic flow increased preferentially with dopexamine, while renal blood flow increased with low doses of dopamine and decreased with nitrates. Combination of dobutamine and enoximone in patients with CHF can increase forearm blood flow more than either drug does alone in patients with CHF (Thuillez et al., 1993). Clearly, in cardiogenic shock the extent to which pharmacological manipulation of regional blood flow is beneficial in increasing O_2 supply and VO_2 in hypoxic areas remains speculative.

Maldistribution of flow at the regional macrocirculatory level as well as at the local microcirculatory level is a characteristic hemodynamic pattern of septic shock (Lang et al., 1984; Thijs et al., 1988; Bersten et al., 1990). It mainly contributes to defective tissue oxygen utilization and finally to oxygen debt despite apparently adequate global $\dot{D}O_2$. Sepsis-induced changes in vascular reactivity could be a major cause of the altered distribution of flow both between and within organs (Nelson et al., 1988; Sibbald et al., 1991).

Redistribution of blood flow during sepsis has been investigated in few studies in humans (Gump et al., 1970; Dhainaut et al., 1987; Dahn et al., 1987; Bowton et al., 1989), while extensively studied in animals. Assessment of splanchnic circulation may be of particular interest since splanchnic oxygen debt presumably contributes to development of multiple organ dysfunction (Carrico et al., 1986).

Otherwise, severe sepsis presumably modifies the impact of adrenergic drugs on regional blood flow, since a depressed vascular responsiveness to vasoactive agent is likely in this setting (Siegel et al., 1967). In this way, administration of a given dose of catecholaminergic agent can by its cardiac effects produce an improvement in global oxygen delivery similar to that obtained in non septic conditions but may result in an altered blood flow redistribution owing to lowered vascular effects. This hypothesis may account for the absence of reduction of renal or splanchnic blood flow observed during vasoconstrictor therapy in experimental endotoxinic shock (Breslow et al., 1987). Interferences of sepsis-modified vasoactive drugs properties with sepsis-induced macrocirculatory maldisturbance have been poorly investigated in humans. Some data indicated that dopamine alone or combined with noradrenaline could increase splanchnic blood flow (Takala et al., 1991). The extent to which this effect is beneficial, in improving splanchnic oxygen balance, and hence in preventing the onset of multiple organ failure, remains unknown. Clearly, further clinical studies are needed to better understand and improve the pharmacological approach of septic shock.

Few studies have examined drug-induced microcirculatory blood flow redistribution in sepsis. In a series of hyperlactatemic septic patients, in whom DO_2 was increased with phentolamine and prostacycline sequentially administered, VO_2 and skin microvascular blood flow were found increased only with prostacyclin (Pittet *et al.*, 1990). It was concluded that phentolamine failed to distribute adequately the increased DO_2 toward hypoxic areas probably because of a detrimental effect on microvascular flow distribution. By contrast, prostacyclin in improving microvascular flow distribution may have increased oxygen uptake in hypoxic tissues. Other evidence of this effect was reported in some septic patients in whom, prostacyclin increased DO_2, VO_2 and oxygen extraction ratio (Bihari *et al.*, 1987).

In summary, interaction between regional or local flow redistributive effects of vasoactive drugs and adaptive or abnormal flow redistribution in shock states cast doubts on the benefits expected from a drug-related increased DO_2. At the bedside, performing an 'oxygen flux test' was proposed to detect a covert tissue oxygen debt (Bihari *et al.*, 1987). Such a debt would be likely when VO_2 increases during the therapy-induced increase in DO_2. Furthermore, the effectiveness of the therapy chosen for the test, in actually improving tissue oxygenation, could justify the use of this therapy for the further care of the patient.

However, some caution must be taken to correctly interpret this test:

(1) A false negative response (unchanged VO_2 despite oxygen debt) may occur if the drug adversely affects blood flow redistribution by itself (Pittet *et al.*, 1990).

(2) A false positive response (increased VO_2 despite absence of oxygen deprivation) may also occur by several mechanisms: (a) there could be a mathematical coupling between DO_2 and calculated VO_2 (independent assessment is thus preferable); (b) external factors could influence oxygen demand during the test (a short time period – 30 min – is needed to minimize these influences); and (c) the agent used could induce an increase in oxygen demand since cAMP accumulation produced by some drugs may increase cellular metabolism (Fellows *et al.*, 1985; Gilbert *et al.*; 1986; Teboul *et al.*, 1992; Teboul *et al.*, 1993).

In patients with stable CHF without elevated blood lactate, VO_2 was observed to increase simultaneously with DO_2 increase after enoximone administration, while in the same patients, VO_2 remained unchanged when dobutamine increased DO_2 by the same magnitude than enoximone did (Teboul *et al.*, 1992). Clearly here, the increased VO_2 with enoximone denoted an increase in oxygen demand rather than an oxygen debt recovery.

Potential thermogenic effects must be taken into account also for the judicious use of catecholamines or PDE inhibitors in critical care settings. In this way, in patients with CHF, following changes in mixed venous oxygen saturation or oxygen extraction ratio may be helpful to detect whether undesirable metabolic effects overrid the beneficial effects on DO_2 of these agents and thereby to adjust rationally drug regimen dose (Teboul *et al.*, 1993).

However in most complex situations, it seems more judicious to combine serial determinations of blood lactate levels with measurements of oxygen-derived variables, both to help in interpreting the oxygen flux test (Vincent *et al.*, 1990a) and to improve the overall management of the critically ill patient (Bakker *et al.*, 1991).

Summary

Optimization of oxygen delivery (DO_2) is a major therapeutic goal in critical care settings. Vasoactive drugs are frequently used for this purpose. In this review we analyse the points of impact on oxygen delivery of the most commonly used vasoactive drugs. Their most important effect is the increase in cardiac output either by enhancing myocardial contractility (inotropic agents) or by reducing left ventricular afterload (vasodilator agents). Their effects on pulmonary gas exchange are complex but, in clinical practice, the overall effect on arterial oxygen content is limited. By contrast, interactions between the blood flow redistribution properties of these agents and the blood flow distribution alteration characterizing shock states make uncertain the benefits expected from the drug-induced increase in DO_2, in terms of peripheral tissue oxygenation. Rational analysis of oxygen consumption/oxygen delivery relationships, combined with serial measurements of blood lactates levels, would help the clinician to assess the effectiveness of vasoactive agents on tissue oxygenation.

References

Bakker J, Coffernils M, Leon M *et al.* (1991) Blood lactate levels are superior to oxygen-derived variables in predicting outcome in human septic shock. *Chest* **99**: 956–62.

Benotti JR, Grossman W, Braunwald E *et al.* (1978) Hemodynamic assessment of amrinone. *New Engl. J. Med.* **299**: 1373–7.

Bersten AD, Gnidec A, Rutledge FS & Sibbald WJ (1990) Hyperdynamic sepsis modifies a PEEP-mediated redistribution in organ blood flows. *Am. Rev. Respiratory Dis.* **141**; 1198–1206.

Bihari D, Smithies M, Gimson A & Tinker J (1987) The effects of vaso-dilation with prostacyclin on oxygen delivery and uptake in critically ill patients. *New Engl. J. Med.* **317:** 397–403.

Bollaert PE, Bauer P, Audibert G *et al.* (1990) Effects of epinephrine on hemodynamics and oxygen metabolism in dopamine-resistant septic shock. *Chest* **98:** 949–53.

Bowton DL, Bertels NH, Prough DS & Stump DA (1989) Cerebral blood flow is reduced in patients with sepsis syndrome. *Crit. Care Med.* **17:** 399–403.

Breslow MJ, Miller CF, Parker SD, Walman AT & Traystman RJ (1987) Effect of vasopressors on organ blood flow during endotoxin shock in pigs. *Am. J. Physiol.* **252:** H291–H300.

Bristow MR, Ginsburg R, Minobe W *et al.* (1982) Decreased catecholamine sensitivity and β-adrenergic receptor density in failing human hearts. *New Eng. J. Med.* **307:** 205–11.

Carrico CJ, Meakins JL, Marshall JC, Fry D & Maier RV (1986) Multiple organ failure syndrome: the gastrointestinal tract: The motor of MOF. *Arch. Surg.* **121:** 196–208.

Colardyn FC, Vandenbogaerde JF, Vogelaers DP & Verbeke JH (1989) Use of dopexamine hydrochloride in patients with septic shock. *Crit. Care Med.* **17:** 999–1003.

Dahn MS, Lange P, Lodbell K *et al.* (1987) Splanchnic and total body oxygen consumption differences in septic and injured patients. *Surgery* **101:** 69–80.

Danek SJ, Lynch JP, Weg JG & Dantzker D (1980) The dependence of oxygen uptake on oxygen delivery in the adult respiratory distress syndrome. *Am. Rev. Respiratory Dis.* **122:** 387–95.

Dantzker D & Gutierrez G (1989) Effects of circulatory failure on pulmonary and tissue gas exchange. In: Scharf S & Cassidy S (eds), *Heart Lung Interactions in Health and Disease*, pp. 983–1019. Dekker, New York.

Desjars P, Pinaud M, Potel G *et al.* (1987) A reappraisal of norepinephrine therapy in human septic shock. *Crit. Care Med.* **15:** 134–7.

Dhainaut JF, Huyghebaert MF, Monsallier JF *et al.* (1987) Coronary hemody-namics and myocardial metabolism of lactate, free fatty acids, glucose, and ketones in patients with septic shock. *Circulation* **75:** 533–41.

Edwards JD (1990) Practical application of oxygen transport principles. *Crit. Care Med.* **18:** S45–8.

Edwards JD, Brown GCS, Nightingale P *et al.* (1989) Use of survivors' cardiorespiratory values as therapeutic goals in septic shock. *Crit. Care Med.* **17:** 1098–103.

Fellows IW, Bennet T & MacDonald IA (1985) The effect of adrenaline upon the cardiovascular and metabolic functions in man. *Clin. Sci.* **69:** 215–22.

Fenwick J. Dodek PM, Ronco JJ *et al.* (1990) Increased concentration of plasma lactate predicts pathologic dependence of oxygen consumption on oxygen delivery in patients with adult respiratory distress syndrome. *J. Crit. Care* **5:** 1–6.

Gage J, Rutman H, Lucido D & LeJemtel TH (1986) Additive effects of dobutamine and amrinone on myocardial contractility and ventricular performance in patients with severe heart failure. *Circulation* **74:** 367–73.

Gilbert EM, Haupt MT, Mandanas RY *et al.* (1986) The effect of fluid loading, blood transfusion, and catecholamine infusion on oxygen delivery and consumption in patients with sepsis. *Am. Rev. Respiratory Dis.* **137**: 873–8.

Gump FE, Price JB Jr, Kinney JM (1977) Whole body and splanchnic blood flow and oxygen consumption measurements in patients with intraperitoneal infection. *Annals Surg.* **171**: 321–28.

Gutierrez G & Pohil RJ (1986) Oxygen consumption is linearly related to O_2 supply in critically ill patients. *J. Crit. Care* **1**: 45–53.

Haupt MT, Bilbert EM & Carlson RW (1985) Fluid loading increases oxygen consumption in septic patients with lactic acidosis. *Am. Rev. Respiratory Dis.* **131**: 912–16.

Installé E, Gonzalez M, Jacquemart JL *et al.* (1987) Comparative effects on hemodynamics of enoximone (MDL, 17, 043), dobutamine and nitroprusside in severe congestive heart failure. *Am. J. Cardiol.* **60**: 46C–52C.

Jardin F, Sportiche M, Bazin M *et al.* (1981) Dobutamine: a hemodynamic evaluation in human septic shock. *Crit. Care Med.* **9**: 329–32.

Jardin F, Genevray B, Brun-Ney D & Margairaz A (1985) Dobutamine: a hemodynamic evaluation in pulmonary embolism shock. *Crit. Care Med.* **13**: 1009–12.

Kox WJ & Brydon C (1991) Improvement of tissue oxygenation with enoximone in septic shock. In Vincent JL (ed.), *Update in Intensive Care and Emergency Medicine*, Vol. 14, Update 1991, pp. 137–43. Berlin, Heidelberg: Springer-Verlag.

Lang CH, Bagby GJ, Ferguson JL & Spitzer JJ (1984) Cardiac output and redistribution of organ blood flow in hypermetabolic sepsis. *Am. J. Phys.* **246**: R331–7.

Lang RM, Carroll JD, Nakamura S *et al.* (1988) Role of adrenoceptors and dopamine receptors in modulating left ventricular diastolic function. *Circ. Res.* **63**: 126–34.

Leier CV (1988) Regional blood flow responses to vasodilators and in inotropes in congestive heart failure. *Am. J. Cardiol.* **62**: 86E–93E.

Leier CV, Heban PT, Huss P *et al.* (1978) Comparative systemic and regional hemodynamic effects of dopamine and dobutamine in patients with cardiomyopathic heart failure. *Circulation* **58**: 466–75.

Lemaire F, Harari A, Rapin M *et al.* (1976) Assessment of gas exchange during VA bypass using the membrane lung. In Zapol W & Qvist J (eds), *Artificial Lungs for Acute Respiratory Failure*, pp. 421–33. New York: Academic Press.

Ludmer PL, Wright RF, Arnold JMO *et al.* (1986) Separation of the direct myocardial and vasodilator actions of milrinone administered by an intracoronary infusion technique. *Circulation* **73**: 130–37.

Lynch JP, Mhyre JG & Dantzker DR (1979) Influence of cardiac output on intrapulmonary shunt. *J. Appl. Physiol.* **46**: 315–22.

Mackenzie SJ, Kapadia F, Nimmo GR *et al.* (1991) Adrenaline in treatment of septic shock: effects on haemodynamics and oxygen transport. *Intensive Care Med.* **17**: 36–9.

Meadows D, Edwards JD, Wilkins RG & Nightingale P (1988) Reversal of intractable septic shock with norepinephrine therapy. *Crit. Care Med.* **16:** 663–6.

Molloy DW, Ducas J, Dobson K *et al.* (1986) Hemodynamic management in clinical acute hypoxemic respiratory failure: dopamine versus dobutamine. *Chest* **89:** 636–40.

Moshenifar Z, Amin D, Jasper AC *et al.* (1987) Dependence of oxygen consumption on oxygen delivery in patients with chronic congestive heart failure. *Chest* **92:** 447–50.

Nelson DP, Samsel RW, Wood LDH, Schumacker PT (1988) Pathological supply dependence of systemic and intestinal O_2 uptake during endotoxemia. *J. Appl. Phys.* **64:** 2410–19.

Parker MM, Shelhamer JH, Bacharach SL *et al.* (1984) Profound but reversible myocardial depression in patients with septic shock. *Ann. Intern. Med.* **100:** 483–90.

Pease RD, Benumof JL & Trousdale FE (1982) PAO_2 and PvO_2 interaction on hypoxic pulmonary vasoconstriction. *J. Appl. Physiol.* **53:** 134–9.

Pittet JF, Lacroix JS, Gunning K *et al.* (1990) Prostacyclin but not phentolamine increases oxygen consumption and skin microvascular blood flow in patients with sepsis and respiratory failure. *Chest* **98:** 1467–72.

Pouleur H, Covell JW & Ross J Jr (1980) Effects of nitroprusside of venous return and central blood volume in the absence and presence of acute heart failure. *Circulation* **61:** 328–37.

Radermacher P, Huet Y, Pluskwa F *et al.* (1988) Comparison of ketanserin and sodium nitroprusside in patients with severe ARDS. *Anesthesiology* **68:** 152–7.

Radermacher P, Santak B, Becker H & Falke KJ (1989) Prostaglandin E_1 and nitroglycerin reduce pulmonary capillary pressure but worsen ventilation-perfusion distribution in patients with adult respiratory distress syndrome. *Anesthesiology* **70:** 601–6.

Ranieri VM, Giuliani R, Eissa NT *et al.* (1992) Oxygen delivery-consumption relationship in septic adult respiratory distress syndrome patients: the effects of positive end-expiratory pressure. *J. Crit. Care* **7:** 150–7.

Regnier B, Safran D, Carlet J & Teisseire (1979) Comparative haemodynamic effects of dopamine and dobutamine in septic shock. *Intens. Care Med.* **5:** 115–20.

Reinhart K, Hannemann L & Kuss B (1990) Optimal oxygen delivery in critically ill patients. *Intensive Care Med.* **16:** S149–55.

Richard C, Ricome JL, Rimailho A *et al.* (1983) Combined hemodynamic effects of dopamine and dobutamine in cardiogenic shock. *Circulation* **67:** 620–6.

Ronco JJ, Phang PT, Walley KR *et al.* (1991) Oxygen consumption is dependent of changes in oxygen delivery in severe adult respiratory distress syndrome. *Am. Rev. Respiratory Dis.* **143:** 1267–73.

Ronco JJ, Fenwick JC, Wiggs BR *et al.* (1993) Oxygen consumption is independent of increases in oxygen delivery by dobutamine in septic patients who have normal or increased plasma lactate. *Am. Rev. Respiratory Dis.* **147:** 25–31.

Russell JA, Ronco JJ, Lockhat D *et al.* (1990) Oxygen delivery and consumption and ventricular preload are greater in survivors than in nonsurvivors of the adult respiratory distress syndrome. *Am. Rev. Respiratory Dis.* **141**: 659–65.

Sandoval J, Long GR, Skood C *et al.* (1983) Independent influence of blood flow rate and mixed venous PO_2 on shunt fraction. *J. Appl. Physiol.* **55**: 1128–33.

Shoemaker WC, Montgomery ES, Kaplan E & Elwyn DH (1973) Physiologic patterns in surviving and nonsurviving shock patients: use of sequential cardiorespiratory variables in defining criteria for therapeutic goals and early warning of death. *Arch. Surgery* **106**: 630–6.

Shoemaker WC, Appel PL & Kram HB (1986) Hemodynamic and oxygen transport effects of dobutamine in critically ill general surgical patients. *Crit. Care Med.* **14**: 1032–7.

Shoemaker WC, Appel PL, Kram HB *et al.* (1988) Prospective trial of supranormal values of survivors as therapeutic goals in high-risk surgical patients. *Chest* **94**: 1176–86.

Shoemaker WC, Appel PL, Kram HB *et al.* (1989) Comparison of hemodynamic and oxygen transport effects of dopamine and dobutamine in critically ill surgical patients. *Chest* **96**: 120–6.

Sibbald WJ, Fox G & Martin C (1991) Abnormalities of vascular reactivity in the sepsis syndrome. *Chest* **100**: 155S–59S.

Siegel JII, Greenspan M & Del Guercio LRM (1967) Abnormal vascular tone, defective oxygen transport and myocardial failure in human septic shock. *Annals Surg.* **165**: 504–17.

Silverman HJ, Slotman G, Bone RC *et al.* (1990) Effects of prostaglandin E_1 on oxygen delivery and consumption in patients with the adult respiratory distress syndrome. Results from the prostaglandin E_1 multicenter trial. *Chest* **98**: 405–10.

Smith GW & Filcek SAL (1989) Dopexamine hydrochloride: a novel dopamine receptor agonist for the acute treatment of low cardiac output states. *Cardiovascular Drug Rev.* **7**: 141–59.

Takala J & Ruokoren E (1991) Blood flow and adrenergic drugs in septic shock. In JL Vincent (Ed). *Update in Intensive Care and Emergency Medicine.* Vol 14 Update 1991, pp. 144–52. Berlin Heidelberg: Springer-Verlag.

Teboul JL, Annane D, Thuillez C *et al.* (1992) Effects of cardiovascular drugs on oxygen consumption/oxygen delivery relationship in patients with congestive heart failure. *Chest* **101**: 1582–7.

Teboul JL, Graini L, Boujdaria R, Berton C & Richard C (1993) Cardiac index versus oxygen-derived parameters for rational use of dobutamine in patients with congestive heart failure. *Chest* **103**: 81–5.

Thijs LG & Groeneveld ABJ (1988) Peripheral circulation in septic shock. *Appl. Cardiopulm. Pathophys.* **2**: 203–14.

Thuillez C, Richard C, Teboul JL *et al.* (1993) Arterial hemodynamics and cardiac effects of enoximone, dobutamine and their combination in severe heart failure. *Am. Heart J.* (in press).

Tuchschmidt J, Fried J, Swinney R & Sharma OMP (1989) Early hemodynamic correlates of survival in patients with septic shock. *Crit. Care Med.* **17**: 719–723.

Tuchschmidt J, Fried J, Astiz M & Rackow E (1992) Elevation of cardiac output and oxygen delivery improves outcome in septic shock. *Chest* **102:** 216–20.

Vermeij CG, Feenstra BWA & Bruining HA (1990) Oxygen delivery and oxygen uptake in postoperative and septic patients. *Chest* **98:** 415–20.

Vincent JL, Van der Linden P, Domb M *et al.* (1987) Dopamine compared with dobutamine in experimental septic shock: relevance to fluid administration. *Anaesthesia Analgesia* **66:** 565–71.

Vincent JL, Carlier E, Berré J *et al.* (1988) Administration of enoximone in cardiogenic shock. *Am. J. Cardiol.* **62:** 419–23.

Vincent JL, Reuse C & Kahn RJ (1989) Administration of dopexamine, a new adrenergic agent, in cardiorespiratory failure. *Chest* **96:** 1233–6.

Vincent JL, Roman A & Kahn RJ (1990a) Oxygen uptake/supply dependency: effects of short term dobutamine infusion. *Am. Rev. Respiratory Dis.* **142:** 2–7.

Vincent JL, Roman A & Kahn RJ (1990b) Dobutamine administration in septic shock: addition to a standard protocol. *Crit. Care Med.* **18:** 689–93.

Voelkel NF (1986) Mechanisms of hypoxic pulmonary vasoconstriction. *Am. Rev. Respiratory Dis.* **133:** 1186–95.

11 The Effects of Sedative Drugs

P. van der Linden and J.-L. Vincent

Introduction

Sedation and analgesia in the intensive care unit (ICU) are often essential for patients' comfort and safety. Most critically ill patients are subjected to pain, stress, and also anxiety from appreciation of the severity of their illness and environmental noise. Moreover, treatment procedures such as endotracheal intubation, mechanical ventilation, tracheal suction, wound dressings, chest and physical therapy, or even toilet can represent additional sources of discomfort.

Various sedative and analgesic agents have been used in the ICU. In the United Kingdom, a recent postal survey (Bion & Ledingham, 1987) showed that 37% of ICUs use opioids alone for routine sedation, and another 60% use an association of an opioid and a benzodiazepine. Etomidate was also very popular until it was found to suppress adrenal steroidogenesis and increase the risk of infection (Watt & Ledingham, 1984). Inhaled agents may be valuable (Kong et al., 1989), but their safety in this context has not been proved and an efficient scavenging of such agents in the ICUs remains difficult. Recently, propofol (2,6-di-isopropylphenol), an intravenous anaesthetic agent with a short half-life, has been also proposed for sedation in intensive care (Newman et al., 1987; Aitkenhead et al., 1989).

The use of loco-regional analgesia has been also recommended. Among the different techniques used to control pain related to trauma or surgical procedures, epidural analgesia is the most frequently used (Lutz & Lamer, 1990). This technique has sometimes been shown to provide better comfort than systemic analgesia and to decrease post-operative complications (Rawal et al., 1984; Yeager et al., 1987). Intermittent injections are used in many centres, but continuous infusion is becoming the preferred method, because it provides a constant level of analgesia, minimizes side-effects, and helps to prevent tachyphylaxis.

The present review will focus on the effects of these agents on tissue oxygen supply–demand relationship and their practical implications.

The Effects of Sedative Agents on Oxygen Demand

Sedation and anaesthesia are considered to decrease whole body oxygen consumption ($\dot{V}O_2$), but the magnitude of this effect is not well-defined. The available studies differ markedly in experimental protocol and the choice of a control reference. Most studies on the effects of anaesthesia on $\dot{V}O_2$ refer to pre-induction values. However, pre-operative $\dot{V}O_2$ is generally higher than resting $\dot{V}O_2$, due to anxiety and pathological conditions. The decrease in $\dot{V}O_2$ observed after induction of anaesthesia is greater if $\dot{V}O_2$ was high before anaesthesia (Shackman et al., 1951). After administration of 0.5 mg kg^{-1} of morphine in critically ill patients, Rouby et al. (1981) observed that $\dot{V}O_2$ decreased by 21% in patients with initially elevated $\dot{V}O_2$ and by only 9% in patients with initially normal $\dot{V}O_2$. Sedation and anaesthesia are frequently associated with a decrease in body temperature, which contributes to reduced $\dot{V}O_2$ (Hall, 1978).

Mechanical ventilation is frequently applied during sedational and analgesia and results in a decrease of the oxygen demand of the respiratory muscles (Nunn & Matthews, 1959). The reduction in stress is followed by a decrease in sympathetic activity (Roisen et al., 1981), and thus in metabolic activity.

Swinamer et al. (1988) showed that routine administration of morphine significantly decreased total energy expenditure in critically ill patients. However, anaesthetic agents do not appear to decrease cell metabolism below the physiologic range and cannot be considered as general metabolic depressants. Mikat et al. (1984) measured whole body O_2 consumption in awake, sleeping and anaesthetized dogs, and observed that deep anaesthesia with either methohexital, thiopental, etomidate or halothane reduced $\dot{V}O_2$ relative to the resting alert state, but increased $\dot{V}O_2$ relative to natural sleep.

During epidural anaesthesia, $\dot{V}O_2$ might also be reduced by the diminished sympathetic tone, as catecholamines play an important role in setting the metabolic rate (Jansky, 1966). $\dot{V}O_2$ levels immediately after surgery have been reported to be lower during regional than during general anaesthesia (Renck, 1969). Reinhart (1991) observed comparable per- and post-operative $\dot{V}O_2$ in patients undergoing infrarenal aortic surgery with thoracic epidural anaesthesia or neuroleptanalgesia, but both groups of patients received analgesia and sedation in the post-operative period.

In a recent study on the effects of various anaesthetic agents on the oxygen supply–demand relationship in a dog model of progressive haemorrhage (Van der Linden et al., 1991b) oxygen demand was assessed by the value of $\dot{V}O_2$ at critical oxygen delivery and by the slope of the supply-independent line (Cain, 1991). Of the anaesthetic agents tested (halothane, enflurane, isoflurane, alfentanil and ketamine), none decreased oxygen demand when compared to a control group. The study of Theye and Michenfelter (1975) also supports the view that anaesthetic agents are not metabolic depressants but that the observed changes in whole body $\dot{V}O_2$ reflect the sum of changes in individual organ consumption resulting from anaesthetic-induced changes in organ function.

The Effects of Sedative Agents on Oxygen Transport

The effects of sedative agents on oxygen transport ($\dot{D}O_2$) are primarily related to their effects on cardiac output. These agents also produce a dose-dependent respiratory depression, which can sometimes decrease PaO_2 and artery oxygen content.

Inhaled Agents

All modern inhaled anaesthetics have comparable dose-dependent negative inotropic properties (Heinrich et al., 1986; Hickey & Eger, 1986) but have different effects on peripheral circulation. Indeed, isoflurane induces more profound peripheral vasodilation than halothane and enflurane (Eger et al., 1970; Stevens et al., 1971; Calverley et al., 1978; Jones, 1984), so that cardiac output is better preserved with this agent. Moreover, isoflurane influences heart rate less than halothane or enflurane, which have parasympathicomimetic properties and direct depressant effects on cardiac tissue conduction (Hickey & Eger, 1986). All inhaled agents also blunt the baroreflex control of heart rate in a dose-dependent fashion (Jones, 1984).

Opioids

With the possible exception of meperidine, opioids are characterized by a remarkable cardiovascular stability. In humans, up to 3 mg kg^{-1} of morphine or 50–100 µg kg^{-1} of fentanyl have little effect on myocardial function (Lowenstein et al., 1972; Lunn et al., 1979; Bovill et al., 1984). Administration of even moderate doses (less than 10 mg i.v.) of morphine may be occasionally associated with hypotension (Drew et al., 1946). The mechanism involved is unclear and probably multifactorial; the underlying disease of the patient and the rate of morphine administration may be important (Bovill et al., 1984). An important cause is probably a decrease in systemic vascular resistance secondary to histamine release (Philbin et al., 1981; Roscow et al., 1982). Another cause may be morphine-induced reduction in venous and arterial tone and decrease in venous return to the heart (Lowenstein et al., 1969, 1972). These vasodilating effects may be due to a direct effect of morphine, as well as histamine, on vascular smooth muscle (Lowenstein et al., 1972; Zelis et al., 1974; Hsu et al., 1979; Rosow et al., 1982). Arterial dilation occurs sooner and is of shorter duration than venodilation (Rosow et al., 1982). Hypotension rarely occurs with fentanyl or it newer derivatives, sufentanil (5–10 times more potent than fentanyl) and alfentanil ($\frac{1}{5}$–$\frac{1}{10}$ less potent than fentanyl), possibly because, unlike morphine, they do not cause histamine release (Rosow et al., 1982).

Except for meperidine, the intravenous injection of opioids produces bradycardia (Liu et al., 1976; Reitan et al., 1978; Bovill et al., 1984). Tachycardia occasionally occurs after administration of morphine, and is then usually associated with facial and upper torso flushing, related to histamine release (Rosow et al., 1982). Opioid-induced bradycardia may be, to some extent, related to the dose (Reitan et al., 1978), and also the speed of injection (Bovill et al., 1984). The mechanism is not fully understood, but stimulation of the central vagal nucleus seems to be involved (Reitan et al., 1978), since it is almost entirely blocked by bilateral vagotomy (Reitan et al., 1978) or pharmacologic vagal block with atropine (Liu et al., 1976). Morphine is also thought to have a direct depressant effect on the sinoatrial node (Urthaler et al., 1975) and to depress the atrioventricular conduction, which may account for some anti-arrhythmic action of the drug (De Silva et al., 1978). Fentanyl is likely to have a similar action.

If adequate analgesia can be obtained relatively easily, sedation and amnesia are more difficult to achieve or require high dosages, which may prolong respiratory depression. Therefore, opioids are often combined with other drugs, like benzodiazepines or droperidol. Surprisingly, Stanley and Webster reported that the intravenous administration of 10 mg diazepam after fentanyl decreased cardiac output and arterial blood pressure, and increased central venous pressure (Stanley & Webster, 1978). Similar results have been found in other studies, irrespective of the dosage or sequence of fentanyl or diazepam administration (Tomischek et al., 1982; Reves et al., 1984), or when fentanyl was associated with midazolam (Heikkila et al., 1984). Significant reduction in arterial blood pressure has also been reported when a high dose of morphine was associated with diazepam (Stanley et al., 1975). The mechanisms by which such combinations result in cardiovascular depression are not clear but may be related to the sympatholytic action of this association. Tomischek et al. (1982) found that the administration of 50 µg kg^{-1} of fentanyl after diazepam significantly decreased plasma concentrations of adrenaline and noradrenaline, when compared to a control group receiving fentanyl alone.

Interestingly, the combination of a major tranquillizer like droperidol with fentanyl, the so-called neuroleptanalgesia, is usually characterized by analgesia, absence of clinically apparent motor activity, suppression of autonomic reflexes, maintenance of cardiovascular stability (Stanley et al., 1975; Stoelting et al., 1975), and amnesia. However, this is not obtained in all patients. The commercial preparation of droperidol and fentanyl (Innovar or Thalamonal) has gained widespread popularity in anaesthesia, probably because it can maintain cardiovascular stability in major surgical procedures (Corssen et al., 1965; Morgan et al., 1974).

Benzodiazepines

The three most common parenteral benzodiazepines used in intensive care are diazepam, lorazepam and midazolam. The low hepatic clearance of diazepam and lorazepam results in terminal elimination half-lives of 20–40 and 10–20 h, respectively (White, 1988). In contrast, midazolam is more rapidly and extensively metabolized by the hepatic microsomal system (Reves et al., 1985), resulting in a shorter elimination half-life of 2–4 h. Therefore, recovery can be more rapidly obtained with midazolam administered either by repeated doses or continuous infusions. When administered alone, benzodiazepines have limited cardiovascular effects (Rao et al., 1973; Reves et al., 1985, 1986). However, they can induce some venodilation, resulting in a decrease of venous return (Reves et al., 1986). Midazolam is also known to decrease peripheral vascular resistance, so that hypotension may occasionally occur after a bolus injection (Reves et al., 1985).

Unfortunately, the combination of benzodiazepines and opioids, even though it can control agitation and decrease the opioid analgesic requirement (Stanley & Webster, 1978), decreases myocardial contractility in isolated muscle experiments (Reves et al., 1984) and causes significant depression of arterial blood pressure and cardiac output (Stanley et al., 1975; Stanley & Webster, 1978; Tomischek et al., 1982; Heikkila et al., 1984).

Etomidate

Etomidate is a carboxylated imidazole-containing compound that is structurally unrelated to any other intravenous anaesthetic. Its clearance rate is 5 times that of thiopental and contributes to a shorter elimination half-life of 2–5 h (White, 1988). Like benzodiazepines, it lacks analgesic properties but possesses anticonvulsant activity. Intravenous injection of etomidate produces rapid loss of consciousness with minimal cardiovascular changes. Studies in normal individuals and in patients with heart disease document the remarkable haemodynamic stability after administration of etomidate (Kessler et al., 1979; Reves et al., 1986). Etomidate does not markedly alter heart rate or cardiac output, although slight decreases in blood pressure might result from a decrease in peripheral vascular resistance (Giese & Stanley, 1983). In dogs, etomidate does not demonstrate negative inotropic effect (Brüssel et al., 1989; Riou et al., 1990). Moreover, the cardiovascular effects of etomidate are not significantly altered by the simultaneous administration of other anaesthetic drugs, such as opioides (Reves et al., 1986).

Propofol

Propofol (2,6-di-isopropylphenol) is the newest short-acting intravenous anaesthetic agent. Pharmacokinetic parameters seem unaltered by renal or hepatic disease, but its clearance is significantly lower in elderly patients (Sebel & Lowdon, 1989). When used as a long-term infusion for sedation in ICU patients, its terminal elimination half-life is significantly prolonged (Albanese *et al.*, 1990). Although propofol may not possess analgesic properties, in contrast to barbiturates agents, it does not appear to decrease the analgesic threshold (White, 1988). Administration of propofol is often associated with marked decreases in arterial blood pressure in humans (Coates *et al.*, 1987; Claeys *et al.*, 1988; Van Aken *et al.*, 1988), which is usually associated with reductions in cardiac output and systemic vascular resistance (Cullen *et al.*, 1987; Lepage *et al.*, 1988; Brüssel *et al.*, 1989). The peripheral effects of propofol have been related to a direct effect of the drug on the vascular smooth muscle. Propofol can also alter the baroreflex activity (Brüssel *et al.*, 1989). Cullen *et al.* (1987) observed that propofol/nitrous oxide anaesthesia does not impair baroreflex sensitivity, but that central sympatholytic and/or vagotonic mechanisms maintain low heart rates despite the decrease in arterial pressure. In addition, propofol had significant negative inotropic properties in animals (Brüssel *et al.*, 1989) and in humans (Mulier *et al.*, 1991). When given as a single bolus, the cardiopressant effects of propofol are more pronounced and more prolonged than those of equipotent doses of thiopental (Mulier *et al.*, 1991). Therefore, propofol may decrease cardiac output and DO_2 both by a reduction in myocardial contractility and by a reduction in cardiac preload associated with its peripheral effects (Lepage *et al.*, 1988).

Ketamine

Ketamine is characterized by unique cardiovascular stimulant properties (White *et al.*, 1982; Tokics *et al.*, 1983) related to a direct central sympathomimetic effect (Ivankowitch *et al.*, 1974). Administration of ketamine is associated with a dose-related increase in heart rate, arterial blood pressure and cardiac index, without change in stroke index (Tokics *et al.*, 1983). The effects of ketamine on myocardial contractility are dose-related (Riou *et al.*, 1989). At low dose, ketamine appears to have a positive inotropic effect, while at high, supratherapeutic concentration, it could have negative inotropic effect related to an inhibition of the sarcoplasmic reticulum function. However, the simultaneous use of other anaesthetic agents, in an attempt to reduce the frequency of emergence reactions, may profoundly alter the cardiovascular effects of ketamine. Indeed, stimulating properties of ketamine are blocked by the addition of barbiturates (Ivankowitch *et al.*, 1974), benzodiazepines or inhaled agents (Lilburn *et al.*, 1978).

Epidural analgesia

Epidural analgesia using local anaesthetic agents is particularly helpful in patients with acute trauma or in the post-operative period. However, marked cardiovascular depression can be associated with epidural anaesthesia alone or in combination with general anaesthesia (Bonica *et al.*, 1972; Reiz *et al.*, 1979). This has been attributed to a reduction in peripheral vascular resistance secondary to diminished sympathetic tone and a decrease in venous return (Bromage, 1967). If upper thoracic segments (T1–T5) are involved in the block, the reduction in sympathetic outflow to the heart may contribute to a reduction in cardiac output and thus $\dot{D}O_2$ (Reiz *et al.*, 1979). Comparing thoracic epidural anaesthesia to neuroleptanalgesia in patients undergoing abdominal aortic surgery, Reinhart *et al.* (1989) observed that epidural anaesthesia was associated with lower cardiac output and mixed venous O_2 saturation ($S\bar{v}O_2$) than neuroleptanalgesia, while $\dot{V}O_2$ was comparable in both groups. As cardiac filling pressures and peripheral vascular resistance were similar in the two groups, the lower cardiac output during epidural anaesthesia was attributed to the negative inotropic and chronotropic effects of the sympathetic blockade. Depression of baroreflex activity has also been reported with epidural anaesthesia, even without blockade of sympathetic efferents to the heart, and has been attributed to enhanced vagal tone (Baron *et al.*, 1986).

Epidural analgesia with opioid agents provides analgesia that is superior to systemic narcotic administration, and has a lesser incidence of side-effects when properly monitored (Lutz & Lamer, 1990). The major advantage of the use of opioids over local anaesthetics for spinal anaesthesia is the absence of motor and sympathetic blockade. However, the most serious side-effect remains respiratory depression. Close monitoring by well-trained nurses is imperative to detect this problem. Because opioids and local anaesthetic agents differ in sites of action, the combination of these agents reduces the dosage requirements for each agent and therefore decrease the potential toxicity.

Among the various other factors that may influence the effects of sedative agents on $\dot{D}O_2$, the underlying clinical status is an important one. Indeed, patients who are stressed because of pain or anxiety can experience a severe decrease in $\dot{D}O2$ when sympatholysis is induced by the sedation. Hypovolaemia may also be hidden by the patient's stress and could also lead to severe hypotension during sedation. Pre-existing cardiovascular diseases and their treatment may also enhance the cardiovascular depression induced by sedative agents (Dauchot *et al.*, 1976).

Effects of Sedative Agents on the $\dot{D}O_2/\dot{V}O_2$ Relationship

The effects of sedative agents on the oxygen supply–demand relationship can be relatively complex. Rouby *et al.* (1981) observed that the administration of $0.5\,\text{mg}\,\text{kg}^{-1}$ of morphine in critically ill patients decreased both $\dot{D}O_2$ and $\dot{V}O_2$, but oxygen extraction ratio did not change, suggesting that the decrease in $\dot{V}O_2$ was caused by a decrease in O_2 demand rather than by an inadequate $\dot{D}O_2$. In patients undergoing aortic surgery, Reinhart *et al.*, (1989) observed that cardiac output and $\dot{D}O_2$ were generally lower during epidural anaesthesia than during neuroleptanalgesia. $S\bar{v}O_2$ was also lower in the epidural group, indicating comparable $\dot{V}O_2$ in both groups. They concluded that the matching of $\dot{D}O_2$ to tissue needs was poorer with epidural anaesthesia than with neuroleptanalgesia.

During experimental endotoxic shock in dogs, the effects of several anaesthetic agents – halothane, enflurane, isoflurane, alfentanil and ketamine – on the $\dot{D}O_2/\dot{V}O_2$ relationship were studied (Van der Linden *et al.*, 1990, 1991a). Intravenous fluids were administered throughout the studying period to maintain cardiac filling pressures at baseline level. In these conditions, $\dot{D}O_2$ was well-maintained but $\dot{V}O_2$ decreased in all anaesthetized groups. Serum lactate increased with all anaesthetic agents, except ketamine (Fig. 11.1). It thus appeared in these experimental conditions, that the decrease in $\dot{V}O_2$ was associated with a worsening of tissue hypoxia, suggesting that the tissue extraction capabilities had been altered by the anaesthetic agents.

Similar conclusions have been proposed by Shibutani *et al.* (1983) who examined the relationship between $\dot{D}O_2$ and $\dot{V}O_2$ in patients undergoing coronary artery bypass graft surgery. They observed that, when $\dot{D}O_2$ was lower than a critical value of $330\,\mathrm{ml\,min^{-1}\,m^{-2}}$, the $\dot{V}O_2$ decreased in proportion to the decrease in $\dot{D}O_2$, while mixed venous O_2 saturation remained relatively high. They suggested that anaesthetic agents may interfere with mechanisms redistributing blood flow to adapt oxygen extraction to the limited oxygen supply.

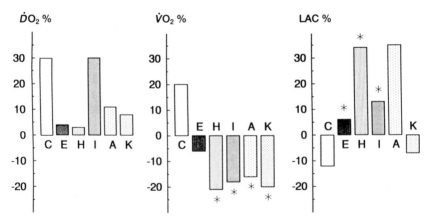

Figure 11.1   Effects of anaesthetic agents on oxygen transport ($\dot{D}O_2$), oxygen consumption ($\dot{V}O_2$) and serum lactate (LAC) during endotoxic shock in the dog. Data represent relative changes observed after 2 h of administration of the anaesthetic agent. C, Control; H; halothane; E, enflurane; I, isoflurane; A, alfentanil; k, ketamine. *$P < 0.05$ versus control group. (Adapted from Van der Linden *et al.*, 1990, 1991a.)

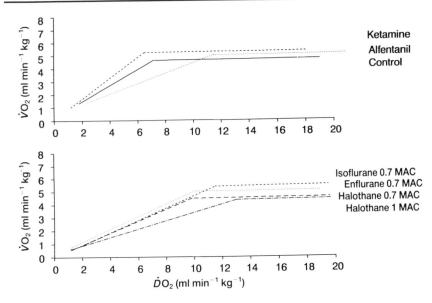

Figure 11.2 Schematic representation of the effects of anaesthetic agents on the $\dot{V}O_2/\dot{D}O_2$ relationship. Critical $\dot{D}O_2$ were control: 7.26 ± 0.55 ml min^{-1} kg^{-1}; alfentanil: 11.54 ± 1.30 ml min^{-1} kg^{-1}; ketamine: 6.56 ± 0.62 ml min^{-1} kg^{-1}; isoflurane: 11.43 ± 1.86 ml min^{-1} kg^{-1}; enflurane: 9.99 ± 1.02 ml min^{-1} kg^{-1}; halothane 0.7 MAC: 9.56 ± 0.82 ml min^{-1} kg^{-1}; and halothane 1 MAC: 1302 ± 2.24 ml min^{-1} kg^{-1}. (Adapted from van der Linden *et al.*, 1991b).

A recent study looked at the effects of the most commonly used anaesthetic agents, i.e. halothane, enflurane, isoflurane, alfentanil and ketamine, on tissue O_2 extraction capabilities on a dog model of progressive haemorrhage (Van der Linden *et al.*, 1991b). In each animal, the oxygen supply/demand relationship was determined from independent measurements of $\dot{D}O_2$ and $\dot{V}O_2$, and the critical O_2 transport ($\dot{D}O_2$crit) was determined from a plot of $\dot{V}O_2$ versus $\dot{D}O_2$. It was observed that all aneasthetic agents but ketamine decreased tissue O_2 extraction capabilities in a dose-related manner. When oxygen supply is acutely curtailed, several central and peripheral vascular mechanisms take place, allowing the organism to adapt its oxygen extraction capabilities to tissue oxygen demand (Cain, 1991; Schlichtig *et al.*, 1991). Alteration of these mechanisms, at the regional or the microcirculatory level, can decrease the oxygen extraction capabilities of the tissues and lead to an abnormal oxygen supply dependency. The deleterious effects observed with most anaesthetic agents are probably in part related to their peripheral vasodilating effects. Determination of systemic vascular resistance at critical point revealed that the most vasodilating agents also had the most deleterious effect on $\dot{D}O_2$crit (Van der Linden *et al.*, 1991b) (Fig. 11.2). The effects of anaesthetic agents on the sympathetic system might also be involved. Among the anaesthetic agents studied, ketamine had the unique property to increase extraction capabilities at low dose and to decrease it at high dose. These effects might be due to the unique centrally mediated sympathomimetic action of this agent while other anaesthetic agents tested all decreased sympathetic activity.

Using a similar model, the effects of three other anaesthetic agents – etomidate, propofol and pentobarbital – on tissue extraction capabilities were also compared (Van der Linden et al., 1993). Each agent was administered as a continuous infusion to maintain a stable level of anaesthesia. In these conditions, etomidate altered tissue O_2 extraction less than did propofol and pentobarbital. An improvement in blood flow distribution might be related to a more appropriate adrenal stress response with etomidate. Indeed, despite comparable effects on vascular tone, the overall cardiovascular response to acute bleeding was better preserved with etomidate than with propofol or pentobarbital.

In summary, most of the routinely used anaesthetic agents can alter tissue O_2 extraction capabilities in a dose-dependent manner by direct vascular effects and or by blunting neurohumoral reflexes. In some clinical circumstances, like sepsis, where the ability of the tissues to extract oxygen can be already altered, the use of anaesthetic agents might aggravate tissue hypoxia by adding its own effects to the underlying defect.

Clinical Implications

In view of the various properties of the different sedative agents available, the choice of an adequate agent remains difficult. There is certainly not one agent of choice for all situations. Some agents, like opioids, provide good analgesia but poor sedation. Others, like benzodiazepines or propofol, provide no analgesia but good sedation. Combination of these two types of agents, by reducing the dose of each agent, decreases the incidence of side-effects, like prolonged respiratory depression. In these conditions, propofol has been found to represent a satisfactory agent which compares favourably with midazolam (Aitkenhead et al., 1989). Recovery of consciousness was more predictable and weaning from mechanical ventilation was achieved significantly faster after discontinuation of propofol than of midazolam (Aitkenhead et al., 1989).

Among the opioids, morphine is probably the most commonly used to provide analgesia in ICU patients. However, alfentanil could be preferable for its remarkable cardiovascular stability and, in particular, its lack of histaminoliberation. Moreover, its rapid elimination and short duration of action could make it more suitable for continuous infusion.

Etomidate produces transient suppression of adrenal steroidogenesis resulting from enzymatic blockade (Fragen et al., 1984). If this phenomenon contraindicated prolonged infusions of etomidate, bolus or short infusions (30–90 min) have been found useful in some conditions (Urquhart & White, 1989).

Despite its undesirable psychomimetic (emergence) reactions, ketamine given as a continuous infusion has been found extremely effective for sedation of mechanically ventilated patients in the ICU (White, 1988).

Finally, epidural analgesia has been shown to be associated with fewer post-operative complications than parenteral administration of analgesic agents (Lutz & Lamer, 1990).

Clearly, the use of sedative agents in the ICU requires careful titration and adequate monitoring. Drug infusions must be titrated to obtain both tranquillity and cooperation from most of the patients. There may be a tendency to give sedative agents at a rate which produces excessive sedation with a risk of delay in the recovery of consciousness and prolonged respiratory depression. Most authors recommend the use of continuous infusion rather than repeated boluses to allow a better control of the clinical effects, a lower total dose requirement and a more rapid recovery (Pathak et al., 1983; Urquhart & White, 1989). Assessment of sedation and adaptation of the rate of infusion must be performed hourly.

Most of the sedative agents used in the ICU will decrease O_2 demand and $\dot{D}O_2$, but the effects on these two parameters might not be proportional. Sedative agents decrease oxygen demand by two mechanisms. First, the abolition of pain and stress decrease sympathetic outflow, and thus the metabolic rate of the cells. Second, sedative agents reduce the organ function, even though they do not decrease cellular metabolism below the physiologic range (Mikat et al., 1984).

Sedative agents can decrease $\dot{D}O_2$ by altering cardiac output both directly by their cardiovascular effects and indirectly by a reduction in the nociceptive stimuli. These effects can be dramatically increased in patients with hypovolaemia or with poor myocardial function. Sedative agents can also alter blood oxygenation by their dose-related respiratory depression effects. When oxygen supply to the tissues is reduced, oxygen extraction ratio must increase to maintain oxygen demand at an adequate level. However, most sedative agents alter tissue O_2 extraction capabilities so that an acute decrease in $\dot{D}O_2$ may not be compensated and tissue hypoxia might develop. This could represent a particular problem in the septic patient. Septic shock is characterized by increased metabolism, decreased tissue extraction capabilities and myocardial depression. In these conditions sedative agents will add their own effects and might worsen tissue hypoxia.

For all these reasons, tissue oxygen balance should be carefully assessed when sedative agents are administered in critically ill patients. Unfortunately there is no single parameter which could directly reflect the adequacy of tissue oxygenation. Measurement of arterial oxygen saturation via pulse oximetry obviously gives no information on the state of tissue oxygenation, but can detect an impairment in arterial oxygenation, related, for example, to respiratory depression. Measurements of blood lactate concentration can detect the presence of tissue hypoxia. Determination of oxygen transport and oxygen consumption requires the use of invasive haemodynamic monitoring to produce measurements of cardiac output and mixed venous oxygen saturation. When some doubt exists about the tissue O_2 extraction capabilities, $\dot{V}O_2$ can be challenged to detect the persistence of tissue hypoxia (Vincent, 1991). In critically ill patients who do not need pulmonary artery catheterization, the continuous measurement of a central vein oxygen saturation has been suggested, using a fibre-optic device incorporated in a central venous catheter (Reinhart, 1991). However, the venous saturation is not the same in the superior vena cava and in the pulmonary artery. This information is, in any case, of limited value in the absence of simultaneous measurement of cardiac output.

Sedation and analgesia in the intensive care unit is essential for patients' comfort and safety. There is no ideal sedative agent, but some agents are better adapted in certain clinical circumstances than others. Adequate sedation and analgesia might also decrease the frequency of complications if proper titration and careful monitoring is performed. Sedative agents, like anaesthetic agents, are expected to reduce both oxygen demand and oxygen delivery. With the possible exception of ketamine, they are all likely to alter the extraction capabilities of the tissues and this limitation cannot be neglected in the critically ill patient.

References

Aitkenhead AR, Willats SM, Park GR et al. (1989) Comparison of propofol and midazolam for sedation in critically ill patients. Lancet 704–9.

Albanese J, Martin C, Lacarelle B et al. (1990) Pharmacokinetics of long term propofal infusion used for sedation in ICU patients. Anesthesiology 73: 214–17.

Baron JF, Decaux-Jacolot A, Edouard A et al. (1986) Influence of venous return on baroreflex control of heart rate during lombar epidural anesthesia in humans. Anesthesiology 64: 188–93.

Bion JF & Ledingham IMcA (1987) Sedation in intensive care – a postal survey. Intensive Care Med. 13: 215–16.

Bonica JJ, Kennedy WF & Gerbershagen HU (1972) Circulatory effects of peridural block. III. Effects of acute blood loss. Anesthesiology 36: 514–18.

Bovill JG, Sebel PS & Stanley TH (1984) Opioid analgesics in anesthesia: with special reference to their use in cardiovascular anaesthesia. Anesthesiology 61: 731–55.

Bromage PR (1967) Physiology and pharmacology of epidural analgesia. Anesthesiology 28: 582–622.

Brüssel T, Theissen JL, Vigfusson G *et al.* (1989) Hemodynamic and cardiodynamic effects of propofol and etomidate: negative inotropic properties of propofol. *Anesthesia Analgesia* **69:** 35–40.

Cain SM (1991) Physiological and pathological oxygen supply dependency. In Gutierrez G & Vincent JL (eds), *Tissue Oxygen Utilization,* pp. 114–23. Berlin, Heidelberg: Springer-Verlag.

Calverley RK, Smith NT & Prys-Roberts C (1978) Cardiovascular effects of enflurane anesthesia during controlled ventilation in man. *Anesthesia Analgesia* **57:** 619–28.

Claeys MA, Gept E & Camus F (1988) Haemodynamic changes during anaesthesia induced and maintained with propofol. *Br. J. Anaesth.* **60:** 3–9.

Coates DP, Christopher RM, Prys-Roberts C & Turtle M (1987) Hemodynamic effects of infusions of the emulsion formulation of propofol during nitrous oxide anesthesia in humans. *Anesthesia Analgesia* **66:** 64–70.

Corssen G, Chodoff P, Domino EF & Khan DR (1965) Neuroleptanalgesia and anesthesia for open-heart surgery. *J. Thorac. Cardiovasc. Surg.* **49:** 901–20.

Cullen PM, Turtle M, Prys-Roberts C *et al.* (1987) Effect of propofol anesthesia on baroreflex activity in humans. *Anesthesia Analgesia* **66:** 1115–20.

Dauchot PJ, Rasmussen JP, Nicholson DH *et al.* (1976) Online systolic time intervals during anesthesia in patients with and without heart disease. *Anesthesiology* **44:** 472–80.

De Silva RA, Verrier RL & Lown B (1978) Protective effect of vagotomic action of morphine sulfate on ventricular vulnerability. *Cardiovasc. Res.* **12:** 167–72.

Drew JH, Dripps RD & Comroe JH (1946) Clinical studies on morphine. II. The effect of morphine upon the circulation of man and upon the circulatory and respiratory response to tilting. *Anesthesiology* **7:** 44–61.

Eger EI II, Smith NT, Stoeltink RK *et al.* (1970) Cardiovascular effects of halothane in man. *Anesthesiology* **32:** 396–403.

Fragen RJ, Shanks CA, Molteni A & Avram MJ (1984) Effects of etomidate on hormonal response to stress. *Anesthesiology* **61:** 652–6.

Giese JL & Stanley TH (1983) Etomidate: a new intravenous anaesthetic induction agent. *Pharmacotherapy* **3:** 251–8.

Hall GM (1978) Body temperature and anaesthesia. *Br. J. Anaesth.* **50:** 39–44.

Heikkila H, Jalonen J, Arola M *et al.* (1984) Midazolam as an adjunct to high dose fentanyl anesthesia for coronary artery bypass graft operation. *Acta Anaesth. Scand* **28:** 683–9.

Heinrich H, Fontaine L, Fösel Th *et al.* (1986) Vergleichende ekocardiographische Untersuchungen zur negativen Inotropie von Halothan, Enfluran und Isofluran. *Anaesthesist* **35:** 465–72.

Hickey RF & Eger EI II (1986) Circulatory pharmacology of inhaled anesthetics. In Miller RD (ed.) *Anesthesia* (2nd edition), pp. 649–66. New York: Churchill-Livingstone.

Hsu HO, Hickey RF & Forbes AR (1979) Morphine decreases peripheral vascular resistance and increases capacitance in man. *Anesthesiology* **50:** 98–102.

Ivankowitch AD, Miletich DJ, Reinmann C *et al.* (1974) Cardiovascular effects of centrally administered ketamine in goats. *Anesthesia Analgesia* **53:** 924–33.

Jansky L (1966) Body organ thermogenesis of the rat during exposure to cold and at maximal metabolic rates. *Fedn. Proc.* **25:** 1297–302.

Jones RM (1984) Clinical comparison of inhalation anaesthetic agents. *Br. J. Anaesth.* **56:** 57S–69S.

Kessler D, Sonntag HL & Donath U (1979) Haemodynamics, myocardial mechanics, oxygen requirements and oxygenation of the human heart during induction of anaesthesia with etomidate. *Anaesthetist* **23:** 717–19.

Kong KL, Wilats SM & Pry-Roberts C (1989) Isoflurane compared with midazolam for sedation in intensive care. *Br. Med. J.* **298:** 1277–80.

Lepage JM, Pinaud ML, Helias JH *et al.* (1988) Left ventricular function during propofol and fentanyl anesthesia in patients with coronary artery disease: assessment with a radionuclide approach. *Anesthesia Analgesia* **67:** 949–55.

Lilburn JK, Moore J & Dundee JW (1978) Attempt to attenuate the cardio-stimulatory effects of ketamine. *Anaesthesia* **32:** 449–55.

Liu WS, Bidwai AV, Stanley TH & Loeser EA (1976) Cardiovascular dynamic after large doses of fentanyl and fentanyl plus N$_2$0 in the dog. *Anesthesia Analgesia* **55:** 168–72.

Lowenstein E, Hallowell P & Levine FH (1969) Cardiovascular response to large doses of intravenous morphine in man. *New Engl. J. Med.* **281:** 1389–91.

Lowenstein E, Whiting RB & Bittar DA (1972) Local and neurally mediated effects of morphine on skeletal muscle vascular resistance. *J. Pharmacol. Exp. Ther.* **180:** 359–67.

Lunn JK, Stanley Th, Eisele J *et al.* (1979) High dose fentanyl anesthesia for coronary artery surgery: Plasma fentanyl concentrations and influence of nitrous oxide on cardiovascular response. *Anesthesia Analgesia* **58:** 390–5.

Lutz LJ & Lamer TJ (1990) Management of postoperative pain: review of current techniques and methods. *Mayo Clin. Proc.* **65:** 584–96.

Mikat M, Peters J, Zindler M & Arndt JO (1984) Whole body oxygen consumption in awake, sleeping and anesthetized dogs. *Anesthesiology* **60:** 220–7.

Morgan M, Lumley J & Gillies DS (1974) Neuroleptanalgesia for major surgery: experience with 500 cases. *Br. J. Anaesth.* **46:** 288–93.

Mulier JP, Wouters PF, Van Aken H *et al.* (1991) Cardiodynamic effects of propofol in comparison with thiopental: assessment with a transesophageal echocardiographic approach. *Anesthesia Analgesia* **72:** 28–35.

Newman LH, McDonald JC, Wallace PGM & Ledingham IMcA (1987) Propofol infusion for sedation in intensive care. *Anaesthesia* **42:** 929–37.

Nunn JF & Matthews RL (1959) Gaseous exchange during halothane anaesthesia: the steady respiratory state. *Br. J. Anaesth.* **31:** 330–40.

Pathak KS, Brown RH, Nash CL & Cascorbi HF (1983) Continuous opioid infusion for scoliosis fusion surgery. *Anesthesia Analgesia* **62:** 841–5.

Philbin DM, Moss J, Akins CW *et al.* (1981) The use of H1 and H2 histamine agonists with morphine anesthesia. *Anesthesiology* **55:** 212–17.

Rao S, Sherbaniuk RW & Prasad K (1973) Cardiopulmonary effects of diazepam. *Clin. Pharmacol. Ther.* **14:** 182–9.

Rawal N, Sjöstrand U, Christoffersson E *et al.* (1984) Comparison of intramuscular and epidural morphine for postoperative analgesia in the grossly obese: influence on postoperative ambulation and pulmonary function. *Anesthesia Analgesia* **63:** 583–92.

Reinhart K (1991) Clinical assessment of tissue oxygenation: value of hemodynamic and oxygen transport related variables. In Gutierrez G & Vincent JL (eds), *Tissue Oxygen Utilization,* pp. 269–85. Berlin: Springer-Verlag.

Reinhart K, Foehring U, Kersting T *et al.* (1989) Effects of thoracic epidural anesthesia on systemic hemodynamic function and systemic oxygen supply-demand relationship. *Anesthesia Analgesia* **69:** 360–9.

Reitan JA, Stangert KB, Wymore ML & Martucci RW (1978) Central vagal control of fentanyl induced bradycardia during halothane anesthesia. *Anesthesia Analgesia* **57:** 31–6.

Reiz S, Nath S, Ponten E *et al.* (1979) Effects of thoracic epidural bloc and the beta-1-adrenoreceptor agonist prenalterol on the cardiovascular response to infrarenal cross-clamping in man. *Acta Anaesth. Scand.* **23:** 395–403.

Renck H (1969) The elderly patient after anaesthesia and surgery. *Acta Anaesth. Scand.* **34 (Suppl.):** 1–136.

Reves JG, Kissin I & Fournier SE (1984) Additive negative inotropic effect of a combination of diazepam and fentanyl. *Anesthesia Analgesia* **63:** 97–100.

Reves JG, Fragen RJ, Vinik RH & Greenblatt DJ (1985) Midazolam: pharmacology and uses. *Anesthesiology* **62:** 310–24.

Reves JG, Flezzani P & Kissin I (1986) Pharmacology of intravenous anaesthetic induction drugs. In Kaplan, J.A. (ed.), *Cardiac Anaesthesia,* pp. 125–50. New York: Grune Stratton.

Riou B, Lecarpentier Y & Viars P (1989) Inotropic effects of ketamine on rat cardiac papillary muscle. *Anesthesiology* **71:** 116–25.

Riou B, Lecarpentier Y, Chemia D & Viars P (1990) In vitro effects of etomidate on intrinsic myocardial contractility in the rat. *Anesthesiology* **72:** 330–40.

Roizen MF, Hornegan RW & Frazer BM (1981) Anesthetic doses blocking adrenergic (stress) and cardiovascular responses to incision – MAC BAR. *Anesthesiology* **54:** 390–8.

Rosow CE, Moss J, Philbin DM & Savarese JJ (1982) Histamine release during morphine and fentanyl anesthesia. *Anesthesiology* **56:** 93–6.

Rouby JJ, Eurin B, Glaser P *et al.* (1981) Hemodynamic and metabolics of morphine in the critically ill. *Circulation* **64:** 53–9.

Schlichtig R, Kramer DJ & Pinsky MR (1991) Flow redistribution during progressive hemorrhage is a determinant of critical O_2 delivery. *J. Appl. Physiol.* **70:** 169–78.

Sebel PS & Lowdon JD (1989) Propofol: a new intravenous anesthetic. *Anesthesiology* **71:** 260–77.

Shackman R, Graber GJ & Redwood C (1951) Oxygen consumption and anaesthesia. *Clin. Sci.* **10:** 219–28.

Shibutani K, Komatsu T, Kubal K *et al.* (1983) Critical level of oxygen delivery in anesthetized man. *Crit. Care Med.* **11:** 640–3.

Stanley TH & Webster LR (1978) Anesthetic requirements and cardiovascular effects of fentanyl-oxygen and fentanyl-diazepam-oxygen anesthesia in man. *Anesthesia Analgesia* **57:** 411–16.

Stanley TH, Bennet GM, Loeser EA *et al.* (1975) Cardiovascular effects of diazepam and droperidol during morphine anesthesia. *Anesthesiology* **44:** 255–8.

Stevens WC, Cromwell TH, Halsey MJ *et al.* (1971) The cardiovascular effects of a new inhalation anesthetic, Forane, in human volunteers at constant arterial carbon dioxide tension. *Anesthesiology* **35:** 8–16.

Stoelting RK, Gibbs PS, Creasser CW & Peterson C (1975) Hemodynamic and ventilatory responses to fentanyl, fentanyl-droperidol, and nitrous oxide in patients with acquired valvular disease. *Anesthesiology* **42:** 319–24.

Swinamer DL, Phang PT, Jones RL *et al.* (1988) Effect of routine administration of analgesia on energy expenditure in critically ill patients. *Chest* **92:** 4–10.

Theye RA & Michenfelter JD (1975) Individual organ contributions to the decrease in whole body oxygen consumption with isoflurane. *Anesthesiology* **42:** 35–40.

Tokics L, Brismar B, Hedenstierna G & Lundh R (1983) Oxygen uptake and central circulation during ketamine anaesthesia. *Acta Anaesth. Scand.* **27:** 318–22.

Tomischek RC, Rosow CE, Schneder RC *et al.* (1982) Cardiovascular effects of diazepam-fentanyl anesthesia in patients with coronary artery disease. *Anesthesia Analgesia* **61:** 217–18.

Urquhart ML & White PF (1989) Comparison of sedative infusions during regional anesthesia: methohexital, etomidate and midazolam. *Anesthesia Analgesia* **68:** 249–54.

Urthaler F, Isobe JH & James TN (1975) Direct and vagally mediated chronotropic effects of morphine studied by selective perfusion of the sinus node of awake dogs. *Chest* **68:** 222–8.

Van Aken H, Meinshausen E, Prien T *et al.* (1988) The influence of fentanyl and tracheal intubation on the hemodynamic effects of anesthesia induction with propofol/N_2O in humans. *Anesthesiology* **68:** 157–63.

Van der Linden P, Gilbart E, Engelman E *et al.* (1990) Comparison of halothane, isoflurane, alfentanil and ketamine in experimental septic shock. *Anesthesia Analgesia* **70:** 608–17.

Van der Linden P, Gilbart E, Engelman E *et al.* (1991a) Adrenergic support during anaesthesia in experimental endotoxin shock: norepinephrine versus dobutamine. *Acta Anaesth. Scand.* **35:** 134–40.

Van der Linden P, Gilbart E, Engelman E *et al.* (1991b) Effects of anesthetic agents on systemic critical O_2 delivery. *J. App. Physiol.* **71:** 83–93.

Van der Linden *et al.* (1993) Comparative effects of etomidate, propofol and pentobarbitol on tissue O_2 extraction capabilities (submitted).

Vincent JL (1991) Advances in the concepts of intensive care. *Am. Heart J.* **121:** 1859–65.

Watt I & Ledingham IMcA (1984) Mortality amongst multiple trauma patients admitted to an intensive therapy unit. *Anaesthesia* **39:** 973–81.

White PF, Way WL & Trevor AJ (1982) Ketamine: its pharmacology and therapeutic uses. *Anesthesiology* **56:** 119–36.

White PF (1988) Clinical pharmacology of intravenous induction drugs. *Int. Anesth. Clin.* **26:** 98–104.

Yeager MP, Glass DD, Neff RK & Brinck-Johnsen, T (1987) Epidural anesthesia and analgesia in high risk surgical patients. *Anesthesiology* **66:** 728–36.

Zelis R, Mansour EJ, Capone RJ *et al.* (1974) The cardiovascular effects of morphine: the peripheral capacitance and resistance vessels in human subjects. *J. Clin. Invest.* **54:** 1247–58.

12   Trauma

G.I.J.M. Beerthuizen & R.J.A. Goris

Introduction

Trauma is the leading cause of death in the first four decades of life, and in the multiple-injuried patient inadequate oxygen supply to the tissues is an acute threat. There are three categories of patients according to severity of injury:

(1) patients with injuries that are interfering with vital functions and therefore threaten life;
(2) patients with injuries not leading to immediate threat to life; and
(3) patients with injuries causing occult damage.

Life-threatening injuries in the first category include airway obstruction and extensive bleeding, both of which directly affect oxygen transport to the tissues. Serious dyspnoea and/or shock reveal a life-threatening condition and immediate intervention is necessary. Patients in the second category will benefit from meticulous physical examination and monitoring. Vital signs, such as blood pressure and arterial saturation are not disturbed, but tissue trauma and progressive blood loss leads to compensatory mechanisms resulting in decreased tissue oxygenation, tissue hypoxia and, if not adequately corrected, cellular death. The third category of patients will require treatment to correct local disturbances of tissue oxygenation.

Pathophysiology

Tissue PO_2

Trauma interferes with tissue oxygenation. This may be because the rate of delivery of oxygen to tissues, the rate of transport of oxygen in tissues or the rate of consumption of oxygen by tissues is disturbed. Figure 12.1 and Table 12.1 show the factors involved in an adequate oxygen supply to tissues. The aim of the circulation is to deliver an adequate volume of oxygen at an adequate partial pressure to replace the oxygen used at the terminal oxidase of the respiratory chain in the mitochondria. This oxygen supply is vital, as

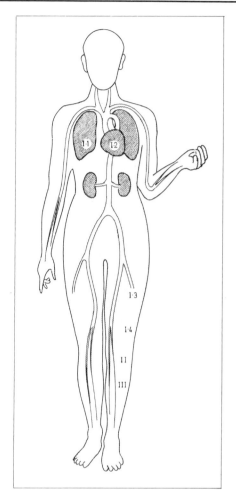

Figure 12.1 Determinants of tissue oxygen pressure. The numbers I.1–I.4, II and III are presented in table 12.1. The heart, lungs, kidneys and arteries indicate the parts of the circulation, which are monitored clinically.

95% of the energy generated by the body normally originates from aerobic pathways, and as the entire oxygen store of the body would support resting needs for 5 min at most (Kreuzer & Cain, 1985).

Until now, only systemic parameters such as arterial blood pressure, central venous pressure, pulmonary arterial pressure and cardiac output have been monitored. In a traumatized patient these parameters are corrected meticulously, but the therapeutic interventions may actually impair tissue perfusion and tissue oxygenation. Direct monitoring of tissue perfusion and/or tissue oxygenation may thus provide a more sensitive method

Table 12.1

I Rate of delivery of oxygen to tissue:
  1 Amount of oxygen in arterial blood
      Oxygen tension in inspired air
      Alveolar ventilation
      Alveolar oxygen partial pressure
      Ventilation/perfusion ratio
      Pulmonary diffusing capacity
      Solubility of oxygen in plasma
      Amount of haemoglobin
      Arterial oxygen saturation
      Arterial oxygen partial pressure
  2 Delivery of arterial blood to tissues
      Cardiac output
      Arterial blood pressure
  3 The microcirculation
      Blood viscosity
      Red blood cell size
      Adherence of cellular blood components
      Arterio-venous shunts
      Number of open capillaries
      Capillary radius
      Capillary flow
      Capillary oxygen content
      Intercapillary distance
  4 Rate at which oxygen leaves the blood
      Affinity of oxygen for haemoglobin
      Rate of dissociation of oxygen from haemoglobin
      Oxygen solubility in plasma
II   Rate of transport of oxygen in tissue
      Krogh's oxygen diffusion coefficient
      Difference in oxygen partial pressure
      Diffusion distance
III Rate of consumption of oxygen by tissue influenced by
      Work
      Drugs
      Hormones (adrenaline, corticosteroids, thyroxine, insulin)
      Temperature of the tissue

for the early detection of tissue hypoxia. Correction of cardiac output and arterial oxygen tension in a traumatized patient does not necessarily ensure normal tissue oxygenation (Niinikoski & Halkola, 1978). Adequacy of tissue oxygenation cannot be predicted solely from measurement of arterial PO_2 since normal values may be associated with inadequate tissue oxygen supply (Kessler et al., 1976). Monitoring PO_2 in the tissue may allow early detection of a disturbance in tissue oxygenation and may indicate how far the various compensatory mechanisms have been mobilized.

Experience with techniques for measuring tissue PO_2 and PCO_2 levels suggests that the measurement of skeletal muscle tissue gas tensions may

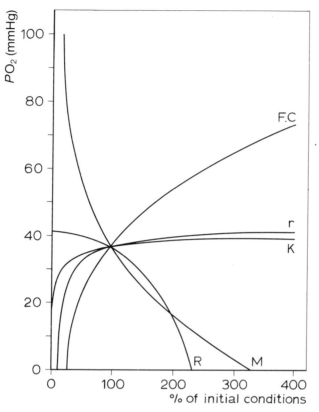

Figure 12.2 The influence of change in myocardial blood flow (F), myocardial oxygen consumption (M), oxygen content of the arterial blood (C), tissue cylinder radius (R), capillary radius (r) and Krogh's diffusion coefficient (K) on myocardial tissue PO_2 (from Rakusan, 1971).

provide an index of peripheral tissue perfusion. Mass spectrometry and tonometry with an implanted silicone rubber tube have shown that during periods of experimentally induced low cardiac output, tissue PO_2 decreases virtually proportionally to decreases in cardiac output (Niinikoski, 1977).

Tissue PO_2 depends upon the balance between rate of oxygen delivery to tissue and rate of oxygen consumption by tissue (Beerthuizen et al., 1990). Each of these in turn depends on cardiac output and its distribution to different organs and on the oxygen content of the blood. Oxygen content of the blood depends on arterial PO_2 (PaO_2), arterial SO_2 (SaO_2) and haemoglobin concentration (Hb). PaO_2 depends on alveolar PO_2 (PAO_2), ventilation/perfusion ratio and pulmonary diffusing capacity. PAO_2 depends on FIO_2 and alveolar ventilation. Oxygen delivery within the muscle depends on the condition of the microcirculation.

Significant elements of capillary behaviour are the number of open capillaries, the presence of non-capillary pathways from artery to vein (shunts) and the range of variation in type, length and flow pattern of the capillary bed (heterogeneity) (Duling, 1980). Creation of greater than normal heterogeneity in flow or its distribution in the peripheral microcirculation has the inevitable consequence of making tissue hypoxic (Shoemaker & Reinhard, 1973).

The final determinant of tissue oxygen tension is the rate at which oxygen leaves the capillary blood and the diffusion of oxygen through the tissue. The rate at which oxygen leaves the blood is a function of the oxyhaemoglobin dissociation curve (related to temperature, pH, carbon dioxide tension and 2,3-diphosphoglycerate concentration), the time required by the haemoglobin to release the oxygen and the oxygen solubility in the plasma. Tissue PO_2 is not solely dependent upon the rate of oxygen consumption by the tissue. If oxygen delivery increases but oxygen consumption increases even more, then tissue oxygen decreases.

Krogh developed the concept of the three-dimensional distribution of oxygen tension in tissue, proposing a theoretical model which consists of a system of parallel capillaries and their surrounding cells, and developing an equation to calculate the oxygen pressure at distance x from the centre of a capillary with a diameter r, which supplies a tissue cylinder with diameter R (Krogh, 1919). Rakusan then went on to show the influence of oxygen consumption, blood flow, arterial oxygen content, radius of tissue cylinder, capillary radius and Krogh's diffusion coefficient on myocardial tissue PO_2 using the 'Krogh cylinder' (Rakusan, 1971) (Fig. 12.2). Tissue oxygen pressure measurements indicate the net result of the simultaneous changes occurring in the factors mentioned above and listed in Table 12.1 and Fig. 12.1. However, they provide no information as to the causes of such changes.

Cellular Changes in Trauma

The majority of 'resting' cellular energy is spent on pumping substances across membranes, either against gradients or faster than passive diffusion would normally allow (Hochachka, 1986). If the cell membranes are rendered more permeable to unwanted substances, the energy and oxygen requirements are increased to keep the ion and other pumps working at a greater rate to maintain a normal consistency of the cytosol. If oxygen delivery is not increased to meet this demand, hypoxia will further deteriorate the cell, increasing the damage. Thus, the mediators of trauma, for example, the monokines, amines, complement factors and arachidonic acid metabolites, increase the need for oxygen by the cell. In the trauma patient oxygen transport and utilization are stressed by an increased metabolic load, in part produced by the need to maintain ionic equilibrium in the face of increased cell membrane permeability. Cellular metabolic disorder, possibly produced by impairment of the phosphocreatinine 'shuttle', gives rise to large transient concentrations of ADP and AMP. Glycolysis, lactic acid production, and depletion of the adenylate pool may result. There is also a loss of autoregulation of the microcirculation, which leads to a need for a greater tissue oxygen pressure to supply oxygen needs.

Under basal conditions, oxygen transport ($\dot{D}O_2$) is approximately $600\,ml\,min^{-1}\,m^{-2}$ and oxygen consumption ($\dot{V}O_2$) $150\,ml\,min^{-1}\,m^{-2}$. Accordingly, only 25% of the available oxygen is extracted by the tissues. A reduction of oxygen delivery triggers compensatory responses to increase oxygen availability to cells. These include activation of the sympatho-adrenal axis, with both neurogenic and humoral catecholamine release, which may augment blood flow to vital organs, increases in oxygen extraction, and decreases in the affinity of haemoglobin for oxygen. Accordingly, more oxygen is released to tissues.

When these compensatory mechanisms fail, a critical oxygen deficit results in progressive impairment of mitochondrial function, the regeneration of high-energy phosphates is decreased and excess lactic acid accumulates (Broder & Weil, 1964; Bland et al., 1985). These are the hallmarks of anaerobic metabolism and its associated tissue injury, which culminates in a potentially fatal outcome. In acute life-threatening trauma, the primary defect is a decrease in effective $\dot{D}O_2$ and therefore decreases in cardiac output and/or arterial oxygen content (CaO_2). As $\dot{D}O_2$ decreases, there is an initial increase in oxygen extraction such that $\dot{V}O_2$ is preserved. However, further curtailment in $\dot{D}O_2$ compromises $\dot{V}O_2$ such that $\dot{V}O_2$ becomes flow-dependent (Chappell et al., 1985; Mohsenifar et al., 1987). Under most clinical circumstances, the absolute $\dot{D}O_2$ and $\dot{V}O_2$ levels do not predict the presence or absence of tissue oxygen deficits (Astiz et al., 1986; Gutierrez et al., 1986).

Oxygen Toxicity

Oxygen toxicity was proven to exist as far back as 1899. J. Lorrain-Smith demonstrated that increasing partial pressures of inspired oxygen produced an increasing incidence of lung injury in animals exposed to varying partial pressures of oxygen for varying periods of time. He showed, for example, that birds, mice, rats and guinea-pigs died in a few days when they were exposed continuously to FIO_2 of 0.7–0.8. Autopsies revealed the lungs to be severely congested with pneumonia-like changes. In contrast, exposure to FIO_2 of 0.4 for a week was harmless (Smith, 1889).

Prolonged continuous exposure to high concentrations of oxygen at atmospheric pressure results in progressive injury to the alveolar epithelium, capillary endothelium and pulmonary interstitial space. The increased permeability of the blood–gas barrier to solute and solvent leads to the formation of non-cardiogenic interstitial and alveolar oedema, atelectasis, hypoxaemia, and hypercapnia and causes the death of the animals from hypoxaemia or respiratory acidosis (Matalon & Egan, 1981; Matalon *et al.*, 1982; Matalon & Cesar, 1985).

Mechanisms involved in oxygen toxicity are enzyme inhibition, free radical formation and peroxidation. High concentrations of oxygen have been shown to inhibit the growth of cultured pulmonary endothelial cells. The inhibition manifests itself 48 h after continuously exposing cultured cells to 60% oxygen. At 95% oxygen the effect is seen within 8 h, and at 40% oxygen there is no evidence of impaired cell growth (Martin & Kachel, 1989). A high concentration of oxygen exposure in rabbits for 3 days not only produces histological damage in the pulmonary artery endothelium, but also causes impairment of vascular reactivity to constricting and relaxing agents. Subcutaneous superoxide dismutase administration prevented oxygen-induced pulmonary artery damage (Obara *et al.*, 1989).

Oxygen Free Radicals

Several studies indicate that oxidants play a major role in producing the microvascular and parenchymal damage associated with reperfusion of ischaemic tissues (McCord, 1985; Granger *et al.*, 1986). The formation of oxygen radicals by xanthine oxidase is considered a fundamental mechanism of tissue injury during reperfusion of ischaemic organs. Neutrophils also appear to play a major role in reperfusion injury. One contributing factor to injury of a traumatized limb might be the formation of oxygen free radicals. In an experimental study in patients undergoing aortic reconstructive surgery, the iliac arterio-venous difference of hypoxanthine and lactate markedly increased immediately post-ischaemia. Plasma hypoxanthine was abundant in the leg on re-oxygenation. The existence of a xanthine oxidase system in skeletal muscle could produce favourable conditions for oxygen radical formation through hypoxanthine degradation, which may contribute to the known muscle tissue injury (Neglen *et al.*, 1989).

Microembolization

Experimental studies have shown that microembolization diminishes the ability of the vascular bed to recruit capillaries and restricts tissue oxygen transport, reducing oxygen consumption. Microembolization may model the defect in tissue oxygen utilization and reactive hyperaemia that have been observed in the clinical states of trauma, suggesting that microembolization may be the mechanism for these defects (Landau *et al.*, 1982).

Neutrophils

In experimental studies it has been shown that white cells play a significant role in the pathophysiology of ischaemic skeletal muscle injury. In an experimental study on skeletal muscle ischaemic injury, Belkin *et al.* (1989) showed a protective effect of neutropenia and suggested a significant role of the white cell in the pathophysiology of ischaemic skeletal muscle injury.

Wound Healing

Poor perfusion and decreased oxygen tension are known to modify healing and resistance to infection. Hypoxia reduces the rate at which leukocytes generate oxygen radicals that are necessary for killing many micro-organisms. In an experimental study it has been shown that resistance to infection with *S. aureus* is oxygen-dependent, particularly when tissue PO_2 is below 40 mm Hg (5.3 kPa) (Jonsson *et al.*, 1988).

Aulick *et al.* (1980) showed that large, non-infected granulating wounds in the goat hindlimb resulted after 12 days in a 70–90% increase in limb blood flow, a 30% increase in limb VO_2, a 30% decrease in arterio–venous O_2 difference and a three-fold increase in glucose uptake and lactate production. The response to a series of α-adrenergic and β-vasodilator stimuli was almost absent, making these legs functionally sympathectomized.

Rosenberg and co-workers monitored oxygen saturation and transcutaneous and subcutaneous oxygen tension in patients undergoing abdominal operations. Subcutaneous PO_2 was 58 mm Hg (7.7 kPa) on the second post-operative night and 61 mm Hg (8.1 kPa) on the third post-operative night. The study showed pronounced intersubject differences in oxygen tensions near the surgical wound in the late post-operative period (Rosenberg *et al.*, 1990).

Ischaemia and Reperfusion

Periods of ischaemia may cause tissue injury directly as a result of events either during the ischaemic period (ischaemic injury) or at reperfusion (reperfusion injury). Total intestinal ischaemia may be followed by reperfusion injury if there is no concomitant congestion and if ischaemic injury is not too extensive (Park *et al.*, 1990). On reperfusion, blood flow is not distributed homogeneously throughout the muscle and the extent of reactive hyperaemia is inversely related to the length of ischaemia. Forrest and co-workers found in an experimental study in dogs, that hyperaemic blood flow reached the maximum rate in the centre portions of the muscle belly, closest to the inflow and did not seem to be related to the distribution of necrosis. Pre-ischaemic blood flow was distributed homogeneously throughout the muscle and on reperfusion, total flow was 6–10 times higher than it was before ischaemia.

Late Effects of Trauma

Tissue oxygen debt has been shown to play an important role in the development of organ failure. Tissue oxygen debt reflected by insufficient $\dot{V}O_2$ appears to be the primary event as well as a major determinant of organ failure and outcome. The initial circulatory failure results in inadequate perfusion of each organ, produces tissue hypoxia, and limits the functional capacity of various vital organs, especially when physiologic demands are increased (Shoemaker *et al.*, 1988). In one study, oxygen tension and collagen deposition were measured in standardized, subcutaneous wounds in post-operative surgical patients. Collagen deposition was found to be directly and significantly proportional to mean wound oxygen tension. Smoking and increasing age were inversely related to wound-tissue PO_2 and collagen deposition. This study showed that major components of wound healing are limited by perfusion and tissue oxygen tension (Jonsson *et al.*, 1991).

Monitoring a Traumatized Patient

The oxygen transport system is of vital importance for the integrity of cellular metabolism, but one or more of the several components of the oxygen transport system may function abnormally in traumatized patients. We can often ascertain on clinical grounds that oxygen transport, both overall and in distribution, is sufficient for tissue needs. For example, a patient admitted with chest pain who is later alert, with normal vital signs and no symptoms, can justifiably be denied invasive monitoring. No laboratory data can confirm the adequacy of oxygen transport more readily than the demonstration of normal function. Normal function provides no quantification and indicates nothing about any reserve that might be present, but it clearly indicates sufficient and adequately distributed oxygen transport.

However, other circumstances require more specific information. The technology of monitoring oxygen transport indicators in traumatized patients is evolving rapidly. As new technologies become available, clinicians must be fully aware of the theoretical background and practical application of the measurements. Absolute values are not as important as trends and the rates of change in variables. Continuous monitoring of oxygen transport indicators may provide an early warning that will allow intervention before tissue hypoperfusion has caused permanent organ damage. With serial measurements, therapeutic trials may be undertaken to determine the often unpredictable optimal patient care. Serial measurements will also help to detect the potentially adverse effects that therapy to improve the function of one organ system may have on another.

Placement of monitoring devices and acquisition of data should not delay therapy but should proceed concomitantly with therapy. During monitoring of a severely traumatized patient, arterial blood pressure, heart rate and urinary production are routinely measured. For more extensive monitoring indwelling central venous catheters are required. Central venous pressure, pulmonary arterial blood pressure, pulmonary capillary wedge pressure and cardiac output can then be determined. If arterial and venous blood-gas analysis is performed, arterial oxygen supply, oxygen extraction and oxygen consumption can be calculated.

However, knowledge of these data still does not allow the determination of tissue oxygenation. When more information about oxygen supply/demand is needed, $P\bar{v}O_2$ is the single most reliable monitor of all the components of that balance. Nevertheless, $P\bar{v}O_2$ tells nothing about unperfused tissues or the distribution of perfusion. Monitoring of $S\bar{v}O_2$ is comparatively useful because it can be monitored continuously, and because its algebraic relations with changes in haemoglobin SaO_2, cardiac output, and $\dot{V}O_2$ are straightforward. Similar quantitative interpretation of $P\bar{v}O_2$ requires more familiarity with the dissociation curve, but $P\bar{v}O_2$ provides a more reliable assessment of the reserve oxygen supply. As opposed to routine collection and analysis of 'profiles', it is often more useful to assess cardiopulmonary status by cautiously applying stress, as by a change in position, volume administration or drug therapy, and observing the response. Monitoring skeletal muscle PO_2 might provide the earliest information about tissue hypoxia.

The Traumatized Patient

In medical practice the clinical condition of the patient still remains the most important criterion for detection of circulatory shock. Extensive bleeding causes a decrease in cardiac output and subsequently a decreased oxygen transport to the tissues. The clinical features are obvious. Extensive bleeding should be treated by emergency thoracotomy and/or laparotomy. In experimental haemorrhagic shock, it has been shown that skeletal muscle PO_2, measured with a recessed needle electrode, decreases early during haemorrhage before arterial blood pressure drops (Kleij et al., 1983). The available studies show that skeletal muscle PO_2 is affected early in developing shock and therefore assessment of skeletal muscle PO_2 in patients might be useful for early detection of shock.

Non-invasive options for monitoring oxygenation include fingertip and ear oximeters, transcutaneous and conjunctival oxygen electrodes. These correlate well with arterial blood oxygenation in haemodynamically stable patients. However, during circulatory shock and especially during cardiac arrest, blood flow is reduced to the skin and conjunctiva to the extent that these measurements become less reliable. More specifically, failure of tissue perfusion precludes reliability and accuracy of such measurements.

During haemorrhage, subcutaneous PO_2 is the first of the PO_2 measurements, and among the first set of haemodynamic variables, to differ significantly from control values. During continuous bleeding, subcutaneous and conjunctival PO_2 fall rapidly, the declines in subcutaneous and conjunctival PO_2 are similar and significantly higher than that found for transcutaneous oxygen tension. After reinfusion of shed blood, subcutaneous oxygen tension is the last of the PO_2 measurements, and among the last set of haemodynamic variables, to return to control values.

Unheated instruments for measuring subcutaneous and conjunctival oxygen tension are reliable indicators of peripheral perfusion during haemorrhage and resuscitation. Subcutaneous oxygen monitoring, in particular, seems capable of assessing early blood loss and adequacy of resuscitation after acute haemorrhage, and may be clinically useful (Gottrup et al., 1989).

In an animal study it has been shown that transcutaneous PO_2 and liver surface PO_2 during hypotensive and normotensive low cardiac output shock, induced by producing normotension during extreme hypovolaemia by an infusion of phenylephrine, were severely decreased as well as cardiac index, oxygen delivery and oxygen consumption. Low transcutaneous PO_2 values during anaesthesia and surgery may correspond to decreased blood volume, blood flow and decreased liver surface PO_2 (Tremper et al., 1989).

In a series of 78 patients with septic shock (40 survivors and 38 non-survivors) at 48 h significant differences were found in cardiac index, oxygen delivery and arterial lactate levels between survivors and non-survivors (Tuchschmidt et al., 1989).

Hartmann and co-workers compared tissue oxygenation in peripheral tissue, measured as transcutaneous PO_2 and subcutaneous PO_2, with oxygenation in gastrointestinal mucosa, measured as intramucosal wall pH, during experimental haemorrhagic shock and resuscitation in pigs. Early indications of shock were decreases in transcutaneous PO_2 and intestinal pH_i. Transcutaneous PO_2 and pH_i in the small intestine and sigmoid colon were the variables that most rapidly indicated blood volume loss. Subcutaneous PO_2, transcutaneous PO_2 and small intestine and sigmoid colon pH_i were correlated to total body oxygen transport. Peripheral tissue perfusion followed intestinal perfusion to some extent (Hartmann et al., 1991).

Subcutaneous PO_2 has been found to be correlated more highly with blood volume lost than transcutaneous PO_2. Furthermore, subcutaneous PO_2 is more sensitive to blood loss than is either cardiac output or transcutaneous PO_2 and, also during the early loss, is more sensitive than mean arterial pressure.

Some organs (e.g. pancreas) appear to lose considerable blood flow with only small loss of blood volume, their blood flow then stabilizes at a low level despite further haemorrhage. Other organs, notably the kidney, appear to be relatively unaffected by substantial loss of blood volume (20–40%), after which, however, their blood flow quite abruptly becomes sensitive to further hypovolaemia. Blood flow-related performance of the kidney (e.g. urine volume) may not adequately predict a developing hazard of peripheral perfusion. Some indicators have been found to be better indices of blood flow in some organs than in others (Gosain et al., 1991).

Calabuig et al. (1990) have shown that after haemorrhagic shock, gall-bladder volume increases, the migrating motor complex decreases and slow wave frequency decreases by 40% in the antrum and 25% in the small bowel. Twenty-four hours after shock these parameters returned to normal. Ischaemic damage to the gastrointestinal tract is postulated as the cause of gall-bladder dysfunction and altered intestinal motility after haemorrhagic shock.

Maintaining an adequate blood flow to all organs requires both sufficient cardiac function and the absence of hypovolaemia. Hypovolaemia is easily masked by the shifting of blood volume from the splanchnic region, kidneys, resting muscles and skin to the central area so that perfusion of the heart and brain remains near normal. No drug or combination of drugs seems to be able to increase myocardial function and maintain the peripheral vascular resistance and the function of all organ systems more than temporarily. Tissues may have maldistribution problems when PaO_2 values are higher than normal.

Very extreme levels of anaemia can be tolerated by most organ systems, provided that perfusion can be maintained. In anaemic hypoxia, the heart is usually the first organ to fail. In hypoxic hypoxia, the circulatory response is similar to hypovolaemia (Bryan-Brown, 1988).

Airway obstruction leads to desaturation of the arterial blood. An adequate ventilation has to be established by creating an adequate airway, treating pneumothorax by inserting chest-tubes and, if necessary, intubation and mechanical ventilation of the injured lung.

Therapy in Traumatized Patients Related to Oxygen Transport

The requirements of the oxygen transport system are:

(1) Haemoglobin (deficit = anaemia)
    Therapy: infusion of red blood cells
(2) Oxygenation (deficit = hypoxia)
    Therapy: increase FiO_2, mechanical ventilation
(3) Flow (deficit = low cardiac output)
    Therapy: infusion of crystalloids, colloids, administration of inotropic drugs

Basically there are three methods of increasing supply to tissues in need:

(1) Recruitment of non-conducting capillaries
(2) Increased diameter of conducting capillaries
(3) Decreased transit time through conducting capillaries

It may well turn out that a decreased transit time of the erythrocyte through a tissue may not give it time to deliver its oxygen load efficiently (Gutierrez, 1986).

Oxygen Tension

It is recommended that PaO_2 should be kept above 70 mm Hg (9.3 kPa) and that any airway manoeuvres, including a high FIO_2, should be used to do this. If a PaO_2 can be maintained above 70 mm Hg (9.3 kPa) the FIO_2 should be reduced to the 0.35–0.40 range. At this PaO_2 the only organ that should need to recruit blood flow in the microcirculation is the heart, as myocardial oxygen extraction is always near the critical level. As the haemoglobin is well over 90% saturated at this oxygen tension, all other organs should be able to function normally without increased cardiac output by extracting more oxygen. Operationally, a higher PaO_2 could be beneficial when some organ system is malfunctioning (e.g. cardiac arrhythmias, depression of the S–T segment, or confusion). On the other hand, unnecessarily high PaO_2 levels may so upset the microcirculation, that small areas of hypoxia arise in tissues due to maldistribution.

Haemoglobin

Two factors should be considered: oxyhaemoglobin dissociation and concentration. For the majority of patients, a normal oxyhaemoglobin dissociation curve would appear to be optimal and a left shift probably best avoided (Gutierrez & Andry, 1989). It appears that the optimum haematocrit for delivering oxygen for the least work is 40–44%. At this level, viscosity and content are in balance (Guyton & Richardson, 1961). Lower haematocrits, produced by isovolaemic haemodilution, may be beneficial if there are restrictions in the cardiovascular system (Messmer et al., 1972). When haematocrit falls below 19% it is not possible to elevate subnormal wound oxygen tensions by fluid loading (Chang et al., 1983). At this level wound healing could be impaired. The restoration of the blood volume would restore wound oxygen tensions to normal at higher haematocrits. The most successful therapy has been to increase tissue O_2 to above normal levels and increase or maintain the circulating blood volume. Pharmacological support of the circulation may cause further damage if the extra cardiac output does not get distributed where it is needed. In conclusion, optimal haemoglobin is probably around normal for most patients, and the PaO_2 should be at least 70 mm Hg (9.3 kPa).

Circulatory Support

The fundamental defect during low flow states of traumatized patients is poor tissue perfusion and decreased oxygen delivery to the cellular and subcellular levels. Therefore, interventions which improve tissue perfusion in order to fulfil systemic and regional oxygen requirements, constitute basic therapeutic goals (Weil & Henning, 1979; Rackow et al., 1988).

The assessment of volume status and subsequent volume expansion is the single most important intervention for treatment of circulatory disturbances, regardless of cause. Volume expansion increases the preload, and thereby augments cardiac output. The specific choice of colloid, crystalloid and electrolyte fluids by the clinician is best based on an understanding of the cause of fluid loss and the severity of the haemodynamic defect in relation to the cardiorespiratory status of the patient. Red cell transfusion augments transport of oxygen to peripheral tissues not only by increasing intravascular volume and therefore preload and cardiac output, but also by increasing oxygen-carrying capacity. However, there are theoretical and practical disadvantages. In stored blood, 2,3-diphosphoglycerate (2,3-DPG) is reduced, the P_{50} is decreased, and hence the affinity of haemoglobin for oxygen is increased (Aberman et al., 1976; Dennis et al., 1978; Woodson, 1979).

An increase in the haematocrit to supernormal levels increases blood viscosity and thereby reduces velocity and volume of blood flow. Clinical studies in various disease states suggest that optimal oxygen availability and survival in patients are in the haematocrit range from 30% to 45%.

Hankeln et al. (1989) compared the cardiopulmonary effects of lactated Ringer's solution with those of 10% hydroxyethylstarch, given in 44 therapeutic interventions in 15 patients by cross-over design. Each agent was given to each patient at least once; seven patients received each agent twice. Infusions were continued until the wedge pressure (WP) had increased to $16 \pm 2\,mm\,Hg$ in trauma patients and $18 \pm 2\,mm\,Hg$ in cardiac patients. Hydroxyethylstarch 10% produced significantly increased cardiac index, left and right ventricular stroke work index, CVP, WP, oxygen delivery, oxygen consumption, and reduced pulmonary vascular resistance index (PVRI). Lactated Ringer's solution increased CVP, WP and PVRI, but did not significantly improve other haemodynamic or oxygen transport variables.

The effects of Dextran 70 with NaCl versus Ringer's acetate on haemodynamics, gas exchange, oxygen transport and survival have been evaluated in a porcine model. This study showed a slight decrease in oxygen delivery for the dextran-treated group compared to the Ringer's acetate group. The superiority of dextran over Ringer's acetate seems to be due to better rheologic effects combined with pharmacologic interactions with granulocytes (Modig, 1988).

In the treatment of burn shock, hourly urinary output and arterial blood pressure have been considered the most important indices of the effectiveness of therapy. Maintenance of optimal tissue perfusion in these patients is essential for survival as well as to prevent morbidity. Large amounts of infusion fluids are needed to resuscitate severely burned patients. Hourly urinary output is commonly used as a parameter for fluid therapy, although its accuracy has been disputed by several authors. In a recent study, skeletal muscle PO_2 was studied as a parameter of tissue perfusion in 13 patients suffering from burns of more than 25% body surface area. After 6, 8, 10, 14, 18, 24, 30, 36 and 48 h routine clinical measurements were performed. Skeletal muscle PO_2 was measured in the quadriceps femoris muscle using a polarographic needle electrode. The relationship between skeletal muscle PO_2 and subsequent resuscitation problems was studied. It was found that skeletal muscle PO_2 did not predict urinary output problems. In patients with clinical shock, the skeletal muscle PO_2 was significantly lower than in patients without clinical shock and skeletal muscle PO_2 preceding clinical shock was significantly lower than during periods without clinical shock. Skeletal muscle PO_2 also decreased before hypotension occurred and enabled early detection of impairment of the circulation. It significantly increased during the period of investigation and was significantly higher 24–30 h post-burn as compared with 6–24 h post-burn (Beerthuizen et al., 1986).

When skeletal muscle PO_2 is normal (>31.5 mm Hg (4.2 kPa)), no shock occurred in a study of critically ill patients. During the study period more patients had one or more periods of shock when at least one of the values was less than 15 mm Hg (2.0 kPa). When skeletal muscle PO_2 was below 22.5 mm Hg (3.0 kPa) the risk of shock was 2.3 times higher. In patients not using inotropic agents, if skeletal muscle PO_2 was below 22.5 mm Hg (3.0 kPa), shock occurred in 73% of the assessments during the subsequent period of 2 h, and always in the period of 4 h before and 6 h after the skeletal muscle PO_2 assessment. It was shown that in critically ill patients, skeletal muscle oxygenation was decreased before clinical shock occurred. The use of inotropes impaired skeletal muscle oxygenation as the skeletal muscle PO_2 was below 22.5 mm Hg (3.0 kPa) in 9 of 10 patients receiving inotropes (Beerthuizen et al., 1989).

In a study by Chang et al. (1983), oxygen partial pressure was measured by using an implanted Silastic catheter in the subcutaneous tissue of the arm in 33 post-operative patients on the day of the operation and the first 5 post-operative days. Tissue hypoxia was a common finding and was most pronounced immediately after abdominal, vascular and cardiac operations. A supplemental bolus of infusion fluid increased low tissue PO_2 in all 19 measurements, implicating hypovolaemia as a common cause of post-operative tissue hypoxia.

The Role of NaHCO$_3^-$

In an animal study, the effects of clinically appropriate doses of NaHCO$_3^-$ on tissue oxygenation was studied when haemorrhagic shock was corrected with hydroxyethylstarch. One group received colloid only while the other group received colloid and bicarbonate. Both groups recovered rapidly haemodynamically, but conjunctival, subcutaneous, and liver tissue PO_2 values returned to baseline more slowly after bicarbonate administration. Arterial plasma lactate remained higher than in the control group at the end of the follow-up period. It was concluded that $NaHCO_3^-$ adjunct has no added beneficial effect on haemodynamics and may be harmful to tissue oxygenation in the treatment of haemorrhagic shock (Makisalo et al., 1989). The use of sodium bicarbonate administration in the treatment of hae-morrhagic shock should be abandoned with regard to oxygen transport to the tissues.

In an experimental study in canine hemorrhagic shock by Iberti et al. (1988) it was shown that there was no statistically significant difference between dogs treated with sodium bicarbonate and those not treated with sodium bicarbonate in any measured haemodynamic, blood-gas or respira-tory gas variable, including heart rate, blood pressure, cardiac output, arterial and venous pH, and bicarbonate levels. Carbon dioxide production was increased in the alkali-treated group and blood lactate levels were significantly higher than in the group treated with NaCl alone, showing persistent tissue hypoxia in hemorrhagic shock treated with sodium bicarbonate.

Adequacy of arterial blood oxygenation and ventilation is determined by arterial blood-gas measurements, but adequacy of peripheral circulation and tissue perfusion is not necessarily assured by the maintenance of blood pressure in the normal range. No patient will ever be saved by a PA catheter; they will only be saved by the therapeutic interventions guided by data provided by the catheter. It is often assumed that normalizing cardiac output will produce normal peripheral tissue perfusion, which is probably no more valid than assuming that normalizing blood pressure will produce normal cardiac output. It is generally accepted that in various clinical syndromes, for example, septic and post-haemorrhagic shock, cardiac out-put may be normal or elevated while tissue perfusion is inadequate. Various methods have been used to describe this maldistribution of peripheral blood flow: peripheral temperature, muscle pH and muscle oxygen tension profiles.

Transcutaneous PO_2 is the PO_2 of heated skin. Normal transcutaneous PO_2 values relative to PaO_2 decrease with patient's age and with most physiologic variables that decrease oxygen transport peripherally. Transcu-taneous PO_2 values also decrease with decreasing cardiac index and PaO_2. To correct tissue hypoxia, oxygen delivery should be increased to a level where oxygen uptake equals oxygen demand and lactic acidosis resolves. For a given level of oxygen demand, the best option is to improve oxygen extraction so that oxygen consumption will be higher for the same level of oxygen transport. This, however, is very difficult. Another approach can consist of further increasing oxygen transport to meet the elevated oxygen demand. Whenever possible, the metabolic needs of the tissues should be restrained.

In an experimental model of haemorrhagic hypovolaemic shock, Dunham *et al.* (1991) showed that the use of oxygen debt and its metabolic consequences of lactic acidaemia and metabolic base deficit were independent variables for the prediction of probability of survival. They also showed that lactic acidaemia and metabolic base deficit are superior as predictors of outcome compared with the conventional haemodynamic variables of blood pressure and cardiac output. A combined prediction from both lactate and base excess appears better to the use of either alone.

References

Aberman A, Cavanilles JM, Michaels SS *et al.* (1976) In vitro changes in blood P50 and erythrocyte 2,3 diphosphoglycerate concentration. *Clin. Chem.* **22:** 1073–7.

Arvidsson D, Rasmussen A, Almqvist P *et al.* (1991) Splanchnic oxygen consumption in septic and hemorrhagic shock. *Surgery* **109:** 190–7.

Astiz ME, Rackow EC & Weil MH (1986) Oxygen delivery and utilization during rapidly fatal septic shock in rat. *Circ. Shock* **20:** 281–90.

Aulick LH, Baze WB, McLeod CG & Wilmore DW (1980) Control of blood flow in large surface wounds. *Ann. Surg.* **191:** 249–58.

Beerthuizen GIJM, Goris RJA, Kley AJ *et al.* (1986) Early detection of burn shock by muscle oxygen pressure assessment. *Bull. Clin. Rev. Burn Inj.* **3:** 29–32.

Beerthuizen GIJM, Goris RJA & Kreuzer FJA (1989) Early detection of shock in critically ill patients by skeletal muscle PO_2 assessment. *Arch. Surg.* **124:** 853–5.

Beerthuizen GIJM, Goris RJA & Kreuzer FJA (1990) Skeletal muscle PO_2 assessment, hemodynamics and oxygen-related parameters in critically ill patients. In Ehrly AM, Fleckenstein W, Hauss J & Huch R (eds), *Clinical Oxygen Pressure Measurement*, Vol. II, Blackwell, Berlin, pp. 77–80.

Belkin M, LaMorte WL, Wright JG & Hobson RW (1989) The role of leukocytes in the pathophysiology of skeletal muscle ischemic injury. *J. Vasc. Surg.* **10:** 14–19.

Bland RD, Shoemaker WC, Abraham E & Choho JC (1985) Hemodynamic and oxygen transport patterns in surviving and nonsurviving postoperative patients. *Crit. Care Med.* **13:** 85–90.

Broder G & Weil MH (1964) Excess lactate: an index of reversibility of shock in human patients. *Science* **143:** 1457–60.

Bryan-Brown DW (1988) Blood flow to organs: parameters for functions and survival in critical illness. *Crit. Care Med.* **16:** 170–8.

Calabuig R, Seggerman RE & Weems WA (1990) Gallbladder and gastrointestinal motility after hemorrhagic shock. *Surgery* **107:** 568–73.

Chang N, Goodon WH III, Gottrup F & Hunt TK (1983) Direct measurement of wound and tissue oxygen tension in postoperative patients. *Ann. Surg.* **197:** 470–8.

Chappell TR, Rubin LJ, Markham RV Jr. *et al.* (1985) Independence of oxygen consumption and systemic oxygen transport in patients with either stable pulmonary hypertension or refractory left ventricular failure. *Am. Rev. Respiratory Dis.* **128:** 30–8.

Dennis RC, Hectman HB, Berger RL *et al.* (1978) Transfusion of 2,3 DPG-enriched red blood cells to improve cardiac function. *Ann. Thorac. Surg.* **26:** 17–19.

Dietrich KA, Conrad SA, Hebert CA *et al.* (1990) Cardiovascular and metabolic response to red blood cell transfusion in critically ill volume-resuscitated nonsurgical patients. *Crit. Care Med.* **18:** 940–4.

Duling BR (1980) Local control of microvascular function: role in tissue oxygen supply. *Ann. Rev. Physiol.* **42:** 373–82.

Dunham CM, Siegel JH, Weireter L *et al.* (1991) Oxygen debt and metabolic acidemia as quantitative predictors of mortality and the severity of the ischemic insult in hemorrhagic shock. *Crit. Care Med.* **19:** 231–44.

Flynn WJ, Cryer HG & Garrison RN (1991) Pentoxifylline restores intestinal microvascular blood flow during resuscitated hemorrhagic shock. *Surgery* **110:** 350–6.

Forrest I, Lindsay TH & Romaschin A (1989) The rate and distribution of muscle blood flow after prolonged ischemia. *J. Vasc. Surg.* **10:** 83–8.

Gosain A, Rabkin J & Reymond JP (1991) Tissue oxygen tension and other indicators of blood loss or organ perfusion during graded hemorrhage. *Surgery* **109:** 523–32.

Gottrup F, Gellett S, Kirkegaard L *et al.* (1989) Effect of hemorrhage and resuscitation on subcutaneous, conjunctival, and transcutaneous oxygen tension in relation to hemodynamic variables. *Crit. Care Med.* **17:** 904–7.

Granger DN, Hollwarth ME & Parks DA (1986) Ischemia-reperfusion injury: Role of oxygen-derived free radicals. *Acta Physiol. Scand.* **548 (Suppl.):** 47.

Gutierrez G (1986) The rate of oxygen release and its effects on capillary O_2 tension: a mathematical analysis. *Respir. Physiol.* **63:** 79–96.

Gutierrez G & Andry JM (1989) Increased hemoglobin O_2 affinity does not improve O_2 consumption in hypoxemia. *J. Appl. Physiol.* **66:** 837–43.

Gutierrez G, Waxley AR & Dantzker DR (1986) Oxygen delivery and utilization in hypothermic dogs. *J. Appl. Physiol.* **60:** 751–7.

Guyton AC & Richardson TO (1961) Effect of hematocrit on venous return. *Circ. Res.* **9:** 157–63.

Hankeln K, Radel C, Beez M *et al.* (1989) Comparison of hydroethyl starch and lactated Ringer's solution on hemodynamics and oxygen transport of critically ill patients in prospective crossover studies. *Crit. Care Med.* **17:** 133.

Hartmann M, Montgomery A, Jonsson *et al.* (1991) Tissue oxygenation in hemorrhagic shock measured as transcutaneous oxygen tension, subcutaneous oxygen tension, and gastrointestinal intramucosal pH in pigs. *Crit. Care Med.* **19:** 205–10.

Hochachka PW (1986) Defence strategies against hypoxia and hypothermia. *Science* **231:** 234–41.

Iberti ThJ, Kelly KM, Gentili DR *et al.* (1988) Effects of sodium bicarbonate in canine hemorrhagic shock. *Crit. Care Med.* **16:** 779–82.

Jonsson K, Hunt TK & Mathes SJ (1988) Oxygen as an isolated variable influences resistance to infection. *Ann Surg.* **208:** 783–7.

Jonsson K, Jensen J, Foodson W, Scheuenstuhl H, Hopf H, Hunt Th (1991) Tissue oxygenation-anemia in relation to wound healing in surgical patients.

Kessler M, Hoper J & Krumme BA (1976) Monitoring of tissue perfusion and cellular function. *Anesthesiology* **45:** 184–97.

Kleij van der AJ, Koning de J, Beerthuizen G *et al.* (1983) Early detection of hemorrhagic hypovolemia by muscle oxygen pressure assessment: preliminary report. *Surgery* **93:** 518–24.

Kreuzer F & Cain SM (1985) Regulation of the peripheral vasculature and oxygenation in health and disease. *Crit. Care Clin.* **1:** 453–70.

Krogh A (1919) The number and distribution of capillaries in muscles with calculations of the oxygen pressure head necessary for supplying the tissue. *J. Physiol. (Lond.)* **52:** 409–15.

Landau SE, Alexander RS, Powers SR *et al.* (1982) Tissue oxygen exchange and reactive hyperemia following microembolization. *J. Surg. Res.* **32:** 38–43.

McCord JM (1985) Oxygen derived free radicals in post-ischemic tissue injury. *New Engl. J. Med.* **312:** 159.

Makisalo HJ, Soini HO, Nordin AJ *et al.* (1989) Effects of bicarbonate therapy on tissue oxygenation during rescuscitation of hemorrhagic shock. *Crit. Care Med.* **17:** 1170–74.

Matalon S & Cesar MC (1985) Effects of oxygen breathing on the capillary filtration coefficient in rabbit lungs. *Microvasc. Res.* **29:** 70–80.

Matalon S & Egan EA (1981) Effects of 100% O_2 breathing on permeability of alveolar epithelium to solute. *J. Appl. Physiol.* **50:** 859–63.

Matalon S, Nesarajah HS & Farhi LE (1982) Pulmonary and circulating changes in conscious sheep exposed to 100% O_2 at 1 ATA. *J. Appl. Physiol.* **53:** 110–16.

Martin WJ & Kachel DL (1989) Oxygen-mediated impairment of human pulmonary endothelial cell growth: Evidence for a specific threshold of toxicity. *J. Lab. Clin. Med.* **113:** 413–21.

Messmer K, Sunder-Plassman L, Klovekorn WP & Hopler K (1972) Circulatory significance of hemodilution: rheologic changes and limitations. *Adv. Microcirc.* **4:** 1–77.

Modig J (1988) Comparison of effects of Dextran-70 and Ringer's acetate on pulmonary function, hemodynamics, and survival in experimental septic shock. *Crit. Care Med.* **16:** 266–71.

Mohsenifar S, Amin D, Jasper AC *et al.* (1987) Dependence of oxygen consumption on oxygen delivery in patients with chronic congestive heart failure. *Chest* **92:** 447–50.

Neglen P, Jabs CM & Eklof B (1989) Plasma metabolic disturbances and reperfusion injury following partial limb ischaemia in man. *Eur. J. Vasc. Surg.* **3:** 165–72.

Niinikoski J. (1977) Tissue oxygenation in hypovolaemic shock. *Ann. Clin. Res.* **9:** 151–6.

Niiniskoski J. & Halkola L (1978) Skeletal muscle PO_2: indicator of peripheral tissue perfusion in haemorrhagic shock. *Adv. Exp. Med. Biol.* **94**: 585–92.

Obara H, Hoshine Y, Mori M *et al.* (1989) Endothelium-dependent relaxation in isolated pulmonary arteries from rabbits exposed to hyperoxia. *Crit. Care Med.* **17**: 780–5.

Park PO, Haglund U, Bulkley GB *et al.* (1990) The sequence of development of intestinal tissue injury after strangulation ischemia and reperfusion. *Surgery* **107**: 574–80.

Rackow EC, Astiz ME & Weil MH (1988) Cellular oxygen metabolism during sepsis and shock. The relationship of oxygen consumption to oxygen delivery. *J. Am. Med. Assoc.* **259**: 1989–93.

Rakusan K (1971) *Oxygen in the Heart Muscle*, p. 39. (Ch. C. Thomas, ed) Springfield, Illinois.

Rosenberg J, Ullstad Th, Larsen PN *et al.* (1990) Continuous assessment of oxygen saturation and subcutaneous oxygen tension after abdominal operations. *Acta Chir. Scand.* **156**: 585–90.

Shoemaker WC & Reinhard JM (1973) Tissue perfusion defects in shock and trauma states. *Surg. Gynecol. Obstet.* **137**: 980–6.

Shoemaker WC, Appel PL & Kram HB (1988) Tissue oxygen debt as a determinant of lethal and nonlethal postoperative organ failure. *Crit. Care Med.* **16**: 1117–20.

Smith JL (1889) Pathological effects due to increase of oxygen tension in air breathed. *J. Physiol.* **24**: 19–35.

Tremper KK, Barker SJ, Hufstedler SM *et al.* (1989) Transcutaneous and liver surface PO_2 during hemorrhagic hypotension and treatment with phenylephrine. *Crit. Care Med.* **17**: 537–40.

Weil MH & Henning RJ (1979) New concepts in the diagnosis and fluid treatment of circulatory shock. *Anaesthesia Analgesia* **58**: 124–32.

Woodson RD (1979) Physiological significance of oxygen dissociation curve shifts. *Crit. Care Med.* **7**: 368–73.

13 Cardiogenic Shock: Pathophysiology, Management and Treatment

R.J. Snell & J.E. Calvin

It is now generally accepted that acute myocardial infarction occurs primarily from intracoronary thrombosis (DeWood *et al.*, 1981), although in a small number of cases coronary artery vasospasm may play a major role (Maseri & Enson, 1968). Knowing the pathophysiological basis of acute myocardial infarction has allowed extensive investigation of thrombolytic agents (which remove the offending clot) in acute myocardial infarction. This form of treatment does reduce mortality and preserves left ventricular (LV) function (GISSI, 1987; International Study of Infarct Survival Collaborative Group (ISIS), 1988; Wilcox *et al.*, 1988). However, despite these approaches large infarctions (usually greater than 40% of muscle loss) do occur (Hands *et al.*, 1989) and contribute directly to cardiac mortality by producing either a low cardiac output state or pulmonary oedema or both.

Cardiogenic shock, the clinical syndrome representing severe pump failure, is defined by the presence of hypotension, altered mental status and oliguria in addition to obvious signs of cardiac failure such as LV dilatation, an S_3 gallop, elevated jugular vein pressure and peripheral or pulmonary oedema. It complicates the clinical course of approximately 5–10% of patients admitted with acute myocardial infarction (Forrester *et al.*, 1976) and the hospital mortality rate using aggressive medical means still exceeds 80% (Forrester *et al.*, 1976).

Earlier clinical suspicion and recognition in combination with therapy based on sound physiological principles is the key to improved mortality.

Pathophysiology of Cardiogenic Shock

Cardiac Abnormalities

The clinical syndrome of cardiogenic shock can result from any one or any combination of the following physiological abnormalities complicating an acute myocardial infarction:

(1) Depressed LV contractility from the infarct itself (Alonso *et al.*, 1973; Parmley *et al.*, 1975; Bertrand *et al.*, 1979; The Multicenter Postinfarction Research Group, 1983; Bigger *et al.*, 1984).
(2) Reduced LV compliance from the infarct (Glantz & Parmley, 1978; Serizawa *et al.*, 1980; Santamore *et al.*, 1981).
(3) Mechanical complications such as severe mitral regurgitation (Buckley *et al.*, 1971; Meister & Helfant, 1972; Gray *et al.*, 1983; Nishimura *et al.*, 1983; Clements *et al.*, 1985) or interventricular septal defect (Meister & Helfant, 1972; Buckley *et al.*, 1971, 1973; Gray *et al.*, 1983; Mann & Roberts, 1988), resulting in acute pump failure, or cardiac rupture, resulting in cardiac tamponade.
(4) Electrical disturbances such as severe bradycardia or tachyarrhythmias.
(5) Depressed ventricular (RV) contractility from RV infarction (Cohn *et al.*, 1974; Lorrell *et al.*, 1979; Calvin, 1991) leading to underfilling of the left ventricle (because of reduced RV stroke output) and reduced LV compliance produced by a direct mechanical ventricular interaction mediated by the pericardium and possibly the interventricular septum (Goldstein *et al.*, 1982; Goto *et al.*, 1985).
(6) Volume depletion (reduced preload) from excessive diuresis or drugs with venodilator capabilities (Loeb *et al.*, 1969).
(7) Depressed myocardial performance by a number of other reversible factors including hypoxaemia, acidosis and cardiac depressing medications (Braunwald *et al.*, 1984; Smith *et al.*, 1988).

Normal Physiological Compensations

Reduced cardiac stroke volume, from whatever reason, can lead to hypotension. Compensatory changes are enacted by the autonomic nervous system to defend against hypotension, and result in tachycardia and profound vasoconstriction. In addition to these vascular compensations the renin–angiotensin system (Errington & Rocha e Silva, 1974) is activated and the release of antidiuretic hormone (ADH) is stimulated resulting in salt and water retention. The heart itself compensates for the depressed stroke volume by (1) dilating to take advantage of its preload reserve and (2) increasing the contractility of uninvolved regions (Bertrand *et al.*, 1979). The former compensation has the compounding effect of increasing LV end-diastolic pressure and pulmonary capillary wedge pressure (PCWP). Filling pressure is also elevated because of the salt and water retention and reduced LV distensibility, giving rise to dyspnoea, tachypnoea and frank pulmonary oedema.

When stroke volume is reduced because of reduced preload or because of primary RV wall infarction, the signs and symptoms of pulmonary congestion (so-called backward failure) are missing. This represents an important clinical entity that can be easily recognized and can often be managed successfully by medical means using volume loading and inotropic agents. It is readily identified by the presence of elevated neck veins, clear chest examination and ST elevation in V_3R and V_4R usually in the setting of an acute inferior or postero-inferior myocardial infarction.

Impact of Low Cardiac Output Upon Oxygen Delivery

The important implication of reduced ventricular stroke volume is depressed cardiac output, for which normal compensations are insufficient, leading to end-organ damage from oxygen deprivation. The use of oxygen transport variables to monitor such patients has not been well-studied in cardiogenic shock. However, they may be of use in assessing the efficacy of medical therapy in such patients. Two studies have demonstrated that oxygen delivery is depressed in such patients with values reported between $310 \pm 89 \, ml \, min^{-1} \, m^{-2}$ (Calvin et al., 1983) and $230 \pm 69 \, ml \, min^{-1} \, m^{-2}$ (Creamer et al., 1990). Treatment with either the afterload reducing agent phentolamine (Calvin et al., 1983) or the use of volume loading and dobutamine can increase oxygen transport to values close to $400 \, ml \, min^{-1} \, m^{-2}$ (Calvin et al., 1983; Creamer et al., 1990). In association with these changes the oxygen extraction ratio falls, oxygen consumption increases slightly, and P_{50} shifts back to the left. Although not completely proven, increasing oxygen transport to values above $400 \, ml \, min^{-1} \, m^{-2}$ may enhance survival (Creamer et al., 1990).

The Clinical and Haemodynamic Subsets of Myocardial Infarction

Any attempt to improve oxygen transport or delivery requires a solid understanding of the patterns of haemodynamic derangement observed during acute myocardial infarction. The first study which related prognosis after myocardial infarction used straightforward clinical signs such as lung crackles, an S_3 and blood pressure (Killip & Kimball, 1967). Mortality ranged from 6% in uncomplicated myocardial infarction to 81% in patients with signs of clinical shock. Forrester and colleagues also developed a similar classification with similar mortalities (Forrester et al., 1976).

With the introduction of flow-directed right heart catheterization in the early 1970s (Forrester et al., 1972; Swan et al., 1976) ventricular function curves could be constructed on such patients. Analysis of such data allowed Forrester and colleagues (Forrester et al., 1976) to develop a new classification based upon cardiac index (CI) and pulmonary capillary wedge pressure (PCWP), which was useful not only for prognosis but also for guiding therapy based on haemodynamic values observed in survivors.

The designated haemodynamic values espoused by the authors also correlated with significant physiological abnormalities such as pulmonary congestion when the PCWP was greater than 18 mm Hg and signs of hypoperfusion when cardiac index was <2.2 litres $min^{-1} m^{-2}$ (Fig. 13.1). It seemed intuitive that if therapy could correct both physiological and haemodynamic abnormalities, prognosis could be improved. The original haemodynamic subgroups are shown in Table 13.1. It is important to note that this classification, although based on ventricular function, does not take into account the independent effects of mechanical defects, RV infarction, degree of coronary artery disease, severe hypertension or co-morbid conditions. Nonetheless, sound principles of therapy can be based upon it.

In this context, we will discuss the haemodynamic management of cardiogenic shock to include the patient with RV infarction, and mechanical defects such as VSD (ventricular septal defect) or mitral regurgitation. Before discussing the management of individual subsets a sound understanding of pharmacological agents is necessary.

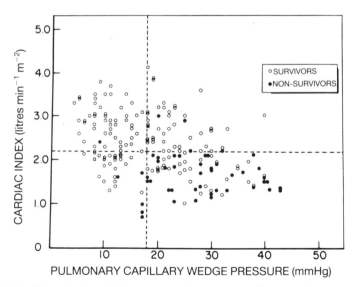

Figure 13.1 The relationship between pulmonary capillary wedge pressure and cardiac index in 200 patients at the time of admission to the Cedar-Sinai Medical Center Myocardial Infarction Research Unit. Dashed lines are placed at the levels of 18 mm Hg for the pulmonary capillary wedge pressure and 2.2 litres $min^{-1} m^{-2}$ for cardiac index. Mortality rate appears to increase as cardiac performance deteriorates as characterized by decreasing CI and increasing PCWP (from Forrester 1976), reprinted with permission.)

Table 13.1   Prognosis after myocardial infarction based upon clinical and haemodynamic parameters

	% Patients	Mortality
Clinical class of acute myocardial infarction (Killip and Kimball (Killip & Kimball, 1967))		
Class 1 – No signs of congestive heart failure	40–50%	6%
Class 2 – S$_3$, pulmonary congestion	30–40%	17%
Class 3 – Acute pulmonary oedema	10–15%	81%
Class 4 – Cardiogenic shock	5–10%	81%
Clinical subsets of acute myocardial infarction (Cedars-Sinai (Forrester *et al.*, 1976))		
(1) No pulmonary congestion or tissue hyperfusion	25%	1%
(2) Pulmonary congestion only	25%	11%
(3) Tissue hypoperfusion only	15%	18%
(4) Tissue hypoperfusion and pulmonary congestion	35%	60%
Haemodynamic subsets (Cedars-Sinai (Forrester *et al.*, 1976))		
Subset 1 PCWP ≤18 mm Hg; CI >2.2 litres min^{-1} m^{-2}	25%	3%
Subset 2 PCWP ≥18 mm Hg; CI >2.2 litres min^{-1} m^{-2}	25%	9%
Subset 3 PCWP ≤18 mm Hg; CI ≤2.2 litres min^{-1} m^{-2}	15%	23%
Subset 4 PCWP ≥18 mm Hg; CI ≤2.2 litres min^{-1} m^{-2}	35%	51%

The Pharmacological Basis for Support of Myocardial Function

To understand the pharmacological activity of the various intravenous inotropic agents now available for the management of myocardial dysfunction, it is necessary to understand the biochemical basis of myocardical contraction and relaxation in the normal and failing heart (Braunwald *et al.*, 1984; Smith *et al.*, 1988).

Each of these inotropic agents is able to increase the inotropic state through their ability to increase cyclic adenosine monophosphate (cAMP) (Fabiato & Fabiato, 1979; Ikemoto, 1982; Chapman, 1983; Kranias & Solaro, 1983; Braunwald *et al.*, 1984). This mediator plays a pivotal role in promoting contraction by its ability to enhance fast calcium movement within the myocardial cell during systole. The enzyme adenylate cyclase regulates intracellular concentration of cAMP (Fig. 13.2). Stimulation of β-receptors on the cell membrane modulates the activity of adenylate cyclase. Phosphodiesterase inhibition can also increase intracellular cAMP by reducing its breakdown.

Increased intracellular cAMP activates protein kinases which catalyse the transfer of phosphates from adenosine triphosphate to intracellular proteins, causing faster calcium movement through slow calcium channels on the cell membrane and the release of intracellular calcium stores. The latter mechanism occurs through activation of a calcium pump in the sarcoplasmic reticulum from the phosphorylation of phospholamban (Fig. 13.2). Increased cytosolic calcium can also be mediated by the sodium–calcium

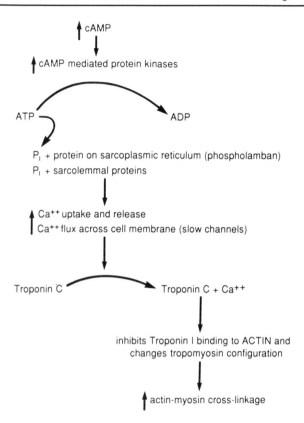

Figure 13.2 Intracellular events mediated by an increase in cyclic AMP. Cyclic AMP-mediated protein kinase phosphorylates proteins on both the sarcoplasmic reticulum and the sarcolemma. It increases calcium uptake and release from the sarcoplasmic reticulum and increases calcium flux across the cell membrane. The interaction of calcium and troponin C changes tropomyosin configuration. This increases actin–myosin cross-linkage.

exchange mechanism at the site of non-gated ionic channels. The increase of cytosolic calcium in conjunction with an adequate supply of ATP allow engagement of actin and myosin myofilaments. As a result, actin is drawn to the centre of the sarcomere, resulting in shortening of myocardial fibres.

The actin–myosin interaction is regulated by the troponin complex which consists of troponin C, troponin I and troponin T. Troponin C contains a specific binding site for calcium which is regulated by troponin I. Tropomyosin, which is bound to the troponin complex by troponin T, prevents actin–myosin interaction. The amount of free cytosolic calcium available determines the extent of binding between calcium and troponin C and the subsequent force of contraction. This binding of calcium to troponin C causes a conformational change in tropomyosin, allowing for the cross-bridging betwen actin and myosin. As tropomyosin withdraws from the space it occupies between the actin and myosin, cross-bridging occurs (Fig. 13.2).

Isovolumic relaxation occurs as the actin–myosin complex dissociates. This is also an energy-requiring process and is mediated by a fall in cytosolic calcium. As a result, calcium dissociates from troponin C and tropomyosin resumes its normal position between actin and myosin. This is an active process regulated by cAMP and phospholambin. Impaired isovolumic relaxation can occur because of impaired uptake of calcium by the sarcoplasmic reticulum, increased calcium affinity for troponin C and a decreased rate of inactivation of actin–myosin cross-bridging.

Understanding the roles of intracellular calcium and cAMP allow a better understanding of how inotropic agents work. Cardiac glycosides increases the amount of cytosolic calcium by inhibiting Na/K^+-ATPase, resulting in a small increase of intracellular sodium which then is exchanged for calcium via the sodium calcium exchange mechanism. $\beta1$-Agonists bind to the β-receptor of the cell (Bristow et al., 1986). Adenylate cyclase activity which is then stimulated, increases the concentration of intracellular cAMP directly. Cyclic AMP then increases calcium entry through slow gate and stimulates the release and uptake of calcium by sarcoplasmic reticulum. Drugs that inhibit phosphodiesterase fraction 3, such as amrinone, retard cyclic AMP degradation and thus increase intracellular cyclic AMP (Benotti et al., 1978).

Parenteral inotropic agents such as the phosphodiesterase inhibitors (e.g. amrinone) and the sympathomimetic amines (e.g. dobutamine, or dopamine or noradrenaline) are preferred over digoxin for treatment of patients with acute heart failure or cardiogenic shock. They are often used in conjunction with vasodilator agents and diuretics to optimize cardiac loading conditions. Digoxin, by its effect on inhibiting the Na^{2+}/K^+ pump (Gysel-Barton & Godfraind, 1979) can increase contractility in the patient with heart failure but not to the extent of the catecholamines (Goldstein et al., 1980) or phosphodiesterase inhibitors. Some reports have actually suggested reduced survival in myocardial infarction patients given digoxin (Moss et al., 1981; Bigger et al., 1985). In general, its use is more widespread in chronic heart failure (The Captopril–Digoxin Multicenter Research Group, 1988).

In these more acute situations, the goal of therapy is to optimize oxygen transport and the clinician must assess the known effects of each inotrope on heart rate, contractility, LV filling pressure, systemic pressure and myocardial oxygen consumption. Specifically, inotropic agents have the potential to aggravate myocardial ischaemia by increasing myocardial oxygen consumption by increasing either pressure work or heart rate. In the presence of ischaemia, therefore, agents with afterload-reducing and only minor chronotropic properties may be desirable (Benotti et al., 1980; Siskind et al., 1986; Wynands, 1989; Moser et al., 1991; Ganz et al., 1991).

It must be pointed out that neither the β-agonists nor the phosphodiesterase inhibitors have been shown to improve survival by themselves. Most clinical studies of these agents have looked at physiological parameters, and strategies have been devised for clinical use based on these physiological effects.

The Use of Catecholamines in Low Cardiac Output States

Catecholamines by their interaction with adrenergic receptors (Ahlquist, 1948; Letkowitz et al., 1983) are frequently used to treat patients with cardiogenic shock, with the main goals being an increase in cardiac index (CI) and blood pressure. With selected agents the PCWP can also be lowered.

Dopamine

Dopamine is a complex drug given the fact that its effects are dose-dependent (Goldberg et al., 1977; Marcus et al., 1987; Wynands, 1989). It is capable of dopaminergic stimulation (Goldberg et al., 1985) with the result-ant effects of increased renal and splanchnic blood flow at low doses of 1–5 $\mu g\,kg^{-1}\,min^{-1}$ (Table 13.2). There is mild β1-agonist (Watanabe, 1983) activity, producing a small increase in stroke volume. At higher doses between 5 and 15 $\mu g\,kg^{-1}\,min^{-1}$, β1-receptor stimulation predominates, resulting in increases in stroke volume, cardiac output and heart rate (HR). Because of its low β2-receptor agonist activity, little peripheral or pulmonary vasodilation occurs. As a result, neither systemic vascular resistance (SVR) nor PCWP change significantly. Doses greater than 15 $\mu g\,kg^{-1}\,min^{-1}$ cause α1-receptor stimulation with the resultant effect of peripheral vasoconstric-tion. Although this helps to maintain or increase blood pressure, it has potential deleterious effects on cardic output and renal blood flow.

Table 13.2 Catecholamine receptors stimulation

Drug	Receptor				
	α_1	α_2	β_1	β_2	DA_1
Adrenaline	+++	+++	+++	0	0
Noradrenaline	+++	+++	+++	0	0
Isoproterenol	0	0	+++	+++	0
Dopamine	++	++[c]	+++[b]	+	+++[a]
Dobutamine	+	0	+++	+	0

α_1 = postsynaptic receptor in vascular smooth muscle; α_2 = presynaptic receptor; β_1 = largely cardiac; β_2 = largely smooth muscle of vasculature and bronchial tree; DA_1 = dopaminergic postsynaptic receptors in renal, splanchnic, cerebral and coronary vessels. + = stimulation; 0 = no effect.
[a] At doses <5 $\mu g\,kg^{-1}\,min^{-1}$.
[b] At doses between 5 and 15 $\mu g\,kg^{-1}\,min^{-1}$.
[c] At doses >15 $\mu g\,kg^{-1}\,min^{-1}$.

Dobutamine

Dobutamine is a synthetic cardioactive sympathomimetic amine that stimu-lates β1-activity predominantly over β2- and α-adrenoceptors (Goldberg *et al.*, 1977; Sonnenblick *et al.*, 1979; Pozen *et al.*, 1981; Marcus *et al.*, 1987; Baim, 1989) (Table 13.2).

In patients with heart failure, dobutamine produces a reduction in sys-temic vascular resistance as cardiac output rises. It has been shown to decrease PCWP and increase stroke work. It can cause increases in HR, although its effect on blood pressure is variable (Sonnenblick *et al.*, 1979; Wynands, 1989).

Dobutamine also increases myocardial oxygen consumption. In a study by Bendersky and colleagues involving patients with chronic heart failure associated with ischaemic heart disease, both coronary sinus flow and myocardial oxygen consumption increased during dobutamine infusion (Bendersky *et al.*, 1981). The investigators reported that overt myocardial ischaemia was a rare occurrence among their patient group. However, in one patient, myocardial lactate extraction changed to lactate production during dobutamine infusion, indicating myocardial ischaemia.

In patients with coronary artery disease, blood flow to the myocardium is compromised. While dobutamine increases blood flow in patients with normal coronary arteries, in patients with coronary artery disease these increases are inhomogeneous. Meyer and colleagues (1976) assessed the influence of dobutamine on coronary blood flow in patients with and with-out coronary artery disease. It was found that dobutamine appeared to increase myocardial perfusion significantly in normal patients, while pro-ducing much smaller increases in mean coronary blood flow and possibly further increasing the inhomogeneity of regional coronary perfusion in some patients with severe coronary artery disease. This finding prompted the authors of the study to suggest that dobutamine be used with caution however, in patients with severe coronary artery disease.

Another study of 18 patients with congestive heart failure complicating coronary artery disease and 7 patients with primary cardiomyopathy deter-mined improved haemodynamics in both groups (Gillespie *et al.*, 1977). However, 22% of the patients with coronary artery disease showed abnormal lactate extraction with doses of dobutamine up to 15 μg kg^{-1} min^{-1}. One experimental study (Vatner & Baig, 1979), using a canine model of coronary artery occlusion, demonstrated evidence of worsening contractile function only when dobutamine increased HR. Another study (Willerson *et al.*, 1976) showed that doses of dobutamine $\geq$20 μg kg^{-1} min^{-1} which increased HR was associated with ST elevation.

In contrast, Gillespie and colleagues (1977) demonstrated in 16 patients with acute moycardial infarction that dobutamine in doses of 1–40 μg kg^{-1} min^{-1} did not increase either ventricular premature beat (VBP) frequency or infarct size measured by CKMB values during the first 7 h of a documented myocardial infarction. Furthermore, Buda and colleagues (1987) demonstrated, using echocardiographic techniques in an experimental model of myocardial infarction, that dobutamine increased the contractility of the non-ischaemic territory and reduced the size of the functional border zone. Therefore, although there is no clear-cut evidence that dobutamine increases infarct size, it should be recognized that in a small percentage of patients with coronary artery disease ischemia may be exacerbated, especially if HR increases significantly. Use of this agent should be guided by close attention to HR changes and possibly markers of ischaemia such as an elevated PCWP or ST segment shift.

Noradrenaline

This is both an α and a β-agonist (Table 13.1). However, it has less $\beta2$–agonist activity. Therefore, it can cause more peripheral vasoconstriction. It may be used to treat a primary decrease in systemic pressure or an exacerbation of right ventricular ischemia and failure. In acute left heart failure it is most commonly used with an $\alpha1$-blocker such as phentolamine to counteract the peripheral vasoconstricting effects which increase LV afterload (Abrams *et al.*, 1973).

Isoproterenol

Isoproterenol (Watanabe, 1983) can be used when a chronotropic response is required in addition to an inotropic effect. Its powerful $\beta1$ effects increase HR significantly, making it useful in treatment of symptomatic bradycardias or complete heart block. However, it is well-known that it produces or aggravates ventricular arrhythmias and can increase myocardial oxygen consumption. Therefore, it is used cautiously in patients with coronary artery disease.

The Role of Phosphodiesterase Inhibitors

Amrinone

Amrinone is a bipyridine guanide that exerts its inotropic effect through inhibition of the enzyme phosphodiesterase III, thereby increasing cyclic adenosine monophosphate (cAMP) and increasing cystolic calcium (Fig. 13.3). In addition to its inotropic properties, amrinone causes vasodilation, both arterial and venous, and thus reduces the systemic vascular resistance and workload (preload and afterload) of the heart.

Intravenous administration of the agent has been shown to increase cardiac output by 30–69% in patients with heart failure, and augment dP/dt without causing significant changes in HR or blood pressure (Benotti *et al.*,

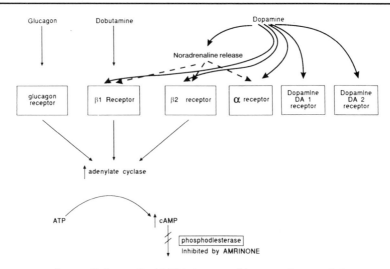

Figure 13.3   Intracellular cyclic AMP is increased by stimulation of glucagon and β_1 and β_2 receptors. Each of these receptors increases adenylate cyclase activity which increases cyclic AMP. Phosphodiesterase inhibitors such as amrinone prevent the breakdown in cyclic AMP.

1978; LeJemtel *et al.*, 1979; Klein *et al.*, 1981). These effects are accompanied by a reduction in LV filling pressure, mean pulmonary and right atrial pressure, and systemic and pulmonary resistance (Fig. 13.4). Amrinone has been shown to reduce PCWP by an average of 27%, while a similar decrease has been reported for SVR. Stroke work is not changed.

Of particular significance is the effect of amrinone on myocardial oxygen consumption. Unlike the sympathomimetic amines, amrinone appears to produce a 20–30% decrease in myocardial oxygen consumption (Benotti *et al.*, 1980; Baim, 1985). An explanation for this phenomenon may lie with the vasodilating capabilities of amrinone. The effect of an inotropic agent on myocardial oxygen consumption depends on its net effect on HR, contractile state and mean systolic wall stress. Unless increased HR and contractile state are offset by decreased wall stress, myocardial oxygen consumption will rise. A reduction in cardiac preload and afterload, achieved through amrinone's vasodilating properties, may produce the necessary fall in resting wall tension required to decrease myocardial oxygen consumption.

Findings from clinical studies appear to support this explanation. In a study by Benotti *et al.* (1980), in which intravenous amrinone was administered to nine patients with ischemic cardiomyopathy, myocardial oxygen consumption fell by 30%, despite a 69% increase in cardiac output. Coronary sinus blood flow decreased by 17% and arterial-coronary sinus oxygen difference fell by 16%.

The beneficial effects upon haemodynamics appear to be sustained better with amrinone than with dobutamine. In a study by Klein *et al.* (1981), comparing these two agents in patients with chronic congestive heart failure,

HEMODYNAMIC EFFECTS OF AMRINONE

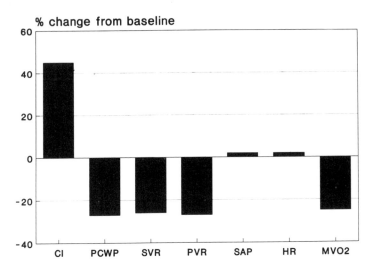

Figure 13.4   The mean effects of haemodynamics produced by intravenous infusion of amrinone from several studies. Amrinone increases cardiac index (CI) and decreases pulmonary capillary wedge pressure (PCWP), systemic vascular resistance (SVR), pulmonary vascular resistance (PVR) and myocardial oxygen consumption (MVO2). Neither systolic arterial pressure (SAP) nor heart rate (HR) are altered.

the haemodynamic effects were found to be comparable. However, the initial increment in cardiac output produced by dobutamine decreased after 8 h of therapy (Fig. 13.3), whereas the increase produced by amrinone was sustained over 24 hours of infusion (Klein *et al.*, 1981). This apparent tachyphylaxis of dobutamine is likely on the basis of β-receptor downregulation (Bristow *et al.*, 1986). Theoretically, this should not occur with amrinone because of its different mechanisms of action. However, one recent study (Maisel *et al.*, 1989) did suggest that β-receptor downregulation occurred with i.v. amrinone. The reason for this observation is unclear. However, overzealous administration of the inotropic drug could have induced a stress response through a reflex mechanism. As a result, circulatory levels of endogenous catecholamines increase and can cause a secondary decrease in β-receptors.

Combination Therapy

Combination therapy with amrinone and dobutamine has been found to decrease PCWP and increase cardiac output to a greater extent than when either of the drugs are used alone. In a study by Gage and colleagues, the effects of amrinone, dobutamine and a combination of the two drugs on positive LV d*P*/d*t* and LV performance were evaluated in 11 patients with chronic congestive heart failure (Gage *et al.*, 1986). When compared to dobutamine alone, the addition of amrinone resulted in further increases in LV dP/dt (from 1202 ± 376 to 1319 ± 419 mm Hg s^{-1}) and cardiac index (from 3.04 ± 0.67 to 3.56 ± 0.78 litres min^{-1} m^{-2}). The combination also induced a further reduction in LV end-diastolic pressure (from 18.2 ± 10.3 to 15.3 ± 11.3 mm Hg) when compared with amrinone alone (Fig. 13.5). It was

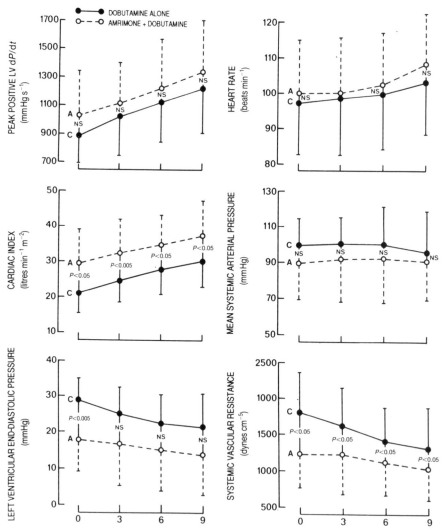

Figure 13.5 The results of combination therapy using dobutamine and amrinone. Increasing doses of dobutamine are administered before and after injection of amrinone. The combination results in further increases in cardiac index and reductions in left ventricular end diastolic pressure and systemic vascular resistance. (Reprinted with permission from Gage *et al.*, 1986.)

concluded that the addition of amrinone to intermediate doses of dobutamine produces greater positive inotropic effect and improvement in LV function than administration of dobutamine alone (possibly at lower metabolic cost to the myocardium).

Common Side-Effects of Inotropic Agents

Arrhythmias and hypotension can occur with either amrinone or dobutamine. Amrinone induces reversible thrombocytopaenia in 2.4–4% of cases and arrhythmias in 3%. Gastrointestinal upset, chest pain and an increase in liver enzymes have been reported on rare occasions (Treadway, 1985).

Dobutamine's side-effect profile is similar to that of amrinone. Premature ventricular beats have been reported to increase in 5% of patients receiving this agent, arrhythmias constituting the most serious side-effect. Occurrence of thrombocytopaenia, however, is rare.

The Role of Vasodilators in Cardiogenic Shock

In the last two decades, vasodilators have taken on a more important role in the treatment of patients with acute heart failure. Patients with reduced pump performance have a critical dependence on the outflow resistance; hence, drugs that relax the peripheral arterial bed and reduce resistance increase stroke volume. Furthermore, the improvement in pump performance is produced by the reduction in myocardial oxygen consumption through reduced systolic pressure or reduced heart size.

In addition to the effect of vasodilators reducing outflow resistance, patients manifesting reduced LV compliance due to acute myocardial ischaemia may benefit from sodium nitroprusside, nitroglycerin and phentolamine (Franciosa et al., 1972; Alderman & Glantz, 1976; Chatterjee et al., 1976a; Berkowitz et al., 1977; Brodie et al., 1977; Miller et al., 1977; Calvin et al., 1983) by virtue of their effects to shift the end-diastolic pressure–volume relationship down and to the right, and hence to mediate an improvement in LV diastolic function. The pericardium appears to be an important modulator of this effect because such shifts are not observed when the pericardium has been surgically removed (Alderman & Glantz, 1976).

Without this effect on LV end-diastolic pressure–volume relationships, much of the benefit observed during the use of vasodilators might be counterbalanced by these agents' effects of reducing venous tone, venous return, and, therefore, LV preload. However, the concomitant shift downward of the LV diastolic pressure–volume relationship observed with these vasodilators both maintains end-diastolic volume and reduces end-diastolic pressure.

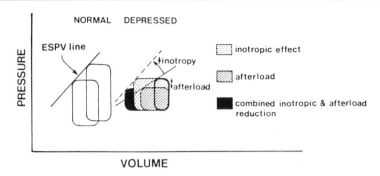

Figure 13.6 The physiological benefits of afterload reduction and increased contractility in patients with depressed ventricular performance using pressure–volume loop analysis. Contractility is defined by the slope of the end-systolic pressure–volume line. An increase in the inotropic state causes an increase in the slope. The physiological result of increased contractility is that the end-systolic point for the pressure–volume curve is shifted to the left, increasing stroke volume (dotted area). Afterload reduction reduces the ejection pressure, assuming that the contractile state has not changed. This will also result in the pressure–volume loop intersecting the end-systolic pressure line at a lower end-systolic volume; hence, stroke volume is also increased (hatched area). Combined therapy increases stroke volume even further (dark area).

Reduction in afterload at a similar preload lowers the pressure at which aortic ejection commences, and converts pressure work to volume work; an increase in stroke volume results, while stroke work may not change significantly (Fig. 13.6).

To gain the maximum benefit from administration of systemic vasodilators the patient must first be adequately volume resuscitated (Pouleur *et al.*, 1980; Packer *et al.*, 1980). In chronic congestive failure, hydralazine mediates an increase in improved forward flow only in those patients with a larger than normal LV preload prior to administration.

Because vasodilators shift LV diastolic pressure–volume relationships downward, thereby reducing wall tension, myocardial O_2 demand is reduced. A decrease in the PCWP with vasodilators will also protect against the development of pulmonary oedema. Concurrently, vasodilators reduce LV afterload, which will be associated with improved stroke volume and O_2 transport when end-diastolic volumes are normal or above normal prior to administration.

Types of Vasodilators

Sodium Nitroprusside

This is an extremely important vasodilator that affects both the arterial and the venous circulation (Pouleur *et al.*, 1980). The side-effects include hypotension from overdose and the accumulation of thiocyanate. The balanced effect on the venous capacitance and arterial resistance vessels results in both afterload reduction and reduction in pulmonary congestion (Franciosa *et al.*, 1972; Palmer & Lasseter, 1975; Chatterjee *et al.*, 1976b). Heart rate, in general, increases and arterial blood pressure is reduced in normal patients; however, in heart failure this is not seen regularly. Nitroprusside is given in a dose between 15 and 400 mg min^{-1} (Table 13.3). Prolonged administration of high doses can result in cyanide toxicity, especially in the presence of renal failure. Thiocyanate levels should be determined under any of these conditions. Acute cyanide poisoning can be treated with amyl nitrite inhalations and intravenous administration of sodium thiosulphate.

Table 13.3 Doses ranges for drugs used in cardiogenic shock

Drug	Usual doses	Intended haemo-dynamic action	Major side-effects
Nitroglycerin	10–200 μg min^{-1}	↓↓ PCWP ↓ ischaemia	hypotension, headache
Nitroprusside	15–40 μg min^{-1}	↓ SAP, afterload, PCWP ↑ CI	Hypotension, thiocyanate toxicity, ↓ PO_2 methaemobloginaemia ischaemia
Phentolamine	0.25–1 μg min^{-1}	↓ SAP, afterload, PCWP ↑ CI	hypotension
Noradrenaline	1–8 μg kg^{-1} min^{-1}	↑ SAP	↑ afterload; variable effect upon cardiac output
Dopamine	1–5 μg kg^{-1} min^{-1} 5–15 μg kg^{-1} min^{-1} >15 μg kg^{-1} min^{-1}	↑ renal blood flow ↑ CI, ↑ SAP ↑ CI, ↑ SAP	↑ HR, arrhythmia
Dobutamine	2.5–15 μg kg^{-1} min^{-1}	↑ CI, ↓ PCWP	↑ HR, arrhythmia (less common) ↑ ischaemia
Amrinone	2.5–10 μg kg^{-1} min^{-1}	↑ CI, ↓ PCWP, ↓ myocardial O_2 consumption	↑ ischaemia (rare)

Intravenous Nitroglycerin

Nitroglycerin i.v. is a commonly used agent in treatment of pulmonary oedema. Nitroglycerin has a profound effect on the venous circulation and therefore results in a reduction in venous return and PCWP (Alderman & Glantz, 1976; Smith *et al.*, 1988). Cardiac output usually is unchanged. The usual dose range is between 30 and 200 μg min^{-1} titrated to a haemodynamic response (usually decreasing PCWP to 14–18 mm Hg and decreasing systolic blood pressure by 10%).

Nitroglycerin may have advantages over diuretics in the treatment of acute pulmonary oedema. Recent studies have demonstrated that furosemide, a potent loop diuretic, can result in a reduction in cardiac output and an elevation in SVR and PCWP within 15–20 min of administration (Francis *et al.*, 1985). Eventually the diuretic effect dominates. It is in this early phase that the use of a venodilator may result in a more immediate reduction in pulmonary venous pressure and congestion.

An Integrated Approach to the Pharmacological Management of Patients With Cardiogenic Shock

The original description by Forrester and colleagues of haemodynamic subsets of myocardial infarction consisted of four groups: (1) patients with normal haemodynamics, (2) patients who have low cardiac output from hypovolaemia, (3) patients with backward failure or pulmonary congestion, and (4) patients with both pulmonary congestion and low cardiac output. It did not specifically take into account patients with mechanical defects such as VSD or papillary muscle rupture, patients with RV infarction or patients with low cardiac output secondary to high LV afterload.

Figure 13.7 provides an algorithm for the use of vasoactive drugs based on a broader spectrum of hemodynamic profiles. Subset 1 represents a patient who is hypovolaemic. This is indicated by a low PCWP in addition to a low cardiac output. This derangement is often based on previous diuretic use, excessive nitrate or morphine administration. In this instance, a volume challenge is the most appropriate choice for therapy. In this setting aloquots of crystalloid or colloid between 100 and 250 ml (Weil & Henning, 1979) to raise the PCWP to between 14 and 18 mm Hg are used. The target range of PCWP must be individualized. Values between 14 and 18 are suggested as an initial target because of previous studies of myocardial patients given either volume for low PCWP or afterload reduction for high PCWP (Crexells *et al.*, 1977). Cardiac output was optimized with this range of filling pressures (Fig. 13.8).

Subset 2 represents a patient who has an elevated afterload indicated by a high blood pressure and depressed cardiac index. The PCWP is optimized between 14 and 18 mm Hg. In this instance, the most appropriate choice for therapy is not an inotropic agent but a vasodilator that has a significant effect on the arterial side of the circulation (i.e. an afterload reducing agent such as nitroprusside, phentolamine or high-dose nitroglycerin). Subset 3 represents a patient that is hypotensive, has a low cardiac index and an elevated PCWP. This patient has depressed inotropy resulting in true cardiogenic shock. The patient could also have a concomitant mechanical defect such as a VSD or papillary muscle rupture which must be excluded. In this instance we use dopamine as our initial drug of choice to restore arterial pressure and

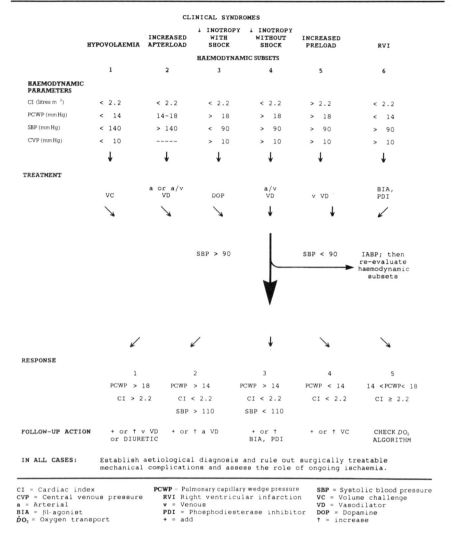

Figure 13.7 Treatment algorithm for patients who have low cardiac outputs states complicating myocardial infarction using volume challenge, inotropic and vasodilator therapy. (See text for explanation.)

maintain coronary perfusion pressure. Agents such as noradrenaline and phenylephrine could also be used and may be more appropriate in the patient with significant tachycardia because they have small chronotropic effects. In most cases, the patient will also require additional agents to decrease the PCWP and increase the cardiac index. If dopamine has resulted in an adequate blood pressure response, vasodilators can be used. In instances where the blood pressure response has been poor the use of dobutamine or amrinone is helpful. If severe hypotension persists the use of an intra-aortic

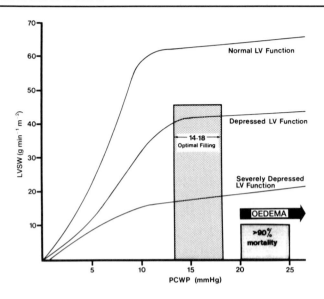

Figure 13.8   Ventricular function curve in acute myocardial infarction. Cardiogenic shock in left ventricular function curve is depressed. Pulmonary oedema formation is noted with pulmonary capillary wedge pressures in excess of 20 mm Hg with high mortality being observed in patients with severely depressed left ventricular function. Optimal filling for such patients appears to be between 14 and 18 mm Hg.

balloon pump (IABP) is useful (McEnany *et al.*, 1978). This technique by itself can salvage approximately 15% of patients but is more useful as a bridge to either definitive surgical correction of a mechanical defect or reperfusion.

Subset 4 represents a patient who is not hypotensive but has a depressed cardiac index and an elevated PCWP. Vasodilators can be used initially in this situation but inotropic agents such as dobutamine or amrinone are often needed if the response to vasodilators is poor or the blood pressure is low. Subset 5 represents the patient who has an elevated PCWP (i.e. backward failure) either because of reduced compliance or poor contractility. In general, these patients are treated with diuretics or venodilators. Underlying myocardial ischaemia manifesting itself as a primary diastolic abnormality may be responsible and should be sought out as a cause. If found, attempts to decrease myocardial O_2 consumption with β-blockers or calcium blockers can help. Finally, subset 6 represents a patient with a predominant RV infarction characterized by an elevated CVP, low PCWP and cardiac index. If the patient is not hypotensive and CVP is >12 mm Hg a β1-agonist (Dell'-Italia *et al.*, 1985) or amrinone can be given. Volume challenge should be attempted if the CVP is <12 mm Hg and the PCWP is less than 15 mm Hg (Benotti *et al.*, 1978; Goldstein *et al.*, 1983; Dell'Italia *et al.*, 1985; Calvin, 1991).

Further volume loading may not be helpful once this range has been achieved. If the patient is or becomes hypotensive, dopamine should be administered.

Figure 13.7 also emphasizes the importance of assessing the response to therapy and subsequent follow-up action. In each situation, haemodynamics should be reassessed. If the systolic blood pressure is lower than 90 mm Hg, consideration of IABP should be given. If the blood pressure is stablized but haemodynamics are not yet optimized, pharmacological agents should be added or increased to achieve the desired end-points.

Once an optimal PCWP and a cardiac index >2.2 litres $min^{-1} m^{-2}$ are achieved, some consideration should be given to the adequacy of oxygen transport. Although, no randomized clinical trials are available that determine the desired target for $\dot{D}O_2$, a goal of 400 ml $min^{-1} m^{-2}$ is recommended. To achieve this one should consider all oxygen transport variables.

Up to now we have considered only cardiac index as an oxygen variable. Other factors such as PaO_2 (gas exchange) and haemoglobin or haematocrit (oxygen-carrying capacity) need to be considered as well. An algorithm depicting clinical decision-making using oxygen transport variables is shown in Fig. 13.9. In

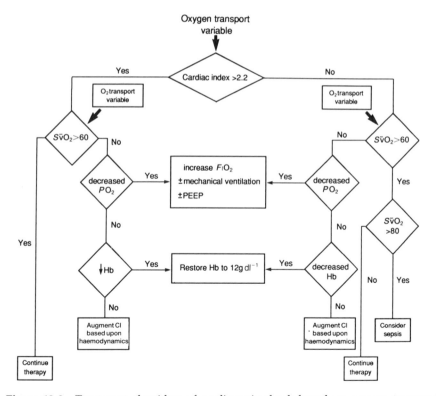

Figure 13.9 Treatment algorithm of cardiogenic shock based on oxygen transport variables.

practice, many of these considerations are being made simultaneously. However, in a logical fashion one needs to ask the following questions:

(1) Has a cardiac index of $2.2\,ml\,min^{-1}\,m^{-2}$ or greater been achieved?
(2) Is a cardiac index of $2.2\,ml\,min^{-1}\,m^{-2}$ or greater adequate?

Question one is easily answered by measurement of the cardiac index by the thermodilution technique. Question two can be answered by measuring the mixed venous O_2 (SvO_2) assessing end-organ function measuring serum lactate. If the SvO_2 is less than 60% the PO_2 and haemoglobin concentration should be measured and optimized if low. The resultant effect of all these strategies is to maintain $DO_2 \geq 400\,ml\,min^{-1}$ in cardiac patients. Although conclusive data are not available to demonstrate improved survival with this approach one study (Creamer et al., 1990) showed better survival when SvO_2 exceeded 60% compared to older studies where this end-point was not used to treat patients.

Measures Aimed at Restoring Myocardial Perfusion

Beyond using supportive therapy aimed at improving cardiac output and optimizing LV preload, the last decade has witnessed major innovations in therapy aimed at restoring myocardial blood flow.

Thrombolytic therapy is now associated with lowered mortalities for myocardial infarction (GISSI, 1987; International Study of Infarct Survival Collaborative Group (ISIS), 1988). The Society for Cardiac Angiography reported in 1985 (Kennedy et al., 1985) a 42% in-hospital mortality rate for cardiogenic shock in patients who were successfully reperfused, representing a significant improvement over earlier observations.

Other studies (O'Neill et al., 1985; Shani et al., 1986; Lee et al., 1988, 1991) have emphasized the need of a comprehensive and aggressive approach to these patients using acute angioplasty, IABP, in addition to thrombolysis. The multicentre registry of angioplasty therapy of cardiogenic shock reported in 1991 on 69 patients with cardiogenic shock. Angioplasty was successful at restoring patency in 49 patients and unsuccessful in 20 patients (Lee et al., 1991). The group where patency was restored with angioplasty had a short-term survival of 69%, versus 20% in the group where patency was not restored. Long-term survival was also improved by successful angioplasty.

Several studies (DeWood et al., 1980; Laks et al., 1986; Phillips et al., 1986; Guyton et al., 1987) have looked at the efficacy of emergency coronary artery bypass surgery in such patients. The combined pool from four surgical series suggest an average in hospital survival of 72.5% (range 58–88%). Coronary artery bypass surgery performed earlier in the course of either shock or the infarction had the best results. The major impediment to the widespread use of this modality is logistical at present including the need for

24 hour availability of comprehensive cardiovascular teams and facilities and inherent time delays.

The use of IABP has been employed in treating cardiogenic shock over the last two decades. Early experience demonstrated it was a useful technique as a bridge to early surgery aimed at reperfusion or correcting mechanical defects. As a sole therapy it is associated with a low salvage rate of approximately 15% (McEnany *et al.*, 1978). More recently DeWood *et al.* (1980) demonstrated that intra aortic balloon pumping alone had an in-hospital mortality of 52%. One-year mortality in such patients was improved if coronary revascularization was performed within 16 hours.

Nonetheless, this technique is the only therapy that can achieve both systolic unloading of the left ventricle and maintenance of coronary perfusion pressure. These two observations result in a lowering of myocardial oxygen demand and an increased myocardial oxygen supply. It is indicated in any patient with cardiogenic shock, especially when the patient is a candidate for other aggressive therapies. The two major contraindications are aortic regurgitation and suspected aortic dissection. Relative contraindications are peripheral vascular disease and a small body habitus.

Mechanical Defects Complicating Myocardial Infarction

Complicating mechanical defects such as interventricular septal defect or papillary muscle rupture are best treated with surgical correction. Early surgical correction in conjunction with pharmacological therapy and IABP results in a survivorship of 50% (Buckley *et al.*, 1973; Errington *et al.*, 1974; Cohn, 1981; Gray *et al.*, 1983; Nishimura *et al.*, 1983; Clements *et al.*, 1985).

An integrated approach to interventional therapy in cardiogenic shock is shown in Fig. 13.10. Once a patient is identified as having cardiogenic shock

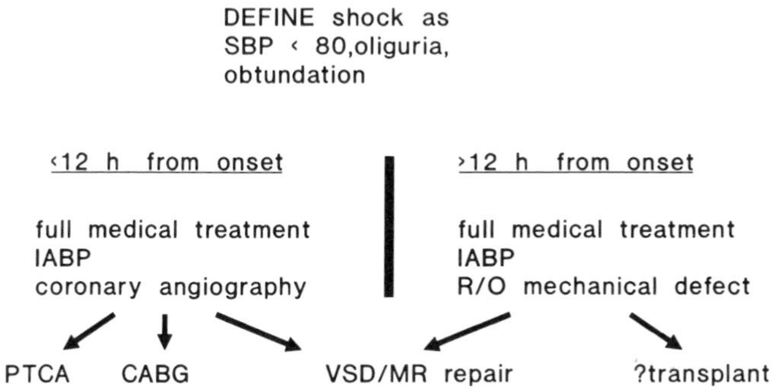

```
                    DEFINE shock as
                    SBP ‹ 80,oliguria,
                    obtundation


    ‹12 h  from  onset       ›12 h  from  onset

    full medical treatment    full medical treatment
    IABP                      IABP
    coronary angiography      R/O mechanical defect

    ↙  ↓  ↘            ↙        ↘
 PTCA    CABG       VSD/MR repair    ?transplant
```

Figure 13.10   An interventional approach to cardiogenic shock defining the roles of reperfusion therapy, repair of mechanical defects and possibly heart transplant. PTCA: pericutaneous transluminal coronary angioplasty; CABG: coronary artery bypass grafting; VSD: ventricular septal defect; MR: mitral valve rupture; R/O: rule out.

the next critical factor is the time from onset of the infarct. When an infarction is less than 6 h to even as long as 12 h consideration should be given to revascularization either in the form of angioplasty or coronary bypass grafting. In addition, identification of a specific mechanical defect mandates repair. Patients who are beyond 12 h should be aggressively supported with a view to potential transplantation.

References

Abrams E, Forrestor JS, Chatterjee K et al. (1973) Variability in response to norepinephrine in acute myocardial infarction. Am. J. Cardiol. **32:** 919–23.

Ahlquist RP (1948) A study of adrenotropic receptors. Am. J. Physiol. **153:** 586–600.

Alderman EL & Glantz SA (1976) Acute hemodynamic interventions shift the diastolic pressure–volume curve in man. Circulation **54:** 662–71.

Alonso DR, Scheidt S & Post M et al. (1973) Pathophysiology of cardiogenic shock: Quantification of myocardial necrosis, clinical, pathologic and electrocardiographic correlation. Circulation **48:** 588–96.

Baim DS (1985) Effects of amrinone on myocardial energetics in severe congestive heart failure. Am. J. Cardiol. **56(3):** B16–B18.

Baim DS (1989) Effect of phosphodiesterase inhibition on myocardial oxygen consumption and coronary blood flow. Am. J. Cardiol. **63:** 23A–6A.

Bendersky R, Chatterjee K, Parmley WW et al. (1981). Dobutamine in chronic ischemic heart failure: alterations in left ventricular function and coronary hemodynamics. Am. J. Cardiol. **48(3):** 554–8.

Benotti JR, Grossman W, Braunwald E et al. (1978) Hemodynamic assessment of amrinone: a new inotropic agent. New Engl. J. Med. **299(25):** 1373–7.

Benotti JR, Grossman W, Braunwald E & Carabello BA (1980) Effects of amrinone on myocardial energy metabolism and hemodynamics in patients with severe congestive heart failure due to coronary artery disease. Circulation **62:** 28–34.

Berkowitz C, McKeever L, Croke RP et al. (1977) Comparative responses to dobutamine and nitroprusside in patients with chronic low output cardiac failure. Circulation **56:** 918–24.

Bertrand M, Rousseau MF, LaBlanche JM et al. (1979) Cineangiographic assessment of left ventricular function in the acute phase of transmural myocardial infarction. Am. J. Cardiol. **43:** 472–80.

Bigger JT, Fleiss JL, Kleiger R et al. (1984) The relationship among ventricular arrhythmias, left ventricular dysfunction, and mortality in the 2 years after myocardial infarction. Circulation **69:** 250–8.

Bigger JT, Fleiss JL, Rolnitsky LAM et al. (1985) Effect of digitalis treatment on survival after acute myocardial infarction. Am. J. Cardiol. **55:** 623–30.

Braunwald E, Sonnenblick EH & Ross JJR (1984) Contraction of the normal heart. In Braunwald E (ed.), Heart Disease, pp. 409–46, Philadelphia: W.B. Saunders.

Bristow MR, Ginsburg R, Umans B *et al.* (1986) Beta-1 and beta-2 adrenergic receptor sub-populations in non-failing and failing human ventricular myocardium: coupling sub-types to muscle contraction and selective beta-1 receptor down-regulation in heart failure. *Circ. Res.* **56:** 297–309.

Brodie BR, Grossman W & McLaurin MT (1977) Effects of sodium nitroprusside on left ventricular diastolic pressure–volume relations. *J. Clin. Invest.* **59:** 59–68.

Buckley MJ, Mundth ED, Daggett WM *et al.* (1971) Surgical therapy for early complication of myocardial infarction. *Surgery* **70:** 814–20.

Buckley MJ, Mundth ED & Daggett WM (1973) Surgical management of ventricular septal defects and mitral regurgitation complicating acute myocardial infarction. *Ann. Thorac. Surg.* **16:** 598–609.

Calvin JE (1991) Optimal right ventricular filling pressures and the role of pericardial constraint in right ventricular infarction in dogs. *Circulation* **84(2):** 852–61.

Calvin JE, Driedger AA & Sibbald WJ (1983) Phentolamine in low cardiac output states: an assessment with ECG-gated cardiac scintigraphy. *Crit. Care Med.* **11(10):** 769–74.

Chapman RA (1983) Control of cardiac contractility at the cellular level. *Am. J. Physiol.* **245:** H535–52.

Chatterjee K, Swan HJC, Kaushik VS *et al.* (1976) Effects of vasodilator therapy for severe pump failure in acute myocardial infarction on short-term and late prognosis. *Circulation* **53:** 797–802.

Clements SD, Story WE, Hurst JW *et al.* (1985) Ruptured papillary muscle, a complication of acute myocardial infarction: Clinical presentation, diagnosis and treatment. *Clin. Cardiol.* **8:** 93–103.

Cohn JN, Guiha NH, Broder MJ & Limas CJ (1974) Right ventricular infarction: Clinical and hemodynamic features. *Am. J. Cardiol.* **33:** 209–14.

Cohn LH (1981) Surgical management of acute and chronic cardiac mechanical complications due to myocardial infarction. *Am. Heart J.* **102:** 1049–60.

Creamer JE, Edwards JD & Nightingale P (1990) Hemodynamic and oxygen transport variables in cardiogenic shock secondary to acute myocardial infarction, and response to treatment. *Am. J. Cardiol.* **65:** 1297–1300.

Crexells C, Chatterjee K, Forrester JS *et al.* (1977) Optimal level of filling pressure in the left side of the heart in acute myocardial infarction. *New Engl. J. Med.* **289:** 1263–6.

Dell'Italia LJ, Starling MR, Blumgardt R *et al.* (1985) Comparative effects of volume loading, dobutamine and nitroprusside in patients with predominant right ventricular infarction. *Circulation* **6:** 1327–35.

DeWood MA, Notske RN, Hensley GR *et al.* (1980) Intra-aortic balloon counterpulsation with and without reperfusion for myocardial infarction shock. *Circulation* **61:** 1105–12.

DeWood MA, Spore J, Nortske R *et al.* (1981) Prevalence of total coronary occlusion during the early hours of transmural myocardial infarction. *New Engl. J. Med.* **303:** 897–902.

Errington ML & Rocha e Silva M, Jr (1974) On the role of vasopressin and angiotensin in the development of irreversible shock. *J. Physiol.* **242:** 119–41.

Fabiato A & Fabiato F (1979) Calcium and cardiac excitation–contraction coupling. *Ann. Rev. Physiol.* **41:** 473–84.

Forrester JS, Ganz W, Diamond G *et al.* (1972) Thermodilution cardiac output determination with a single flow-directed catheter. *Am. Heart J.* **83:** 306–11.

Forrester JS, Diamond G, Chatterjee K & Swan HJC (1976) Medical therapy of acute myocardial infarction by application of hemodynamic subsets. *New Engl. J. Med.* **295:** 1356–62; 1404–13.

Franciosa JB, Buiha NM, Limas CJ *et al.* (1972) Improved left ventricular function during nitroprusside infusion in acute myocardial infarction. *Lancet* **1:** 650–4.

Francis GS, Siegel RM, Goldsmith SR *et al.* (1985) Acute vasoconstrictor response to intravenous furosemide in patients with chronic congestive heart failure. *Ann. Intern. Med.* **103:** 1–5.

Gage J, Rutman J, Lucido D & LeJemtel TH (1986) Additive effects of dobutamine and amrinone on myocardial contractility and ventricular performance in patients with severe heart failure. *Circulation* **74(2):** 367–73.

Ganz W, Watanabe I, Kanamasa K *et al.* (1991) Does reperfusion induce myocardial necrosis? *Circulation* **83:** 1459–60.

Ghysel-Barton J & Godfraind T (1979) Stimulation and inhibition of the sodium pump by cardioactive steroids in relation to their binding sites and their inotropic effect on guinea-pig isolated atria. *Br. J. Pharmacol.* **66:** 175–84.

Gillespie TA, Ambos HD, Sobel BE & Roberts R (1977) Effects of dobutamine in patients with acute myocardial infarction. *Am. J. Cardiol.* **39:** 588–94.

GISSI, Gruppo Italiano Per Lo Studio Della Streptochi-Nasi Nell 'Infarto Miocardico (1987). Long-term effects of intravenous thrombolysis in acute myocardial infarction: Final report of the GISSI study. *Lancet* **2(2):** 871–4.

Glantz SA & Parmley WW (1978) Factors which affect the diastolic pressure–volume curve. *Circ. Res.* **42(2):** 171–80.

Goldberg LI & Rafzer SI (1985) Dopamine receptors. Applications in clinical cardiology. *Circulation* **72:** 245–8.

Goldberg LJ Hsleh YY & Resnekov L (1977) Newer catecholemines for treatment of heart failure and shock: an update for dopamine and a first look at dobutamine. *Prog. Cardiovasc. Dis.* **19:** 327–40.

Goldstein JA, Vlahakes GJ, Verrier ED *et al.* (1982) The role of right ventricular systolic dysfunction and elevated intrapericardial pressure in the genesis of low output in experimental right ventricular infarction. *Circulation* **65:** 513–22.

Goldstein JA, Vlahakes GJ, Verrier ED *et al.* (1983) Volume loading improves low cardiac output in experimental right ventricular infarction. *J. Am. Coll. Cardiol.* **2:** 270.

Goldstein RA (1985) Clinical effects of intravenous amrinone in patients with congestive heart failure. *Am. J. Cardiol.* **56(3):** B16–B18.

Goldstein RA, Passamani ER & Roberts R (1980) A comparison of digoxin and dobutamine in patients with acute infarction and cardiac failure. *New Engl. J. Med.* **303:** 846–50.

Goto Y, Yamamoto J, Saito M *et al.* (1985) Effects of right ventricular ischemia on left ventricular geometry and the end-diastolic pressure–volume relationship in the dog. *Circulation* **72(5):** 1104–14.

Gray RJ, Sethna D & Matloff JM (1983) The role of cardiac surgery in acute myocardial infarction with mechanical complications. *Am. Heart J.* **106:** 723–8.

Guyton RA, Arcidi JM, Jr, Langford DA *et al.* (1987) Emergency coronary bypass for cardiogenic shock. *Circulation* **76 (Suppl. V):** V22–7.

Hands ME, Rutherford JD, Muller JE *et al.* (1989) The in-hospital development of cardiogenic shock after myocardial infarction: incidence, predictors of occurrence, outcome and prognostic factors. *J. Am. Coll. Cardiol.* **14:** 40–6.

Ikemoto N (1982) Structure and function of the calcium pump protein of sarcoplasmic reticulum. *Ann. Rev. Physiol.* **44:** 297–317.

International Study of Infarct Survival Collaborative Group (ISIS) (1988) Randomised trial of intravenous streptokinase, oral aspirin, both, or neither among 17 187 cases of suspected acute myocardial infarction: ISIS-2. *Lancet* **2(1):** 349–60.

Kennedy JW, Gensini GG, Timmis GC *et al.* (1985) Acute myocardial infarction treated with intracoronary streptokinase: A report of the Society for Coronary Angiography. *Am. J. Cardiol.* **55:** 871–5.

Killip T & Kimball JT (1967) Treatment of myocardial infarction in a coronary care unit: A two year experience with 250 patients. *Am. J. Cardiol.* **20:** 457–64.

Klein NA, Siskind SJ, Frishman WH *et al.* (1981) Hemodynamic comparison of intravenous amrinone and dobutamine in patients with chronic congestive heart failure. *Am. J. Cardiol.* **48(1):** 170–5.

Kranias EG & Solaro J (1983) Coordination of cardiac sarcoplasmic reticulum and myofibrillar function by protein phosphorylation. *Fedn. Proc.* **42:** 33–8.

Laks H, Rosenbranz E & Buckberg GD (1986) Surgical treatment of cardiogenic shock after myocardial infarction. *Circulation* **74 (Suppl. III):** III-11–III-15.

Lee L, Bates ER, Pitt B *et al.* (1988) Percutaneous transluminal coronary angioplasty improves survival in acute myocardial infarction complicated by cardiogenic shock. *Circulation* **78:** 1345–51.

Lee L, Erbel R, Brown T *et al.* (1991) Multicenter registry of angioplasty therapy of cardiogenic shock: Initial and long-term survival. *J. Am. Coll. Cardiol.* **17(3):** 599–603.

LeJemtel TH, Keung E, Sonnenblick EH *et al.* (1979) Amrinone: a new on-glycosidic, non-adrenergic cardiotonic agent effective in the treatment of intractable myocardial failure in man. *Circulation* **59(6):** 1098–104.

Letkowitz RJ, Stadel JM & Caron MG (1983) Adenylate cyclase-coupled beta adrenergic receptors: Structure and mechanisms of activation and desensitization. *Ann. Rev. Biochem.* **52:** 159–86.

Loeb HS, Pietas RJ, Tobin JR & Gunnar RM (1969) Hypovolemia in shock due to acute myocardial infarction. *Circulation* **40:** 653–9.

Lorrell B, Leinbach RC, Pohost GM *et al.* (1979) Right ventricular infarction: Clinical diagnosis and differentiation from cardiac tamponade and pericardial constriction. *Am. J. Cardiol.* **43:** 465–71.

McEnany MT, Kay HR, Buckley MJ *et al.* (1978) Clinical experience with intra-aortic balloon pump support in 728 patients. *Circ. Suppl.* **58(3):** I-124–I-132.

Maisel AS, Wright M, Carter SM *et al.* (1989) Tachyphylaxis with amrinone therapy: association with sequestration and down-regulation of lymphocyte beta-adrenergic receptors. *Ann. Intern. Med.* **110:** 195–201.

Mann JM & Roberts WC (1988) Acquired ventricular septal defect during acute myocardial infarction: Analysis of 38 unoperated necropsy patients and comparison with 50 unoperated necropsy patients without rupture. *Am. J. Cardiol.* **62:** 8–19.

Marcus FI, Opie LH & Sonnenblick EH (1987) Digitalis, sympathomimetics and inotropic dilators. In Opie LH (ed.), *Drugs in the Heart (2nd edn)*, pp. 91–110. Philadelphia: W.B. Saunders.

Maseri A & Enson Y (1968) Mixing in the right ventricle and pulmonary artery in man: evaluation of ventricular volume measurements from indicator washout curves. *J. Clin. Invest.* **47:** 848–59.

Meister SG & Helfant RH (1972) Rapid bedside differentiation of ruptured interventricular septum from acute mitral insufficiency. *New Engl. J. Med.* **287:** 1024–5.

Miller RR, Awan NA, Joye JA *et al.* (1977) Combined dopamine and nitroprusside therapy in congestive heart failure. *Circulation* **55:** 881–4.

Moser KM, Cantor JP, Olman M *et al.* (1991) Chronic pulmonary thromboembolism in dogs treated with tranexamic acid. *Circulation* **83:** 1371–9.

Moss AJ, Davis HT, Conard DL *et al.* (1981) Digitalis associated cardiac mortality after myocardial infarction. *Circulation* **64:** 1150–6.

Naccarelli GV, Gray EL, Doughtery AH *et al.* (1984) Amrinone: acute electrophysiologic and hemodynamic effects in congestive heart failure. *Am. J. Cardiol.* **54(6):** 600–4.

Nishimura RA, Schaff HV, Shuh C *et al.* (1983) Papillary muscle rupture complicating acute myocardial infarction: Analysis of 17 patients. *Am. J. Cardiol.* **51:** 373–7.

O'Neill W, Erbel R, Laufer N *et al.* (1985) Coronary angioplasty therapy of cardiogenic shock complicating acute myocardial infarction. *Circulation* **72:** III–309.

Packer M, Miller J, Medina N *et al.* (1980) Importance of left ventricular chamber size determining the response of hydralazine in severe chronic heart failure. *New Eng. J. Med.* **303:** 250–1.

Palmer RP & Lasseter KC (1975) Sodium nitroprusside. *New Engl. J. Med.* **292:** 294–7.

Parmley WW, Tomoda H, Diamond G *et al.* (1975) Dissociation between indices of pump performance and contractility in patients with coronary artery disease and acute myocardial infarction. *Chest* **67(2):** 141–6.

Phillips SJ, Zeff RH, Skinner JR *et al.* (1986) Reperfusion protocol and results in 738 patients with evolving myocardial infarction. *Ann. Thorac. Surg.* **4:** 119–25.

Pouleur H, Covell JW & Ross J (1980) Effects of nitroprusside on venous return and central blood volume in the absence and presence of acute heart failure. *Circulation* **61:** 328–37.

Pozen RG, DiBianco R, Katz RJ *et al.* (1981) Myocardial metabolic and hemodynamic effects of dobutamine in heart failure complicating coronary artery disease. *Circulation* **63(6):** 1279–85.

Santamore WP, Carey R, Goodrich D & Bove AA (1981) Measurement of left and right ventricular volume from implanted radiopaque markers. *Am. J. Physiol* **249:** H896–H900.

Serizawa T, Carbello BA & Grossman W (1980) Effect of pacing-induced ischemia on left ventricular diastolic pressure–volume relations in dogs with coronary stenoses. *Circ. Res.* **46(3):** 430–9.

Shani J, Rivera M, Greengart A *et al.* (1986) Percutaneous transluminal coronary angioplasty in cardiogenic shock. *Am. Coll. Cardiol.* **7:** 149A.

Siskind SJ, Sonnenblick EH, Forman R *et al.* (1986) Acute substantial benefit of inotropic therapy with amrinone on exercise hemodynamics and metabolism in severe congestive heart failure. *Circulation* **74(2):** 367–73.

Smith TW, Braunwald E & Kelly RA (1988) Management of heart failure. In Braunwald E (ed), *Heart Disease*, pp. 485–543. Philadelphia: W.B. Saunders.

Sonnenblick EH, Frishman WH & LeJemtel TH (1979). Dobutamine: A new synthetic cardioactive sympathetic amine. *New Engl. J. Med.* **300(1):** 17–22.

Swan HJC, Ganz W, Forrester JS *et al.* (1976) Catheterization of the heart in man with the use of a flow directed balloon-tipped catheter. *New Engl. J. Med.* **283:** 447–51.

The Captopril-Digoxin Multicenter Research Group (1988) Comparative effects of therapy with captopril and digoxin in patients with mild to moderate heart failure. *J. Am. Med. Assoc.* **259:** 539–44.

The Multicenter Postinfarction Research Group (1983) Risk stratification and survival after myocardial infarction. *New Engl. J. Med.* **309:** 331–6.

Treadway G (1985) Clinical safety of intravenous amrinone – a review. *Am. J. Cardiol.* **56(3):** B39–B40.

Vatner SF & Baig H (1979) Importance of heart rate in determining the effects of sympathomimetic amines on regional myocardial function and blood flow in conscious dogs with acute myocardial ischemia. *Circ. Res.* **45:** 793–803.

Watanabe AM (1983) Recent advances in knowledge about beta-adrenergic receptors: Application to clinical cardiology. *J. Am. Coll. Cardiol.* **1:** 82–9.

Weil MH & Henning RJ (1979) New concepts in the diagnosis and fluid treatment of circulatory shock (Thirteenth Annual Becton, Dickinson and Company Oscar Schwidetsky Memorial Lecture). *Anesthesia Analgesia* **58(2):** 124–32.

Wilcox RG, Olsson CG, Skene AM *et al.* (1988) Trial of tissue plasminogen activator for mortality reduction in acute myocardial infarction (Anglo-Scandinavian Study of Early Thrombolysis (ASSET)). *Lancet* **2(1):** 525–30.

Willerson JT, Hutton I, Watson JT *et al.* (1976) Influence of dobutamine on regional myocardial blood flow and ventricular performance during acute and chronic myocardial ischemia in dogs. *Circulation* **53(5):** 828–33.

Wynands JE (1989) Amrinone: Is it the inotrope of choice? *J. Cardiothor. Anaesth.* **3:** 45–57.

14 Septic Shock

Kevin M. Chan and Edward Abraham

Introduction

Overview

Sepsis and septic shock are a major cause of mortality in the intensive care setting. More than 300 000 cases of Gram-negative bacteraemia are reported annually in the United States, with shock developing in approximately 40% of the cases (Bone et al., 1989a; Tuchschmidt et al., 1991). Mortality from septic shock has remained between 30 and 60% over the past 20 years, even with advances in antibiotic therapy, critical care and haemodynamic monitoring (Rackow et al., 1988; Tuchschmidt et al., 1991). Approximately 40% of septic shock episodes are caused by Gram-negative aerobic bacilli. However, Gram-positive organisms as well as fungi increasingly account for a significant proportion of cases (Rackow et al., 1988; Ziegler et al., 1991). In most studies, Escherichia coli is the predominant Gram-negative organism, followed by the Klebsiella group and then the Pseudomonas group (Rackow et al., 1988; Tuchschmidt et al., 1991). Staphylococcus aureus, S. epidermidis, as well as Streptococcus and Candida species are on the rise as iatrogenic causes of sepsis (Rackow et al., 1988; Tuchschmidt et al., 1991).

Definition

Bacteraemia is defined as the presence of viable bacteria in the circulating blood, while sepsis is defined as the presence of various pus-forming or other pathogenic organisms and/or their 'toxins' in the blood or tissues (Bone, 1991). This is suggested by a presumed site of infection, associated with tachycardia, tachypnoea, and hyperthermia or hypothermia. The 'sepsis syndrome' has further been defined by Bone et al. as representing a systemic response associated with infection, and is diagnosed by sepsis with evidence of altered function (Bone, 1991; Bone et al., 1989a). In an effort to standardize terminology, the 'sepsis syndrome' has been defined as hypothermia (temperature $< 35.6°C$ or $> 38.3°C$), tachycardia (heart rate > 90 beats min^{-1}), tachypnoea (> 20 breaths min^{-1}), and evidence of inadequate organ perfusion, including one or more of the following: PaO_2

< 75 mm Hg (10 kPa), altered cerebral function, elevated lactate disseminated intravascular coagulation (DIC), or oliguria (< 0.5 ml kg^{-1}) (Bone et al., 1989a; Bone, 1991). It is important to note that a positive blood culture or hypotension is not required in this definition. Septic shock is defined by Bone as the sepsis syndrome with hypotension (systolic blood pressure < 90 mm Hg or a reduction of systolic blood pressure of > 40 mm Hg from baseline) (Bone et al., 1989a; Bone, 1991). Others would not require hypotension for a shock state to exist, but rather would consider septic shock to be a condition where infection is coupled with severe tissue hypoperfusion, leading to a total body oxygen debt (Sprung, 1991). Reported mortality from septic shock ranges from 40% to 90% with 43% mortality recently reported in a multicentre trial examining the efficacy of corticosteroids in sepsis (Bone et al., 1989a). This is important prognostically since the mortality of patients with the 'sepsis syndrome', but without shock, was reported as only 13% (Bone et al., 1989a). Therefore, an important goal is to identify septic patients early in the course of disease and to prevent further progression to the shock state.

Haemodynamic Changes With Sepsis and Septic Shock

Cardiac Output in Sepsis

Cardiac output in septic shock can be initially reduced by peripheral pooling of blood, but after the initial volume resuscitation, a hyperkinetic state ensues with an increased or normal cardiac output and a reduced systemic vascular resistance (Siegel et al., 1967; Vincent & Van der Linden, 1990). The reduction in vascular tone is in contrast to hypovolaemic or cardiogenic shock where an increased tone is present.

A reduction in myocardial contractility has long been demonstrated in various septic models (Siegel et al., 1967; Lang et al., 1984; Parrillo et al., 1985; Rackow et al., 1987; Suffredini et al., 1989; Parrillo, 1990; Vincent & Van der Linden, 1990). Although cardiac output appears high, stroke volume is reduced due to the presence of tachycardia (Tuchschmidt et al., 1991) In addition, in sepsis, the left ventricular stroke work index is often diminished (Rackow et al., 1987; Tuchschmidt et al., 1991). This myocardial depression appears early and is directly proportional to the severity of the sepsis (Vincent & Van der Linden, 1990). Suffredini et al. demonstrated the relationship between endoxotaemia and myocardial dysfunction by showing reduced ejection fractions in human subjects infused with endotoxin (Suffredini et al., 1989). A study by Parrillo et al. confirmed the presence of a myocardial depressant factor in sepsis, but failed to demonstrate a relationship between the amount of myocardial dysfunction and mortality (Parrillo et al., 1985). In contrast, other studies showed that patients capable of maintaining cardiac output by increasing heart rate and left ventricular stroke volume are more likely to survive (Parker *et al.*, 1989). Proposed causes for myocardial dysfunction in sepsis include the development of myocardial oedema, membrane alterations of myocardial cells leading to abnormal ion fluxes and contraction, and the circulation of various 'myocardial depressant substances' including cytokines such as tumor necrosis factor (TNF). (Parrillo *et al.*, 1985; Tuchschmidt *et al.*, 1991; Vincent & Van der Linden, 1990).

Oxygen Debt

Tissue oxygen requirements rise, often more than 50% above normal, during sepsis, reflecting a hypermetabolic state (Rackow *et al.*, 1988). Despite the increased cardiac output and concomitant increase in delivery of oxygen ($\dot{D}O_2$) to the periphery, it has been found that oxygen debt, as defined by decreased intracellular oxygen tension and a shift from aerobic to anaerobic metabolism, still occurs. This may result in the development of lactic acidosis. Therefore, the problem in sepsis often is not the delivery of substrate (i.e. oxygen), but rather the inability to utilize oxygen and other substrates brought to the cells.

Oxygen extraction (OER) is the amount of oxygen obtained from blood by the tissues and is represented by the fraction of oxygen consumption/oxygen delivery ($\dot{V}O_2/\dot{D}O_2$). In normal humans, OER lies between 0.25 and 0.35 at rest and is able to increase to greater than 0.80 with exercise (Dantzker *et al.*, 1991). This mechanism enables $\dot{V}O_2$ to remain independent of $\dot{D}O_2$ over a wide range of $\dot{D}O_2$ values. As oxygen delivery in the normal individual decreases or metabolic demand outstrip supply, OER increases to offset the relative reduction in delivery. At critical delivery levels, when the OER is maximum, $\dot{V}O_2$ finally becomes dependent on $\dot{D}O_2$ and begins to fall. For example, during exercise, metabolic demands eventually reach a point where $\dot{D}O_2$ or OER are not sufficient to match metabolic requirements. This is termed the anaerobic threshold and the OER at this level has been found to be approximately 0.60 (Dantzker *et al.*, 1991). Similar maximal increases in OER, to approximately 0.6–0.7 have been found in models where cardiac output and oxygen delivery are reduced through haemorrhage (Smith & Abraham, 1986). In laboratory studies in animals, OER has achieved values between 0.65 and 0.75 with reductions in $\dot{D}O_2$ (Dantzker *et al.*, 1991; Lister, 1991).

During sepsis and in ARDS, oxygen consumption is dependent on oxygen delivery at relatively low levels of OER. This finding may be due to peripheral shunting of blood-transported oxygen and impaired oxygen extraction. Two alterations may be important in sepsis: microvascular occlusion and loss of autoregulatory ability (Groenveld *et al.*, 1987; Dantzker, 1989). Peripheral leukocyte plugging, platelet aggregation, microthrombi and endothelial damage may cause microembolization of small vessels (Groeneveld *et al.*, 1987; Rackow *et al.*, 1988; Vincent & Van der Linden,

1990, Dantzker, 1989). This causes loss in the capillary cross-sectional area and interferes with nutrient capillary recruitment, thereby reducing maximal oxygen extraction (Dantzker, 1989). Microvascular embolization, in an animal model, caused reduced $\dot{V}O_2$ as $\dot{D}O_2$ decreased, producing supply dependency (Dantzker, 1989). Several mediators associated with infection, particularly tumour necrosis factor and platelet activating factor, are capable of activating complement and the coagulation cascade, and may play an important role in producing peripheral microemboli.

The decreased ability to autoregulate vascular tone also can be caused by damage to the endothelium and underlying smooth muscle (Groeneveld et al., 1987; Dantzker, 1989). Mediators of sepsis, including complement activation, platelet aggregating factor and oxygen radical production, cause damage to resistance vessels which may result in $\dot{D}O_2/\dot{V}O_2$ mismatch. Clinical studies correlated a reduction in systemic vascular resistance (SVR) as a marker for abnormal autoregulation with loss of oxygen extraction ability (Dantzker, 1989).

The severe tissue inflammation and interstitial oedema of sepsis contribute to impairment of oxygen diffusion from the capillary bed to the tissues (Groeneveld et al., 1987; Dantzker, 1989; Vincent & Van der Linden, 1990). This is most likely compounded by increased capillary flow secondary to the underlying hyperdynamic state, and results in deficient oxygen extraction by failing to provide enough time for oxygen equilibration between red cells and extravascular cells (Dantzker, 1989).

Maldistribution of Blood Flow

Maintenance of tissue oxygen consumption is partially dependent on the interaction of local vasodilating influences and central and humorally mediated vasoconstriction. Appropriate matching of cellular oxygen needs and oxygen delivery would result in maximal extraction. In sepsis, there is often a maladministration of flow with excessive flow to areas of low metabolic demands and low flow to areas of high oxygen need. (Siegel et al., 1967; Rackow et al., 1988; Vincent & Van der Linden, 1990). Normally, the skin, kidneys, carotid baroreceptors and adrenal glands have high flow rates relative to metabolic demands (Lister, 1991). These organs therefore, under normal conditions, have low OER (skin 0.05, kidneys 0.07), with the heart and brain found to have high OER at 0.60 and 0.33 respectively (Lister, 1991). During sepsis, splanchnic, renal and skin perfusion is compromised and poor matching of oxygen delivery and consumption occurs (Lister, 1991).

Further studies have demonstrated marked increases in splanchnic flow to the liver in sepsis, with a disproportionately higher oxygen consumption in the splanchnic bed when compared to non-septic patients (Dahn et al., 1987). An increase of 40–70% in blood flow to the heart, spleen, adrenal glands and small intestine with a greater than sixfold increase in hepatic flow was found in septic rats (Lang *et al.*, 1984). Blood flow to pancreas, stomach and skeletal muscle was consistently compromised, by 24%, 39% and 52% respectively, in the same study (Lang *et al.*, 1984). Regional increases in shunting have been demonstrated, with flow through splanchnic arterio-venous shunts increasing from 18.6% to 36.5% in canine sepsis (Archie, 1977). Kidney shunting also increased from 4% to 18.6% in endotoxic dogs in the same study (Archie, 1977).

Finally, there also is evidence that circulating mediators in infection affect intracellular metabolism and oxygen utilization. Endotoxic shock produces marked dysfunction in hepatic oxidative metabolism (Bautista & Spitzer, 1990). Similarly, Haupt and co-workers have shown that the plasma from septic patients can alter hepatocyte Krebs' cycle function (Haupt *et al.*, 1987).

Cardiorespiratory Measurements

In septic patients, the cardiac output may be initially reduced due to venous pooling and increased capillary permeability leading to relative intravascular hypovolaemia (Weil & Nishijama, 1978). In this setting, fluid resuscitation produces the 'classic' haemodynamic profile of sepsis with increased cardiac output and a severe reduction in systemic vascular resistance, secondary to peripheral vasodilation and shunting of blood flow. Pulmonary pressures rise due to pulmonary vasoconstriction resulting in elevated right ventricular pressures (Vincent & Van der Linden, 1990). Pulmonary hypertension and a reduced right ventricular ejection fraction are more severe in non-survivors (Vincent & Van der Linden, 1990). A preterminal state has been defined and is characterized by a reduction in cardiac output, elevation in SVR and increasing lactic acidosis with eventual death (Tuchschmidt *et al.*, 1991). However, there is recent data indicating that this low cardiac state is relatively rare, occurring in less than 15% of septic patients (Parrillo, 1990).

In septic patients, as well as in those with the adult respiratory distress syndrome (ARDS), numerous studies have demonstrated $\dot{V}O_2$ dependence through a wide range of $\dot{D}O_2$ manipulations (Danek *et al.*, 1980; Haupt *et al.*, 1985; Gilbert *et al.*, 1986; Bihari *et al.*, 1987; Lenz *et al.*, 1987; Wolf *et al.*, 1987; Tuchschmidt *et al.*, 1989; Vincent *et al.*, 1990; Edwards, 1991). This has been termed 'pathologic supply dependency' and implies that in the septic state, a higher $\dot{D}O_2$ is required to meet oxidative metabolic needs (Fig. 14.1) (Lister, 1991). Septic patients are unable to extract oxygen normally and, even though $\dot{D}O_2$ may be increased in this state, the tissue needs are increased even more, leading to a state of relative tissue hypoxia. Classically, this is often manifest by low or normal arterio-venous O_2 saturation differences (Tuchschmidt *et al.*, 1991). This implies that sepsis is a state of increased oxidative demand with cellular utilization dysfunction, and therapy should be aimed at correcting oxygen extraction or increasing oxygen delivery.

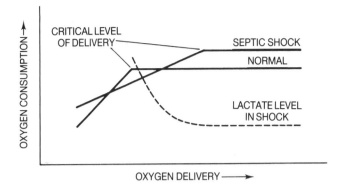

Figure 14.1 Pathologic oxygen supply dependency as seen in patients with sepsis. Critical levels of oxygen delivery required to meet tissue oxygen requirements are higher in the setting of septic shock. (Reprinted by permission from Tuchschmidt *et al.*, 1991.)

Artifacts in $\dot{V}O_2$ calculations using the Fick equation can occur, due to the use of a common factor in both $\dot{D}O_2$ and $\dot{V}O_2$ calculations, the so-called 'coupling' of data (Rackow *et al*, 1988; Lister, 1991; Weg, 1991). The coupling effect has been discounted by Weg and other authors who showed continued dependency by regression analysis and by independent measurements both by the Fick method and by direct measurement (Weg, 1991). Recent studies continue to present $\dot{V}O_2$ independence by direct measurement (Ronco *et al.*, 1991; Vermeji *et al.*, 1991).

Lactate as a Marker

Lactic acid is used as a marker of anaerobic metabolism and high levels of blood lactate are associated with a poor prognosis in patients with shock (Weil & Afifi, 1970; Vitrek & Cowley, 1971; Castagneto *et al.*, 1983; Vincent *et al.*, 1983; Kaufman *et al.*, 1984; Rashkin *et al.*, 1985; Groeneveld *et al.*, 1987; Astiz *et al.*, 1988). The hyperdynamic phase of septic shock is often accompanied by normal or reduced oxygen extraction, normal or reduced oxygen consumption, and lactic acidaemia, despite increased cardiac index, oxygen delivery and presumed elevated tissue oxygen demand (Groeneveld *et al.*, 1987). This tendency to maintain an increased cardiac output as oxygen consumption falls is indirect evidence of a progressive impairment of cellular oxidative metabolism (Castagneto *et al.*, 1983). Gilbert and Haupt demonstrated that in patients with sepsis, elevated lactate levels were associated with a clinically demonstrable oxygen debt (Haupt *et al.*, 1985; Gilbert *et al.*, 1986). In these studies, manipulations to increase oxygen delivery led to increases in oxygen consumption only when lactate levels were high, signifying an increased and unmet tissue oxygen need (Haupt *et al.*, 1985; Gilbert *et al.*, 1986). In patients with ARDS, Rashkin *et al.* (1985) found that oxygen delivery greater than $8\,\mathrm{ml}\,\mathrm{min}^{-1}\,\mathrm{kg}^{-1}$ was associated with improved survival and normal lactate levels, while patients with lower delivery levels developed lactic acidosis and were non-survivors. In septic patients, Tuchschmidt *et al.* (1989) determined the critical oxygen delivery level, above which tissue oxygen needs were met and no lactate produced, to be $15.0\,\mathrm{ml}\,\mathrm{min}^{-1}\,\mathrm{kg}^{-1}$ (Fig. 14.2). Other studies demonstrated the critical level of $\dot{D}O_2$ in sepsis to be between 6.4 and $20\,\mathrm{ml}\,\mathrm{min}^{-1}\,\mathrm{kg}^{-1}$ before lactate levels rise (Danek *et al.*, 1980; Jan *et al.*, 1980; Tuchschmidt *et al.*, 1989). These studies, showing a requirement for higher $\dot{D}O_2$ levels to meet tissue oxygen requirements in sepsis, even if the increased metabolic demands are accounted for, support the hypothesis that peripheral shunting of blood-transported oxygen occurs in this setting (Kaufman *et al.*, 1984; Astiz *et al.*, 1987; Rackow *et al.*, 1988).

Maximizing Oxygen Delivery and Consumption in Sepsis

Therapeutic Options

As discussed previously, oxygen consumption ($\dot{V}O_2$) is primarily flow-limited and often displays pathologic supply dependency in septic shock. (Rackow *et al.*, 1988; Vincent & Van der Linden, 1990). Therefore, therapy should be aimed at correcting tissue hypoxia, to a level where $\dot{V}O_2$ equals

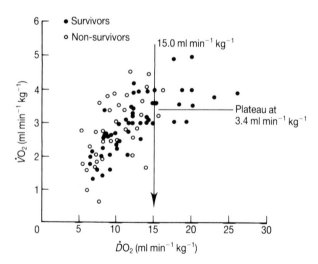

Figure 14.2 Clinical oxygen delivery ($\dot{D}O_2$) levels in patients with septic shock. At $\dot{D}O_2$ values greater than $15\,\mathrm{ml}\,\mathrm{min}^{-1}\,\mathrm{kg}^{-1}$, no further increases in $\dot{V}O_2$ were present. (Reprinted by permission from Tuchschmidt *et al.*, 1989.)

oxygen demand and lactic acidosis resolves. For a given level of oxygen demand, two options can be considered: either to improve oxygen extraction so that $\dot{V}O_2$ will be higher for the same level of oxygen transport, or increase $\dot{D}O_2$ further so that $\dot{V}O_2$ will be higher for a given level of oxygen extraction.

The first option is the most difficult since, in order to improve oxygen extraction, autoregulatory phenomena, vasodilation, peripheral oedema, and microthrombi would have to be reversed pharmacologically. Vasoconstrictors would be considered first to improve maldistribution of blood flow. Unfortunately, noradrenaline does not improve the peripheral distribution of blood flow, and the adrenergic stimulation of dopamine may reduce perfusion to vital organs, thereby reducing oxygen extraction (Vincent & Van der Linden, 1990). Cyclo-oxygenase inhibitors have been shown to improve peripheral blood flow in septic shock; however, no conclusive clinical studies have been completed (Vincent & Van der Linden, 1990).

The second option, of increasing oxygen transport to elevate oxygen consumption and meet metabolic demands, is more easily attainable and has been studied extensively. Shoemaker and Bland and colleagues examined physiologic and oxygen transport patterns in post-operative patients (Shoemaker et al., 1973; Bland et al., 1985). They demonstrated that non-survivors had persistent evidence of decreased myocardial performance as seen by a reduced cardiac index (CI) and left ventricular stroke work index (LVSWI) (Bland et al., 1985). Additionally, increased pulmonary pressures and decreased $\dot{D}O_2$, despite maintenance of normal arterial oxygenation and haemoglobin values, were present in non-survivors (Shoemaker et al., 1973; Bland et al., 1985). Abraham et al. (1984b) confirmed these findings in septic shock by correlating survival patterns to a higher CI, LVSWI, $\dot{D}O_2$ and $\dot{V}O_2$ before episodes of hypotension occurred. The elevation in $\dot{D}O_2$ and CI represent a response to an increase in tissue metabolic needs. The increase in the $\dot{V}O_2$ of survivors reflects better attainment of tissue metabolic demands of sepsis than that achieved by the non-survivors.

Shoemaker and co-workers also examined the hypothesis that the median values of survivors of life-threatening post-operative conditions, rather than the normal indices of unstressed patients, are the appropriate haemodynamic goals of critically ill patients. They successfully demonstrated that optimization of $CL > 4.5$ litres min^{-1} m^{-2}, $\dot{D}O_2 > 550$ ml min^{-1} m^{-2}, and $\dot{V}O_2 > 170$ ml min^{-1} m^{-2}, reduced morbidity and mortality in critically ill post-operative patients (Shoemaker et al., 1982, 1988). Edwards et al. (1989) also demonstrated that maintaining adequate delivery and consumption of oxygen increased the survival of patients with multiple-organ failure after sepsis. Tuchschmidt confirmed these findings by retrospectively correlating a higher CI and $\dot{D}O_2$ at 48 h post-septic shock in survivors versus non-survivors (Tuchschmidt et al., 1989).

Therefore, in order to increase survival in septic patients, oxygen delivery should be elevated to meet the tissue metabolic demands, in light of an inadequate oxygen extraction. This is accomplished by maximizing arterial oxygen saturation, haemoglobin concentration and cardiac output.

Oxygen Saturation

Frequent monitoring of arterial blood PaO_2 is necessary in septic patients. Supplemental oxygen is required in order to maximize alveolar to pulmonary capillary gas exchange, with the goal of maintaining an arterial oxygen saturation at or above 90%. In cases of severe respiratory alkalosis, which often occurs in early sepsis, maintenance of a PaO_2 > 60 mm Hg (8 kPa) is more important than the higher saturation, due to the leftward shift of the oxygen–haemoglobin dissociation curve. Further progression of the sepsis syndrome leads to tachypnoea, with ventilatory work increasing as much as ten to twentyfold (Schuster, 1990). During cardiorespiratory failure, the $\dot{V}O_2$ of the respiratory muscles may increase to 25% of total body $\dot{V}O_2$ and diaphragmatic blood flow to 20% of total cardiac output (Griffel *et al.*, 1990). Consequently, the early introduction of mechanical ventilation and sedation reduces oxygen consumption and may be beneficial in the $\dot{D}O_2$–$\dot{V}O_2$ relationship (Schuster, 1990; Vincent & Van der Linden, 1990; Tuchschmidt *et al.*, 1991). Elective intubation also offers less risk in the haemodynamically stable patient and allows for the delivery of higher levels of oxygen with positive end-expiratory pressures.

Optimal Haematocrit

Arterial oxygen content is also determined by the haemoglobin concentration. The optimal haematocrit for oxygen delivery in critically ill patients is unknown, but data suggest no benefit for haematocrits greater than 33% in septic patients. Czer and Shoemaker (1978) demonstrated that $\dot{V}O_2$ was dependent on $\dot{D}O_2$ in critically ill post-operative patients when haematocrit values were below, but not above 33%. They found that maximal survival rates occur in patients with pretransfusion haematrocit values between 27% and 33%, with the optimal haematocrit values between 27% and 33%, with the optimal haematocrit value being 33% (Czer & Shoemaker, 1978). Capillary red cell flow is optimized at a haematocrit of 30–33% (Dietrich *et al.*, 1990). Haematocrit values between 42% and 45% have been found to optimize delivery and consumption in non-septic dogs (Steffes *et al.*, 1991).

Optimal haematocrit range for constant oxygen supply is different for various organs (Fan *et al.*, 1980). In the normal brain, a reduction of haematocrit to 30% increases blood flow and tissue oxygenation (Dantzker, 1989). During periods of experimentally induced canine shock, whole body $\dot{V}O_2$ is optimal at a haematocrit of 45% while optimal cardiac haematocrit is 25%

(Jan *et al.*, 1980). However, in the same study, total body $\dot{V}O_2$ remained constant over a wide range of haematocrit variations between 25% and 45% (Jan *et al.* 1980). Fan *et al.* (1980) demonstrated that the heart and brain accommodate haematocrit variations well, with maintenance of $\dot{D}O_2$ between haematocrits of 20% and 65%; while liver, intestine, and kidney maintained constant $\dot{D}O_2$ through a narrower range of 30–55%. The diversity in optimal haematocrit is due to interorgan variability in adjustments to haemodilution and haemoconcentration. Enhanced $\dot{V}O_2$ may be seen with haemodilution through the dispersal of aggregated red blood cells, improved blood rheology, and an increase in capillary permeability–surface area. Similarly, the higher viscosity that accompanies an elevated haematocrit may offset the improvement in oxygen content and delivery (Jan *et al.*, 1980; Gilbert *et al.*, 1986).

Gilbert *et al.* (1986) and Abraham *et al.* (1984a) illustrated the use of blood transfusions to increase cardiac output and the oxygen-carrying capacity, thus oxygen delivery, in critically ill patients. Elevations in $\dot{V}O_2$ followed these manipulations in septic patients, confirming unmet tissue oxygen needs. Steffes *et al.* (1991) demonstrated the benefits of increasing the oxygen-carrying capacity in surgical septic patients, through blood transfusions alone. Their study verified a proportional relationship between $\dot{D}O_2$ and $\dot{V}O_2$ when blood transfusion was used to augment delivery in the face of an unchanging cardiac output (Steffes *et al.*, 1991). However, other studies have concluded that red cell transfusions in septic patients, already volume resuscitated, fail to improve $\dot{V}O_2$ (Conrad *et al.*, 1989; Dietrich *et al.*, 1990). Haemoglobin in these studies ranged from $8.2\,g\,dl^{-1}$ to $10.5\,g\,dl^{-1}$. Their data suggest that the supply dependency of $\dot{V}O_2$ is mediated primarily through improvement in the flow component of $\dot{D}O_2$ rather than through the oxygen-carrying capacity (Conrad *et al.*, 1989). However, these patients were adequately volume resuscitated and augmented with full inotropic support, and these interventions may have fulfilled tissue oxygen demands prior to red cell transfusion (Dietrich *et al.*, 1990). Additionally, a subset of septic shock patients with OER < 0.24, did demonstrate a significant response in $\dot{V}O_2$ with a rise in CaO_2 from an increase in haematocrit (Conrad *et al.*, 1989).

Volume Resuscitation

Cardiac output is a central determinant of oxygen transport and perfusion. Septic patients may be relatively volume-depleted, and volume repletion should be a priority in the resuscitation of these patients. As noted previously, the end-points for volume resuscitation are improvement of $\dot{D}O_2$ and $\dot{V}O_2$, either to correct dependency of $\dot{V}O_2$ on $\dot{D}O_2$, or to achieve levels of $\dot{D}O_2$ and $\dot{V}O_2$ correlating with survival (Shoemaker *et al.*, 1988; Edwards *et al.*, 1989). Intravascular volume expansion with colloids significantly

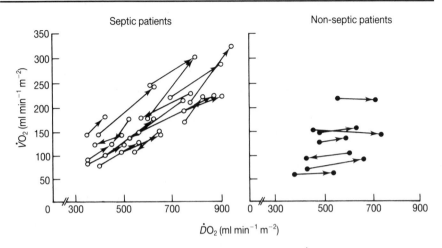

Figure 14.3 The dependence of oxygen consumption ($\dot{V}O_2$) on oxygen delivery ($\dot{D}O_2$) in septic and non-septic patients. The arrows represent the directional change after volume loading. No relationship between $\dot{D}O_2$ and $\dot{V}O_2$ was present in non-septic patients. In contrast, $\dot{V}O_2$ increased with $\dot{D}O_2$ in the setting of sepsis. (Reprinted by permission from Wolf *et al.*, 1987.)

increases CI, $\dot{D}O_2$ and $\dot{V}O_2$ in septic patients (Fig. 14.3) (Abraham *et al.*, 1984a; Haupt *et al.*, 1985; Wolf *et al.*, 1987). Presumptively, this is secondary to improved oxygen supply to tissues on the basis of an increased CI through the Frank–Starling effect (Abraham *et al.*, 1984a). Fluids are administered to maximize cardiac output without causing pulmonary oedema and elevated filling pressures. Rackow *et al.* (1987) demonstrated that a pulmonary artery occlusion pressure of greater than 15 mm Hg was rarely associated with a further increase in LVSWI. Crystalloids or colloids may be used to accomplish this goal and advocates for either exist. Rackow *et al.* (1983) compared albumin, hydroxyethylstarch, and 0.9% sodium chloride as treatment for circulatory shock. Two to four times the volume of saline was required, as compared to albumin or hydroxyethylstarch, in order to achieve the same haemodynamic end-points. In addition, 87% of the saline-resuscitated patients developed pulmonary oedema versus 22% in the albumin/hydroxyethylstarch groups (Rackow *et al.*, 1983). A later study by the same group, found that lung and extravascular water was not increased with crystalloids as compared with colloid infusion during sepsis in rats (Rackow *et al.*, 1989). The distribution of colloids remains intravascular due to their inability to permeate through vascular membranes. It also increases intravascular volume by providing an elevated colloid oncotic pressure and allows for haemodynamic improvement for 24–36 h. Crystalloids distribute throughout the intravascular and extravascular compartments with a resultant reduction in intravascular oncotic pressure, which may account for this study's increased incidence of pulmonary oedema.

Inotropic Support

If further support to optimize CI, $\dot{V}O_2$ and $\dot{D}O_2$ is necessary after adequate fluid and red blood cell loading, the addition of an inotropic agent may be beneficial. The initial stimulus for the use of catecholamines was the α-adrenergic vasoconstrictor action by which blood pressure is increased (Ruiz et al., 1979). Subsequently, the use of β-agonists such as noradrenaline, metaraminol bitartrate, and isopropterenol hydrochloride were favoured for their inotropic effects (Ruiz et al., 1979).

Dobutamine is a synthetic catacholamine with predominantly β1-adrenergic effects, and is currently favoured as the first line inotrope to improve tissue perfusion in patients who are not severely hypotensive. It has been found to be an effective inotropic agent in cardiac failure and in septic patients with myocardial dysfunction (Jardin et al., 1981; Regnier et al., 1979). In septic shock dobutamine infusion produced significant improvement in cardiac index (2.9–3.9 litres min^{-1} m^{-2}), stroke index (32–37 ml m^{-2}), and mean arterial pressure (69–83 mm Hg) without a change in systemic vascular resistance (Jardin et al., 1981). $\dot{V}O_2$ was also improved (132–140 ml min^{-1} m^{-2}), demonstrating unmet tissue oxygen needs (Jardin et al., 1981). Vincent et al. (1990) described significant improvement in $\dot{V}O_2$ in septic patients (139–167 ml min^{-1} m^{-2}) only when lactate levels were elevated (Figs 14.4 and 14.5). The

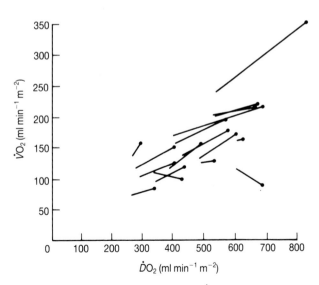

Figure 14.4 Changes in oxygen consumption ($\dot{V}O_2$) and oxygen delivery ($\dot{D}O_2$) induced by dobutamine in septic patients with increased blood lactate. $\dot{V}O_2$ increased with $\dot{D}O_2$ in septic patients with tissue hypoxia, as demonstrated by lactic acidosis. (Reprinted by permission from Vincent et al., 1990.)

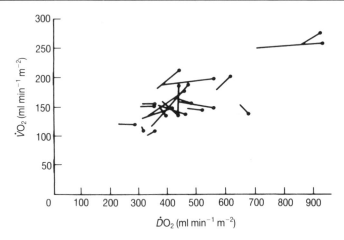

Figure 14.5   Changes in oxygen consumption ($\dot{V}O_2$) and oxygen delivery ($\dot{D}O_2$) induced by dobutamine in septic patients without increased blood lactate. No relationship between $\dot{D}O_2$ and $\dot{V}O_2$ was present in the absence of lactic acidosis. (Reprinted by permission from Vincent *et al.*, 1990.)

tissue perfusion effects of dobutamine were compared to those of dopamine by Shoemaker *et al.* (1991). Dobutamine produced significantly greater cardiac index (34% versus 23%), $\dot{D}O_2$ (36% versus 23%), and $\dot{V}O_2$ (20% versus 14%) at comparable doses (Shoemaker *et al.*, 1991). Usual doses of dobutamine in sepsis are up to $10\,\mu g\,kg^{-1}\,min^{-1}$, but higher doses, to $20\,\mu g\,kg^{-1}\,min^{-1}$ can be used if $\dot{D}O_2$ continues to improve and hypotension and tachycardia (due to excessive β actions of dobutamine) do not become limiting.

Catecholamines can increase $\dot{V}O_2$ by direct metabolic effects on cells, and arguments have been made that dobutamine may elevate $\dot{V}O_2$ based on this effect (Gilbert *et al.*, 1986). However, the influence of limited doses of dobutamine on $\dot{V}O_2$ in congestive heart failure (CHF) has been minimal, and the non-dependency of $\dot{V}O_2$ in CHF and septic patients, without elevated lactate levels, provides evidence against this (Vincent *et al.*, 1990).

Dobutamine also elevates pulmonary shunting minimally when compared to dopamine (16% versus 27%), and reduces right and left ventricular filling pressures (14% and 28% respectively) (Regnier *et al.*, 1979). Dobutamine is therefore useful in the management of septic shock when cardiac dysfunction is present, filling pressures are elevated, severe peripheral vasoconstriction is prominent, or marked pulmonary shunting exists (Regnier *et al.*, 1979; Jardin *et al.*, 1981). For these reasons, dobutamine is the preferred inotrope for augmentation of tissue oxygen delivery to achieve optimal haemodynamic goals. Combination therapy with dopamine or noradrenaline is occasionally beneficial in cases of severe cardiac dysfunction and reduced SVR. In particular, in hypotensive septic patients, noradrenaline or dopamine may be required initially to achieve adequate blood pressure. Dobutamine can then be added to further enhance DO_2 and optimize tissue perfusion.

Dopamine hydrochloride is useful in cases of severe hypotension because of its β and α, as well as its dopaminergic effects. Dopaminergic effects predominate at low doses (3 μg kg^{-1} min^{-1}) of the drug with a favourable increase in renal blood flow. Higher rates (4–10 μg kg^{-1} min^{-1}) of infusion cause a mixed β- and α-adrenergic response with elevated rates (> 10 μg kg^{-1} min^{-1}) predominantly producing α-adrenergic changes with peripheral vaso-constriction. Dopamine increases venomotor tone, therefore decreasing peripheral pooling of blood and increasing venous return (Regnier et al., 1979; Vincent and Van der Linden, 1990). It also has a chronotropic as well as an inotropic effect and may be partly efficient even if hypovolaemia is present (Jardin et al., 1981). Consequently, dopamine acts favourably in sepsis by increasing blood pressure by improving myocardial performance in combination with an increase in systemic vascular resistance (Bollaert et al., 1990).

Noradrenaline is primarily a peripheral vasoconstrictor and is useful in cases of severe septic shock with extremely low resistance, or in shock refractory to other catecholamine therapy (Desjars et al., 1987; Bollaert et al., 1990; Redl-Wenzl et al., 1990). Desjars et al. (1987) illustrated this advantage in patients with refractory shock on maximal dopamine therapy. Mean arterial pressure increased (48–62 mm Hg), SVRI increased (700–899 dyne s cm^{-5} m^{-2}) and heart rate decreased (142–136 beats min^{-1}), without a change in cardiac index (Desjars et al., 1987). Redl-Wenzl and colleagues showed that mean arterial pressures can be increased by 30% and creatinine clearance improved from 73 to 114 ml min^{-1} with concomitant use of renal dose dopamine (i.e. 3 μg kg^{-1} min^{-1}) (Redl-Wenzl et al., 1990). They further demonstrated that the adverse effects of increased afterload with resultant reduction in cardiac output, DO_2 and VO_2 are not present during therapy with noradrenaline in refractory shock (Redl-Wenz et al., 1990). Patients unable to tolerate dopamine, secondary to severe tachycardia, may benefit by a substitution to noradrenaline due to its vasoconstrictive but less prominent chronotropic effects. Also, because an important component of dopamine's action is indirect, through release of noradrenaline from pre-synaptic nerve terminals, many septic patients do not respond well to this agent since they have depleted endogenous catecholamine stores. Use of a direct acting adrenergic agent, such as noradrenaline, in these patients may improve their haemodynamic profile. For this reason, noradrenaline has been recommended as the first agent to be used in septic patients who remain hypotensive after volume resuscitation.

Adrenaline with its combination α- and β-adrenergic effects, has also been documented to be useful in refractory shock (Bollaert et al.,1990). Dopexa-mine, a catecholamine with dopaminergic and β2-agonist action is currently under investigation (Kruse & Carlson, 1991). However, its utility appears to be limited in septic, hypotensive patients because of tachycardia and vaso-dilation associated with its use.

Other Agents

The use of inotropes to increase oxygen delivery and oxygen consumption has been questioned. Gilbert and colleagues found that $\dot{D}O_2$ and $\dot{V}O_2$ were directly related in septic patients when dobutamine was administered, regardless of lactate levels (Gilbert et al., 1986). These results suggested that catecholamines may exert a direct effect on oxidative metabolism. In order to eliminate this variable, the use of vasodilating agents to increase $\dot{D}O_2$ and $\dot{V}O_2$ has been examined (Holcroft et al., 1986; Bihari et al., 1987; Bone et al., 1989b; Vincent et al., 1990).

Prostacyclin (PGI_2) is a potent vasodilator that antagonizes the effects of thromboxane-A_2, inhibits platelet aggregation and suppresses leukocyte adherence to damaged endothelium (Bihari et al., 1987). Inhibition of these effects may reverse maldistribution of blood flow in patients with sepsis or ARDS, therefore, improving $\dot{D}O_2$ and $\dot{V}O_2$. Bihari demonstrated that prosta-cyclin infusion produced an increase in $\dot{D}O_2$ (375 versus 492 ml min^{-1} m^{-2}) as a consequence of increases in CI (median increase of 25%) in patients with ARDS (Bihari et al., 1987). This was associated with an increase in $\dot{V}O_2$, particularly in non-survivors and patients with elevated lactate levels (Bihari et al., 1987). These results, showing improvement in $\dot{D}O_2$ and $\dot{V}O_2$ with the administration of PGI_2, suggest that this agent may be useful in treating septic patients, particularly those with abnormalities in peripheral oxygen utilization. Unfortunately, because of the intense vasodilatory properties of PGI_2, use of this substance may be limited in septic patients, particularly those with severe hypotension.

PGE_1 is another prostaglandin that attenuates the inflammatory response in ARDS and sepsis. Holcroft et al. (1986) found that there was an improvement in survival of post-operative ARDS patients in those who received PGE_1 compared to placebo (71% versus 35%). A multicentre trial by Bone et al. (1989b) concluded that PGE_1 did not enhance survival in ARDS patients after a 7-day infusion of the agent. However, further exam-ination of the data by Silverman et al. (1990) found significant increases in $\dot{D}O_2$ in the PGE_1-died and PGE_1-survived groups (25% and 34%, respectively) as well as corresponding higher $\dot{V}O_2$ values (17% and 15% respectively). Although survival was not enhanced with therapy, volume resuscitation was not optimized prior to PGE_1 administration and supra-normal goals as determined by Shoemaker et al. (CI > 4.5 litres min^{-1} m^{-2}, $\dot{D}O_2 > 550$ ml min^{-1} m^{-2}, and $\dot{V}O_2 > 170$ ml min^{-1} m^{-2}) were not obtained until the fourth day in the PGE_1-died group (Silverman et al., 1990). Hence, PGE_1 may be a useful ancillary agent after optimization of metabolic goals with fluids and blood products, and may even establish an improved outcome if these goals are met prior to PGE_1 use (Shoemaker, 1990; Silverman *et al.*, 1990).

Summary

Patients with sepsis are at an increased risk of mortality if they progress into a septic shock state. Oxygen metabolism in the septic patient is deranged, so that even if cardiac output is elevated, there is peripheral maldistribution of blood flow resulting in decreased oxygen extraction and an abnormal relationship between oxygen delivery and consumption. This results in a peripheral tissue oxygen debt, often leading to anaerobic metabolism with lactic acidosis. The aims of therapy, therefore, are to maximize oxygen delivery and consumption in order to meet cellular metabolism requirements. By achieving supranormal values of CI, $\dot{D}O_2$ and $\dot{V}O_2$, morbidity and mortality are improved in septic patients. These goals can be achieved by oxygen supplementation, fluid loading, the addition of red blood cells to increase oxygen-carrying capacity, and the use of inotropes and vasodilating prostaglandins.

References

Abraham E, Shoemaker WC & Cheng PH (1984a) Cardiorespiratory responses to fluid administration in peritonitis. *Crit. Care Med.* **12:** 664–8.

Abraham E, Bland RD, Cobo JC & Shoemaker WC (1984b) Sequential cardiorespiratory patterns associated with outcome in septic shock. *Chest* **85:** 75–9.

Archie JP (1977) Anatomic arterial–venous shunting in endotoxic and septic shock in dogs. *Ann. Surg.* **186:** 171–6.

Astiz ME, Rackow EC, Falk JL *et al.* (1987) Oxygen delivery and consumption in patients with hyperdynamic septic shock. *Crit. Care Med.* **15:** 26–8.

Astiz ME, Rackow EC, Kaufman B *et al.* (1988) Relationship of oxygen delivery and mixed venous oxygenation to lactic acidosis in patients with sepsis and acute myocardial infarction. *Crit. Care Med.* **16:** 655–8.

Bautista AP & Spitzer JJ (1990) Superoxide anion generation by in situ perfused rat liver: effect of in vivo endotoxin. *Am. J. Physiol.* **259:** G907–12.

Bihari D, Smithies M, Gimson A & Tinker J (1987) The effects of vasodilation with prostacyclin on oxygen delivery and uptake in critically ill patients. *New Engl. J. Med.* **317:** 397–403.

Bland RD, Shoemaker WC, Abraham E & Cobo JC (1985) Hemodynamic and oxygen transport patterns in surviving and non-surviving postoperative patients. *Crit. Care Med.* **13:** 85–90.

Bollaert PE, Bauer P, Audibert G *et al.* (1990) Effects of epinephrine on hemodynamics and oxygen metabolism in dopamine resistant septic shock. *Chest* **98**: 949–53.

Bone RC (1991) Sepsis, the sepsis syndrome, multi-organ failure: a plea for comparable definitions. *Ann. Intern. Med.* **114**: 332–3.

Bone RC, Fisher CJ, Clemmer TP *et al.* (1989a) Sepsis syndrome: a valid clinical entity. *Crit. Care Med.* **17**: 389–93.

Bone RC, Slotman G, Maunder R *et al.* (1989b) Randomized double-blind, multicenter study of prostaglandin E_1 in patients with the adult respiratory distress syndrome. *Chest* **96**: 114–19.

Castagneto M, Biovannini I, Boldrini G *et al.* (1983) Cardiorespiratory and metabolic adequacy and their relation to survival in sepsis. *Circ. Shock* **11**: 113–30.

Conrad SA, Dietrich KA, Hebert CA & Romero MD (1989) Failure of RBC transfusion alone to improve $\dot{V}O_2$ in septic shock. *Circ. Shock* **27**: 346.

Czer LSC & Shoemaker WC (1978) Optimal hematocrit value in critically ill postoperative patients. *Surg. Gynecol. Obstet.* **147**: 363–8.

Dahn MS, Lange PL, Lobdell K *et al.* (1987) Splanchnic and total body oxygen consumption differences in septic and injured patients. *Surgery* **101**: 69–80.

Danek SJ, Lynch JP, Weg JG & Dantzker DR (1980) The dependence of oxygen uptake on oxygen delivery in the adult respiratory distress syndrome. *Am. Rev. Respiratory Dis.* **122**: 387–95.

Dantzker D (1989) Oxygen delivery and utilization in sepsis. *Crit. Care Clin.* **5(1)**: 81–98.

Dantzker DR, Foresman B & Gutierrez G (1991) Oxygen supply and utilization relationships: a re-evaluation. *Am. Rev. Respiratory Dis.* **143**: 675–9.

Desjars P, Pinaud M, Potel G *et al.* (1987) A reappraisal of norepinephrine therapy in human septic shock. *Crit. Care Med.* **15**: 134–7.

Dietrich KA, Conrad SA, Hebert CA *et al.* (1990) Cardiovascular and metabolic response to red blood cell transfusion in critically ill volume-resuscitated nonsurgical patients. *Crit. Care Med.* **18**: 940–4.

Edwards JD (1991) Oxygen transport in cardiogenic and septic shock. *Crit. Care Med.* **19**: 658–63.

Edwards JD, Brown GC, Nightingale P *et al.* (1989) Use of survivors' cardiorespiratory values as therapeutic goals in septic shock. *Crit. Care Med.* **17**: 1098–103.

Fan FC, Chen RYZ, Schuessler GB & Chien S (1980) Effects of hematrocrit variations on regional hemodynamics and oxygen transport in the dog. *Am. J. Physiol.* **238**: H545–52.

Gilbert EM, Haupt MT, Mandanas RY *et al.* (1986) The effect of fluid loading, blood transfusion, and catecholamine infusion on oxygen delivery and consumption in patients with sepsis. *Am. Rev. Respiratory Dis.* **134**: 873–8.

Griffel MI, Astiz ME, Rackow EC & Weil MH (1990) Effect of mechanical ventilation on systemic oxygen extraction and lactic acidosis during early septic shock in rats. *Crit. Care Med.* **18**: 72–6.

Groenveld JAB, Kester ADM, Nauta JJP & Thijs LG (1987) Relation of arterial blood lactate to oxygen delivery and hemodynamic variables in human shock states. *Circ. Shock* **22**: 35–53.

Haupt MT, Gilbert EM & Carlson RW (1985) Fluid loading increases oxygen consumption in septic patients with lactic acidosis. *Am. Rev. Respiratory Dis.* **131:** 912–16.

Haupt MT, Balaan MR & Carlson RW (1987) Changes in oxidative metabolism in rat liver mitochondrial preparations following the addition of serum of patients with advanced sepsis. *Crit. Care Med.* **15:** 442.

Holcroft JW, Vassar MJ & Weber CJ (1986) Prostaglandin E_1 and survival in patients with the adult respiratory distress syndrome. *Ann. Surg.* **203:** 371–8.

Jan KM, Heldman J & Chien S (1980) Coronary hemodynamics and oxygen utilization after hematocrit variations in hemorrhage. *Am. J. Physiol.* **239:** H326–32.

Jardin F, Sportiche M, Bazin M *et al.* (1981) Dobutamine: a hemodynamic evalution in human septic shock. *Crit. Care Med.* **9:** 329–32.

Kaufman BS, Rackow EC & Falk JL (1984) Relationship between oxygen delivery and consumption during fluid resuscitation of hypovolemic and septic shock. *Chest* **85:** 336–40.

Kruse JA & Carlson RW (1991) Vasoactive drugs to support oxygen transport in sepsis. *Crit. Care Med.* **19:** 144–6.

Lang CH, Bagby GJ, Ferguson JL & Spitzer JJ (1984) Cardiac output and redistribution of organ blood flow in hypermetabolic sepsis. *Am. J. Physiol.* **246:** R331–7.

Lenz K, Laggner A, Druml W *et al.* (1987) Hemodynamic characterization of sepsis. *Prog. Clin. Biol. Res.* **236B:** 129–38.

Lister G (1991) Oxygen supply/demand in the critically ill. In Taylor RW & Shoemaker WC (eds), *Critical Care: State of the Art*, pp. 311–350. Fullerton, CA: Society of Critical Care Medicine.

Parker MM, Shelhamer JH & Natanson C (1989) Responses of left ventricular function in survivors and non-survivors of septic shock. *J. Crit. Care* **4:** 19.

Parrillo JE (1990) Cardiovascular pattern during septic shock. In Parrillo JE (Moderator), *Septic Shock in Humans: Advances in the Understanding of Pathogenesis, Cardiovascular Dysfunction, and Therapy. Ann. Intern. Med.* **113:** 227–9.

Parrillo JE, Burch C, Shelhamer JH *et al.* (1985) A circulating myocardial depressant substance in humans with septic shock. *J. Clin. Invest.* **76:** 1539–53.

Rackow EC, Falk JL, Fein A *et al.* (1983) Fluid resuscitation in circulatory shock: a comparison of the cardiorespiratory effects of albumin, hetastarch, and saline solutions in patients with hypovolemic and septic shock. *Crit. Care Med.* **11:** 839–50.

Rackow EC, Kaufman BS, Falk JL *et al.* (1987) Hemodynamic response to fluid repletion in patients with septic shock: evidence for early depression of cardiac performance. *Circ. Shock* **22:** 11–22.

Rackow EC, Astiz ME & Weil MH (1988) Cellular oxygen metabolism during sepsis and shock. *J. Am. Med. Assoc.* **259:** 1989–93.

Rackow EC, Astiz ME, Schumer W & Weil MH (1989) Lung and muscle water after crystalloid and colloid infusion in septic rats: effect on oxygen delivery and metabolism. *J. Lab. Clin. Med.* **113:** 184–9.

Rashkin MC, Bosken C & Baughman RP (1985) Oxygen delivery in critically ill patients. *Chest* **87:** 580–4.

Redl-Wenzl EM, Armbruster C, Edelmann G et al. (1990) Noradrenaline in the high output-low resistance state of patients with abdominal sepsis. Anaesthesist **39;** 525–9.

Regnier B, Safran D, Carlet J & Teisseire B (1979) Comparative haemodynamic effects of dopamine and dobutamine in septic shock. Intensive Care Med. **5:** 115–20.

Ronco JJ, Phang T, Walley KR et al. (1991) Oxygen consumption is independent of changes in oxygen delivery in severe adult respiratory distress syndrome. Am. Rev. Respiratory Dis. **143:** 1267–73.

Ruiz CE, Weil MH & Carlson RW (1979) Treatment of circulatory shock with dopamine. J. Am. Med. Assoc. **242:** 165–8.

Schuster DP (1990) A physiologic approach to initiating, maintaining and withdrawing mechanical ventilatory support during acute respiratory failure. Am. J. Med. **88:** 268–78.

Shoemaker WC (1987) Circulatory mechanisms of shock and their mediators. Crit. Care Med. **15:** 787–94.

Shoemaker WC (1990) Was the magic bullet aimed in the right direction? Chest **98:** 257.

Shoemaker WC, Montgomery ES, Kaplan E & Elwyn DH (1973) Physiologic patterns in surviving and non-surviving shock patients. Arch. Surg. **106:** 630–6.

Shoemaker WC, Appel PL, Waxman K et al. (1982) Clinical trial of survivors cardiorespiratory patterns as therapeutic goals in critically ill postoperative patients. Crit. Care Med. **10:** 398–403.

Shoemaker WC, Appel PL, Kram HB, Waxman K & Lee TS (1988) Prospective trial of supranormal values of survivors as therapeutic goals in high risk surgical patients. Chest **94:** 1176–86.

Shoemaker WC, Appel PL & Kram H (1991) Oxygen transport measurements to evaluate tissue perfusion and titrate therapy: dobutamine and dopamine effects. Crit. Care Med. **19:** 672–88.

Siegel JH, Greenspan M & Del Guercio LRM (1967) Abnormal vascular tone, defective oxygen transport and myocardial failure in human septic shock. Ann. Surg. **163:** 504–16.

Silverman HJ, Slotman F, Bone RC et al. (1990) Effects of prostaglandin E_1 on oxygen delivery and consumption in patients with the adult respiratory distress syndrome. Chest **98:** 405–10.

Smith M & Abraham E (1986) Conjunctival oxygen tension monitoring during hemorrhage. J. Trauma **26:** 217–26.

Sprung CL (1991) Definitions of sepsis – have we reached a consensus? Crit. Care Med. **19:** 849–51.

Steffes CP, Bender JS & Levinson MA (1991) Blood transfusion and oxygen consumption in surgical sepsis. Crit. Care Med. **19:** 512–17.

Suffredini AF, Fromm RE, Parker MM et al. (1989) The cardiovascular response of normal humans to the administration of endotoxin. New Engl. J. Med. **321:** 280–7.

Tuchschmidt J, Fried J, Swinney R & Sharma OP (1989) Early hemodynamic correlates of survival in patients with septic shock. Crit. Care Med. **17:** 719–23.

Tuchschmidt J, Oblitas D & Fried JC (1991) Oxygen consumption in sepsis and septic shock. *Crit. Care Med.* **19:** 664–71.

Vermeij CG, Feenstra BWA, Adrichem WJ & Bruining HA (1991) Independent oxygen uptake and oxygen delivery in septic and postoperative patients. *Chest* **99:** 1438–43.

Vincent JL & Van der Linden P (1990) Septic shock: particular type of acute circulatory failure. *Crit. Care Med.* **18:** S70–4.

Vincent JL, Dufaye P, Berre' J et al. (1983) Serial lactate determinations during circulatory shock. *Crit. Care Med.* **11:** 449–51.

Vincent JL, Roman A, De Backer D & Kahn RJ (1990) Oxygen uptake and supply dependency: effects of short-term dobutamine infusion. *Am. Rev. Respiratory Dis.* **142:** 2–7.

Vitrek V & Cowley RA (1971) Blood lactate in the prognosis of various forms of shock. *Ann. Surg.* **173:** 308–13.

Weg JG (1991) Oxygen transport in ARDS and other acute circulatory problems: relationship of oxygen delivery and oxygen consumption. *Crit. Care Med.* **19:** 650–7.

Weil MH & Afifi AA (1970) Experimental and clinical studies on lactate and pyruvate and indicators of the severity of acute circulatory failure (shock). *Circulation* **41:** 989–1001.

Weil MH & Nishijima H (1978) Cardiac output in bacterial shock. *Am. J. Med.* **64:** 920–2.

Wolf YG, Shamay C, Perel A & Manny J (1987) Dependence of oxygen consumption on cardiac output in sepsis. *Crit. Care Med.* **15:** 198–203.

Ziegler EJ, Fisher CJ, Sprung CL et al. (1991) Treatment of gram-negative bacteremia and septic shock with HA-1A human monoclonal antibody against endotoxin. *New Engl. J. Med.* **324:** 429–36.

15 The Adult Respiratory Distress Syndrome

Luis Ortiz and Guillermo Gutierrez

Introduction

The adult respiratory distress syndrome (ARDS) is a leading cause of acute respiratory failure in both medical and surgical patients. From the time of its description by Ashbaugh *et al*. (1967), ARDS has been associated with a high mortality rate. Approximately 30–70% of the patients with this syndrome die, in spite of an increasing awareness of the mechanisms of acute lung injury and of the introduction of novel forms of therapy, monitoring and support (Fowler *et al*., 1985).

Hypoxaemia is a well-recognized feature of ARDS, but the inability of the lungs to provide for adequate gas exchange is seldom the cause of mortality, since more patients with ARDS die as the result of the multiple systems organ failure syndrome (MSOF) than from hypoxaemia itself (Villar *et al*., 1991). It appears, however, that the development of MSOF may be related to peripheral tissue hypoxia, which tends to go undetected by current monitoring techniques. This occult tissue hypoxia is likely to be related to abnormalities in local oxygen delivery, as well as to a defect in oxygen extraction by the peripheral tissues (Gutierrez & Pohil, 1986). The purpose of this chapter is to provide an overview of the pathophysiology of ARDS, given from the perspective of impairments in oxygen transport, as well as an appraisal of the current therapeutic strategies.

Definition of ARDS

From a clinical viewpoint, ARDS can be defined as the presence of pulmonary oedema with normal hydrostatic pressure in the pulmonary microvasculature. From this definition one can infer that fluid moves from the pulmonary capillaries into the gas exchange areas of the lung as the result of increased endothelial permeability. Although discrepancies remain, the following are widely accepted clinical requirements for the diagnosis of ARDS (Petty, 1981; Fowler *et al*., 1983; Pepe, 1986):

(1) Acute onset of severe respiratory dysfunction, excluding patients whose respiratory failure develops slowly from the progression of a chronic pulmonary disease.

(2) Rapid roentgenographic appearance of bilateral alveolar infiltrates involving all regions of the lung. This criterion serves to exclude patients with respiratory failure secondary to localized pathology.
(3) A pulmonary artery occlusion pressure (PAOP) < 16 mm Hg. This criterion serves to exclude patients in whom pulmonary oedema is of cardiogenic origin.
(4) Decreased lung compliance resulting in 'stiff' lungs. The total static thoracic compliance, defined as the ratio of tidal volume to plateau airway pressure should be $\leq 50\,ml\,cm^{-1}\,H_2O$.
(5) Hypoxaemia at high concentration of inspired oxygen, defined as an arterial $PO_2 \leq 60\,mm\,Hg$ (8 kPa) while breathing an inspired O_2 fraction (FiO_2) ≥ 0.50.

It has been proposed that these criteria should be broadened to include patients with milder degrees of lung dysfunction, as well as to identify clinical disorders that may eventually determine patient outcome (Murray et al., 1988). Furthermore, the recognition of functional dysfunction in organs other than the lung should be included in the definition of ARDS, to help establish the real incidence and prognosis of this syndrome (Matthay, 1990).

Pulmonary Pathology of ARDS

ARDS is characterized by diffuse alveolar damage that is non-specific in character. The pathological changes seen with ARDS represent a limited and stereotypical reaction of the lung to a variety of insults.

The histopathologic appearance of the lung depends on the duration of the process, the extent and the location of the injury, and the ability of the lung to repair itself. For all practical purposes, diffuse alveolar damage has been divided into two discrete but overlapping stages (Katzenstein & Askin, 1990). Initially there is the early acute exudative stage that occurs within the first week of the injury. It is characterized by endothelial cell-swelling, prominent interstitial oedema, and the appearance of hyaline membranes. Also seen is denudation of epithelial basement membrane and hyperplasia of alveolar cells. Some vascular changes such as fibrin thrombi, medial hypertrophy and vessel obliteration also can be identified. This early stage is followed by an organizing or proliferative stage, in which phagocytosis of the hyaline membrane is prominent and proliferation of fibroblasts results in lung fibrosis. This fibrosing process is more marked in the interstitium but it can be generalized. This sequence of events may vary depending upon a variety of conditions, such as broncho-aspiration, sepsis, oxygen toxicity, barotrauma, etc. that can complicate the clinical course of ARDS.

Clinical Manifestations of ARDS

The clinical manifestations of ARDS are variable, but the onset is usually abrupt following the initiating event. Prospective studies have shown that 80% of patients that ultimately develop ARDS, will do so during the first 24 h after experiencing a predisposing insult (Fowler *et al.*, 1985). The time frame for ARDS development is shorter in patients with sepsis, generally after 6 h (Weinberg *et al.*, 1984). During this latent period, the patient may be asymptomatic and the chest roentgenogram is either normal, or without diffuse bilateral infiltrates. This phase is followed by the progressive development of severe hypoxaemia that is usually associated with hyperventilation. It is also accompanied by radiographic changes compatible with the accumulation of fluid in the perivascular and interstitial lung tissue. This hypoxaemia is refractory to increased levels of inspired oxygen and it often requires the endotracheal intubation and mechanical ventilation of the patient to assure adequate oxygenation.

The physical examination is non-specific in ARDS. Crackles are prominent but have little discriminatory value. In prospective studies, the physical examination was found to be useful in discriminating cardiogenic from non-cardiogenic pulmonary oedema in only 40% of the cases (Pepe, 1986).

Pathophysiology of ARDS

The alveolar-capillary membrane is the primary site of injury in ARDS and extensive damage to the lung microvasculature is virtually universal in established ARDS (Wiedemann *et al.*, 1990). Endothelial damage has been assessed from tracer studies of the endothelial barrier by measuring the production of Von Willebrand factor (Carvahlo *et al.*, 1982) and alterations in the release of angiotensin-converting enzyme (Johnson *et al.*, 1985).

The large inflammatory reaction generated during the early stages of ARDS implicate the inflammatory system, with its diverse components of cellular and humoral mechanisms, as the principal culprit of this syndrome. Knowledge of the role of the neutrophil in ARDS evolved from the recognition that hypoxaemia following dialysis was associated with complement activation and polymorphonuclear sequestration in lung capillaries (Craddock *et al.*, 1977). The analysis of pathologic studies in patients with ARDS demonstrated a large accumulation of polymorphonuclear cells in the alveoli (Bachofen & Weibel, 1977) a finding that was later confirmed by the use of broncho-alveolar lavage in humans and animals (Lee *et al.*, 1981; Rinaldo *et al.*, 1984).

The confirmation by Zimmerman *et al.* (1983) of activated polymorphonuclear cells in patients with ARDS, gave further credence to the notion that this cell plays a critical role in ARDS. It has been hypothesized that a given stimulus activates complement, which in turn generates a chemotactic response trapping and activating polymorphonuclear cells in the pulmonary capillaries with resulting endothelial damage. The validity of this hypothesis has been weakened by the finding of Tate and Repine (1983), who demonstrated the presence of ARDS in neutropenic patients. Subsequent studies also have been unable to confirm the finding that activation of complement predicts the onset of ARDS (Weinberg *et al.*, 1984). An alternative hypothesis that might explain the presence of ARDS in neutropenic patients, is that the macrophage, not the neutrophil, is responsible for the endothelial damage. Alveolar macrophages have a longer life than the polymorphonuclear neutrophils, as well as similar cytotoxic capabilities. The macrophage has the advantage of being an immune regulator cell, producing large amounts of mediators (cytokines) that function as agents for intercellular communication. The macrophage is also a principal source of cytokines, which by their potent autocrine, paracrine and endocrine effects can amplify the inflammatory response. It appears that tumour necrosis factor (TNF), among the many monokines released by macrophages, plays a major role in the pathogenesis of ARDS. Released in response to endotoxin, TNF initiates a chain of events that lead to the sepsis syndrome (Mathison *et al.*, 1988), including the sequestration of neutrophils in the lung, as well as oedema and haemorrhage in other organs (Tracey *et al.*, 1988; Ferrari *et al.*, 1989). Other cytokines implicated in the development of ARDS are interleukin-8 (IL-8), that modulates the chemotactic action over the polymorphonuclear, and endothelin, which, once produced by the endothelium, can trigger a severe vasoconstrictive response (Inoue *et al.*, 1989).

The role of bacterial lipopolysaccharide (endotoxin) in ARDS has been widely documented. Brigham and Meyrick (1986) showed that endotoxin can be a priming agent for the activation and release of cytotoxic products by the neutrophil and macrophage. Moreover, endotoxin exerts a direct effect on the pulmonary endothelia cell (Brigham *et al.*, 1987) as well as on the systemic circulation, altering local vascular responsiveness to endothelial-dependent relaxing factors. This may play an important role in microvascular impairment, resulting in a defect of oxygen extraction and tissue hypoxia (Nelson *et al.*, 1987).

Abnormalities of Pulmonary Gas Exchange in ARDS

The ventilation–perfusion ratio ($\dot{V}/\dot{Q}$) of alveolar units, that is, an alveolus with its associated capillary, is the principal determinant of the degree of oxygenation of blood at the end of the pulmonary capillary (West, 1985). The $\dot{V}/\dot{Q}$ ratio varies from zero, in those alveolar units that are perfused but not ventilated, to infinity, in those alveolar units that are ventilated but not

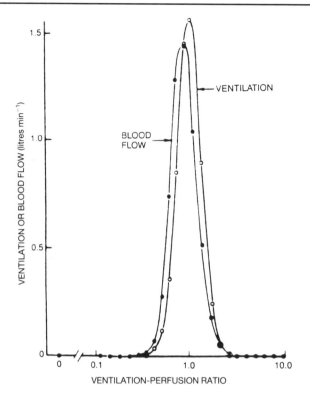

Figure 15.1 Ventilation–perfusion relationship. Distribution of ventilation–perfusion ratios in a normal subject, measured by the multiple inert gas technique. Most units demonstrate ratios of 1 due to good coupling of the ventilation and perfusion. (From Wagner *et al.*, 1974, with permission.)

perfused. In normal individuals one can find $\dot{V}/\dot{Q}$ ratios varying from 0.6 to about 3, but the vast majority of alveolar units involved on gas exchange will have a $\dot{V}/\dot{Q}$ ratio of 1, the result of a perfect match between local ventilation and perfusion. This can be appreciated in the diagram shown in Fig. 15.1 (Wagner *et al.*, 1974).

Under pathologic conditions the balance between ventilation and perfusion is easily disrupted and the $\dot{V}/\dot{Q}$ ratio becomes abnormal, allowing a predominance of alveolar units with either a high or a low $\dot{V}/\dot{Q}$ ratio. In extreme conditions, venous blood returning from the circulation passes through the lung without coming in contact with alveolar gas. This constitute 'physiologic' shunt, a condition normally found in blood emanating from the bronchial and thebesian veins that drain directly into the arterial side. Blood not exposed to the alveoli has a low PO_2 and, when mixed with well-oxygenated blood coming from other lung units, it will decrease the PO_2 of the mixture. Under physiologic conditions, the amount of blood shunted is minimal, and so is the drop in PO_2 from end-capillary to arterial blood. However, increases in shunt bring about large discrepancies in PO_2 between end-capillary and arterial blood. Another important characteristic of the hypoxaemia secondary to right-to-left shunt is its resistance to correction by increasing the fraction of inspired oxygen. The reason for this lack of reversal of hypoxaemia with increases in FIO_2, is that no matter how high alveolar O_2 concentration rises, it will not affect blood that does not come in contact with the alveolus. On the other hand, blood leaving partially ventilated alveolar units also will have a low PO_2. This condition is defined as a $\dot{V}/\dot{Q}$ abnormality, in contrast to shunt, and is represented by $\dot{V}/\dot{Q}$ ratios between zero and one. However, given the sigmoidal shape of the oxy-haemoglobin curve with its flat segment at high levels of PO_2, any level of $\dot{V}/\dot{Q}$ inequality in a given patient can be completely eliminated by raising the inspired oxygen fraction to 1.0. This property has an important clinical application, since one can calculate the degree of shunt responsible for the patient's hypoxaemia by administering an FIO_2 of 1.0 and monitoring the arterial PO_2. The equation defining the shunt fraction is:

$$\text{Shunt fraction} = \frac{CcO_2 - CaO_2}{CcO_2 - C\bar{v}O_2}$$

where CcO_2, CaO_2 and $C\bar{v}O_2$ are the end-capillary, arterial and mixed venous O_2 contents. Since we cannot measure CcO_2 directly, this parameter is calculated by assuming a haemoglobin saturation of 1.0 and an end-capillary PO_2 equal to the PO_2 computed from the alveolar air equation. For example, a patient is breathing pure oxygen ($FIO_2 = 1.0$), with arterial gases showing $PO_2 = 140\,mm\,Hg$ (18.7 kPa), O_2 saturation $= 0.99$, and $PCO_2 =$ mm Hg (4 kPa). Mixed venous gases show $PO_2 = 26\,mm\,Hg$ (3.5 kPa), O_2 saturation $= 0.5$, and $PCO_2 = 46\,mm\,Hg$ (6.1 kPa). The total haemoglobin concentration is $15\,g\,dl^{-1}$. Since the $FIO_2 = 1.0$, we can calculate the shunt fraction. First we calculate the alveolar PO_2, or PAO_2,

$$PAO_2 = FIO_2 \times (Pb - 47) - 1.25 \times PACO_2$$

where Pb is the barometric pressure. In this case,

$$PAO_2 = 1.0 \times (760 - 47) - 1.25 \times 30 = 676\,mm\,Hg\,(90\,kPa)$$

Then we calculate the various O_2 contents, beginning with end-capillary blood:

$$CcO_2 = 1.34 \times Hb \times O_2 \text{ saturation} + 0.003 \times PAO_2$$

or

$$CcO_2 = 1.34 \times 15 \times 1.00 + 0.003 \times 676 = 22.13\,ml\,O_2\,dl^{-1}\,blood$$

The arterial and mixed venous O_2 contents are:

$$CaO_2 = 1.34 \times 15 \times 0.99 + 0.003 \times 140 = 20.32 \, ml \, dl^{-1}$$
$$C\bar{v}O_2 = 1.34 \times 15 \times 0.50 + 0.003 \times 26 = 10.13 \, ml \, dl^{-1}$$

and the shunt fraction equals

$$(22.13 - 20.32)/(22.13 - 10.13) = 0.15 \, or \, 15\%$$

If the patient had been on an FiO_2 other than 1.0, the above calculation would have been labelled 'venous' admixture' instead of shunt.

Microatelectasis and the accumulation of fluid contribute to the loss of the elastic properties of the lung in ARDS, resulting in lung tissue with low compliance and decreased functional residual capacity. As the accumulation of fluid progresses, the alveoli will lose volume while remaining perfused. This leads to an increase in right-to-left intrapulmonary shunt. By this mechanism, shunt becomes the predominant gas exchange abnormality in patients with ARDS (Dantzker, 1986), a phenomenon that is illustrated in Fig. 15.2.

Use of Positive End-Expiratory Pressure to Treat Shunt

The notion that right-to-left shunt is the principal mechanism of hypoxia in patients with ARDS has several implications. As previously discussed,

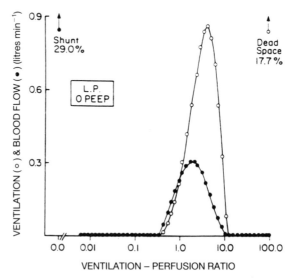

Figure 15.2 Shunt as the predominant mechanism of abnormal gas exchange in ARDS. Blood flow is found mostly in shunt units in a patient with ARDS and receiving no PEEP, as determined by the multiple inert gas elimination technique. Notice that some blood flow is found in units with high $\dot{V}/\dot{Q}$ ratios. (From Dantzker *et al.*, 1979, with permission.)

arterial PO_2 will increase little with increases in FIO_2, a phenomenon that is better appreciated as the shunt fraction increases. On the other hand, even small increases in PaO_2 in these patients is beneficial, since they are usually coupled to significant increases in haemoglobin saturation. The reason is that low levels of arterial PO_2 correspond to the steep portion of the oxy-haemoglobin dissociation curve, and a small rise in PO_2 will increase arterial oxygen content. Since arterial oxygen content is an important determinant of oxygen delivery, a progressive increase in the fraction of inspired oxygen is always warranted as an initial therapeutic manoeuvre. However, the preferred therapy for these patients is the institution of positive end-expiratory pressure (PEEP), a ventilatory manoeuvre that results in decreases in the shunt fraction and improved PO_2 (Dantzker, 1986). This is illustrated in Fig. 15.3, where the levels of shunt and $\dot{V}/\dot{Q}$ inequalities were measured in a patient before and after the initiation of PEEP using the multiple inert gases method. It is clear from the top figure that the major gas exchange disturbance was pulmonary shunt, since ventilated units had a near normal $\dot{V}/\dot{Q}$ relationship. The application of PEEP resulted in a decrease in the shunt fraction from 43.8% to 14.2%.

The application PEEP to correct the hypoxaemia of ARDS has been a standard practice for over two decades. Gregory *et al.* (1971) demonstrated its value in increasing arterial PO_2 while allowing a reduction in FIO_2. PEEP increases mean airway pressure, allowing the recruitment of pre-viously hypoventilated alveoli as the intra-alveolar fluids spreads over a larger surface area. This same effect will restore the functional residual capacity towards a normal value, improving the length–tension char-acteristics of the respiratory muscles. No evidence exists that the use of PEEP will decrease the extravascular lung water, in fact, it may even accelerate the rate at which it accumulates. However, a redistribution of the fluid in the alveoli towards a more compliant location in peribronchial areas has been shown to occur. A progressive, stepwise, increase in the PEEP leads to a reduction in the percentage of cardiac output that perfuse non-ventilated units. Similar results have been observed with increases in tidal volume (Dantzker *et al.*, 1980).

The cardiopulmonary interactions resulting from the application of PEEP may lead to right ventricular dysfunction and a decrease in cardiac output, an effect that can be corrected by fluid infusion (Marini *et al.*, 1989). This effect is also illustrated in Fig. 15.3, where the patient's cardiac output decreases as higher levels of PEEP are applied. Another possible untold effect of PEEP is the overdistention of lung tissues resulting in further alveolar damage. An alternative ventilatory manoeuvre is to apply inverse ratio ventilation, where the inspiratory time is prolonged (Marcy & Marini, 1991). This has the advantage of improving pulmonary gas exchange at lower PEEP and peak inspiratory pressures. Patients often do not tolerate this mode of ventilation and require heavy sedation.

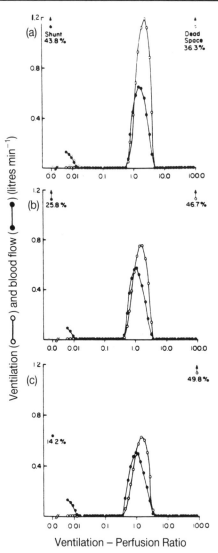

Figure 15.3   The effect of positive end-expiratory pressure (PEEP) on the ventilation–perfusion distribution in a patient with ARDS. (a) $Q_T = 9.0$ litres min^{-1}, 0 cm PEEP; (b) $Q_T = 5.1$ litres min^{-1}, 12 cm PEEP; (c) $Q_T = 4.5$ litres min^{-1}, 16 cm PEEP. The applications of increasing levels of PEEP led to a decrease in the intrapulmonary shunt from 43.8% to 14.2%. It should be noticed that a 50% reduction in cardiac output occurred concomitantly while the dead space increased. (From Dantzker *et al.*, with permission.)

Other Possible Causes of Hypoxaemia in ARDS

Arterial PO_2 is markedly dependent on changes in mixed venous PO_2 and clinical conditions resulting in a low mixed venous PO_2 also may lead to worsening hypoxaemia. Decreases in mixed venous PO_2 are the result of conditions where O_2 demand is greater than O_2 delivery and the tissues are forced to increase the fraction of O_2 extracted from capillary blood. These conditions include increased metabolic activity, decreased haemoglobin O_2 saturation or haemoglobin concentration, and decreased cardiac output.

Abnormalities of Peripheral Gas Exchange in ARDS

The awareness that a large number of patients with ARDS die of MSOF, rather than of hypoxaemia, and that local tissue hypoxia plays an important role in the pathogenesis of MSOF, has led to the recognition that generalized activation of inflammation occurs in both entities (Dorinsky & Gadek, 1989). Furthermore, ARDS also appears to be associated with peripheral gas exchar.ge abnormalities manifested as an abnormal relation between systemic oxygen uptake ($\dot{V}O_2$) and systemic oxygen delivery ($\dot{D}O_2$).

The Relationship between Oxygen Delivery and Oxygen Uptake

The relationship of systemic $\dot{D}O_2$ to $\dot{V}O_2$ was initially explored by Stainsby and Otis (1964) in canine skeletal muscle. They found that $\dot{V}O_2$ changes in a non-linear, or biphasic manner with progressive reductions in $\dot{D}O_2$. This is illustrated in Fig. 15.4, where $\dot{V}O_2$ is shown as a function of $\dot{D}O_2$. This

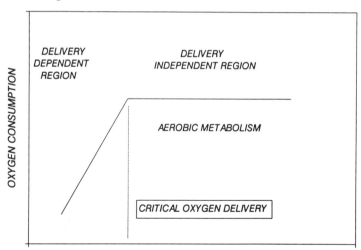

OXYGEN DELIVERY

Figure 15.4 Idealized representation of the relationship between oxygen delivery ($\dot{D}O_2$) and oxygen consumption ($\dot{V}O_2$). $\dot{V}O_2$ is illustrated as a function of $\dot{D}O_2$. On the $\dot{D}O_2$ independent region, aerobic metabolism is adequate to supply energy requirements and $\dot{V}O_2$ remains constant. Below the critical $\dot{D}O_2$ there is a dependency of $\dot{V}O_2$ on $\dot{D}O_2$, and the difference between the plateau $\dot{V}O_2$ and measured $\dot{V}O_2$ has to be provided by anaerobic metabolism.

function has two regions, one where $\dot{V}O_2$ remains constant for a wide range of $\dot{D}O_2$ values and the other where $\dot{V}O_2$ is dependent on $\dot{D}O_2$. In the region of constant $\dot{V}O_2$ or '$\dot{V}O_2$ plateau', aerobic metabolism supplies the energy required by cellular metabolism. The constancy of $\dot{V}O_2$ is the result of microvascular adaptations that increase the fraction of oxygen extracted by the tissues from capillary blood. This can be expressed as the oxygen extraction ratio, defined as $OER = \dot{V}O_2/\dot{D}O_2$. If we continue to decrease $\dot{D}O_2$, a condition eventually results where aerobic energy production becomes less than that required by cellular metabolism. At that level of $\dot{D}O_2$, defined as the 'critical' $\dot{D}O_2$ ($\dot{D}O_2$crit), the tissues are forced to recruit anaerobic sources of energy (Gutierrez, 1991). With the notable exception of diving mammals, in whom the diving reflex helps them redirect cardiac output to vital organs while decreasing metabolic requirements in other tissues, mammals lack regulatory mechanisms to allow adaptive decreases in energy requirements during hypoxia (Hochachka, 1986). Therefore, once $\dot{D}O_2$ falls below the $\dot{D}O_2$crit, $\dot{V}O_2$ becomes oxygen supply-dependent and anaerobic sources of energy must be used if the tissues are to survive hypoxia.

The biphasic nature of the $\dot{D}O_2$–$\dot{V}O_2$ relationship has been confirmed in numerous experimental studies in animals. These experiments initially implied that $\dot{D}O_2$crit was a fixed quantity that could be useful as an index of anaerobic metabolism in critically ill patients. However, subsequent studies showed that $\dot{D}O_2$crit was not a fixed quantity, but that it varied according to the metabolic needs of the tissues for oxygen and also with factors that affect the oxygen transport system, such as hypothermia (Gutierrez et al., 1986) and the position of the oxyhaemoglobin dissociation curve (Warley & Gutierrez, 1988).

Oxygen Delivery and Oxygen Uptake in ARDS

In contrast to animal studies, clinical investigations in critically ill patients, including those with ARDS, have shown a linear relationship between $\dot{D}O_2$ and $\dot{V}O_2$, one lacking a critical $\dot{D}O_2$. The exception has been the work of Shibutani et al. (1983), who pooled data obtained from anaesthetized patients prior to undergoing cardiopulmonary bypass and found a biphasic $\dot{D}O_2$–$\dot{V}O_2$ relationship.

Danek et al. (1980) measured $\dot{D}O_2$, $\dot{V}O_2$ and mixed venous PO_2 in 20 patients with ARDS and 12 others with various diseases. In all but one of the patients, the $\dot{D}O_2$–$\dot{V}O_2$ relationship was linear, even at $\dot{D}O_2$ levels of 50 ml min^{-1} kg^{-1}, three times the $\dot{D}O_2$ of normal subjects at rest (Fig. 15.5). This finding has been confirmed repeatedly by other investigators (Mohsenifar et al., 1983; Lorente et al., 1991). Gutierrez and Pohil (1986) fitted six different mathematical functions to the $\dot{D}O_2$–$\dot{V}O_2$ data pairs obtained in individual patients with respiratory failure. They concluded that a linear function was

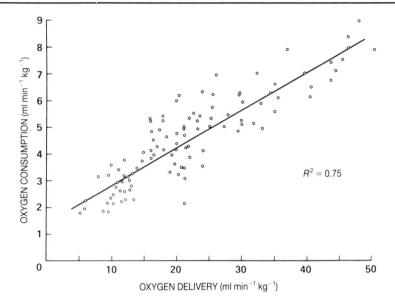

Figure 15.5 The relationship of O_2 delivery to O_2 uptake in patients with ARDS. The data demonstrate a linear relationship between $\dot{D}O_2$ and $\dot{V}O_2$ in all but one of 12 patients with ARDS, even when $\dot{D}O_2$ was 3 times that of normal subjects at rest. (From Danek *et al.*, 1980, with permission.)

an accurate representation of the $\dot{D}O_2$–$\dot{V}O_2$ relationship in acutely ill patients, regardless of their diagnosis. In a recent study, Clarke *et al.* (1991) corroborated the finding that a linear function is the best descriptor of the $\dot{D}O_2$–$\dot{V}O_2$ relationship in critically ill patients. Incidentally, these patients were subjected to increases in $\dot{D}O_2$ produced by vasoactive drugs and plasma expansion, but the presence of a $\dot{V}O_2$ 'plateau' could not be established.

Pathologic Oxygen Supply Dependence

Several theories have been proposed to explain the discrepancy between experimental studies, displaying a non-linear, biphasic $\dot{D}O_2$–$\dot{V}O_2$ relationship with a clearly defined critical $\dot{D}O_2$, and clinical studies, showing a linear function. Perhaps the most plausible hypothesis is that advanced by Kreuzer and Cain (1985), who proposed that the linear dependency of $\dot{V}O_2$ on $\dot{D}O_2$ in patients with ARDS can be explained by a combination of decreased ability of the tissues to extract O_2 from blood, and greater basal metabolic requirements for O_2, resulting in a higher than normal $\dot{V}O_2$ plateau (Fig. 15.6). According to this hypothesis, levels of $\dot{D}O_2$ that in normal subjects are sufficient to sustain aerobic metabolism (solid line), are inadequate for patients with ARDS (dashed line). Therefore, these patients

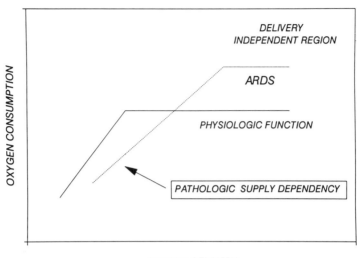

Figure 15.6 Pathologic supply dependency in ARDS. A linear relationship between oxygen consumption ($\dot{V}O_2$) and oxygen delivery ($\dot{D}O_2$) is found in critically ill patients. This may be explained by a combination of greater basal metabolic requirements and a decreased ability of the tissues to extract O_2 from blood.

have a wider range of $\dot{D}O_2$ values where $\dot{V}O_2$ is O_2 supply dependent, a condition defined as pathologic O_2 supply dependency. Support for this hypothesis can be found in the study by Gutierrez and Pohil (1986) (Fig. 15.7), who noted that changes in $\dot{V}O_2$ in one group of patients (group A), were dependent on $\dot{D}O_2$, whereas in the other group (group B) $\dot{V}O_2$ varied little with alterations in $\dot{D}O_2$. The ability of a given patient to maintain $\dot{V}O_2$ constant depended on the capacity of the tissues to extract oxygen from blood. Patients with O_2 supply dependency (Group A) had a 70% mortality rate and included patients with disease entities capable of disrupting microvascular control, peripheral blood distribution, or tissue gas exchange, such as ARDS, sepsis, and acute haemorrhage. Group B patients, who maintained $\dot{V}O_2$ relatively constant, had a mortality rate of only 30%, and for the most part they had cardiac failure, although some of them also carried the diagnosis of ARDS. Another study supporting the concept of pathologic O_2 supply dependency in critically ill patients, with its corollary of a hidden O_2 debt, is that of Bihari *et al.* (1987). They noted that the infusion of prostacyclin, a potent vasodilator, increased $\dot{D}O_2$ in 27 critically ill patients with respiratory failure. In 13 of these patients, all of whom died during the course of their illness, increases in $\dot{D}O_2$ were accompanied by increases in $\dot{V}O_2$, suggesting a hidden O_2 debt.

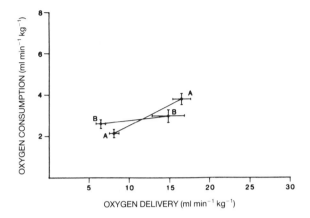

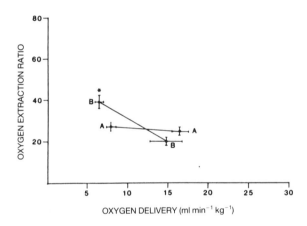

Figure 15.7 Mortality as determined by pathologic O_2 supply dependency. The relationship of oxygen consumption ($\dot{V}O_2$) to oxygen delivery ($\dot{D}O_2$) and oxygen extraction ratio (OER) was measured in two groups of critically ill patients. Group A exhibited O_2 supply dependency and had a mortality of 70%. Group B maintained constant VO_2 by increases in OER. This group had a mortality of only 30%. (From Gutierrez & Pohil, 1986, with permission.)

Is Oxygen Supply Dependency in ARDS Patients a Pathologic Condition?

The theory of pathologic O_2 supply dependency has been challenged by several clinical studies. Annat *et al.* (1986) measured $\dot{D}O_2$ in eight mechanically ventilated patients with ARDS using the expired gas method, instead of calculating it by the Fick equation, the procedure commonly used in most intensive care units. They lowered cardiac output and $\dot{D}O_2$ by the institution of PEEP and found no decreases in $\dot{V}O_2$ or increases in blood lactate. They concluded that these patients with ARDS were capable of increasing O_2 extraction to meet cellular O_2 requirements. Furthermore, they did not find a higher $\dot{V}O_2$ plateau in these patients, since their basal $\dot{V}O_2$ was not different from that of patients with non-ARDS respiratory failure.

It appears that critically ill patients, including those without ARDS, will exhibit a linear $\dot{D}O_2$–$\dot{V}O_2$ relationship. Dorinsky et al. (1988) measured $\dot{V}O_2$ and $\dot{D}O_2$ in patients with ARDS, as well as in patients with respiratory failure unrelated to ARDS. They found that $\dot{V}O_2$ was a linear function of $\dot{D}O_2$ in both groups. Furthermore, they noted greater OER in patients with ARDS over a similar range of $\dot{D}O_2$, and concluded that O_2 supply dependency was not unique to patients with ARDS. In a more recent study, Ronco et al. (1991) measured $\dot{V}O_2$ by the expired gases method in 17 patients with ARDS, and increased $\dot{D}O_2$ by blood transfusion. They found no changes in $\dot{V}O_2$, even in those patients with elevated blood lactate ($n = 10$), concluding that O_2 supply dependency in ARDS patients may be a methodological artifact produced by the computation of $\dot{V}O_2$ and $\dot{D}O_2$ from shared variables, such as cardiac output and arterial O_2 content.

It is possible that the discrepancy between animal and clinical studies may be related to the temporal characteristics of clinical data collection, during which the patient's basal energy requirements change. Experimental protocols usually consist of subjecting a healthy animal preparation for a short time to graded reductions in $\dot{D}O_2$. Under these conditions, basal $\dot{V}O_2$ should remain constant and $\dot{D}O_2$ is the manipulated variable. In contrast, in a clinical study, in which data are collected over a protracted period of time, basal $\dot{V}O_2$ will go up or down according to the metabolic needs of the patient. Therefore, at certain times the patient may experience decreases in $\dot{D}O_2$ below the critical point. At other times, however, arterial oxygenation and cardiac output may be adequate, but $\dot{D}O_2$ will increase in response to agitation, fever, or exercise. In the former case $\dot{V}O_2$ is dependent on $\dot{D}O_2$, whereas in the latter it is $\dot{D}O_2$ that depends on $\dot{V}O_2$. The end-result of this variation in $\dot{V}O_2$ and $\dot{D}O_2$ is a linear $\dot{D}O_2$–$\dot{V}O_2$ relationship.

Dantzker et al. (1991) examined the concept of O_2 supply dependency from a physiological perspective by compiling data from critically ill patients, as well as data from normal subjects during exercise. They noted that exercise produces large increases in $\dot{D}O_2$ and OER until an anaerobic threshold is reached. In contrast, the O_2 transport system appears to be unable to substantially increase systemic OER as a way of maintaining aerobic metabolism when faced with decreases in $\dot{D}O_2$. As a result, the critical OER in normal humans may lie close to the normal resting OER, and a $\dot{V}O_2$ plateau may be difficult to establish. Therefore, the linear interaction between $\dot{D}O_2$ and $\dot{V}O_2$ in ARDS may represent the normal physiological behaviour of the system, rather than an abnormality in O_2 extraction capacity. Increase in OER during exercise may be related to the redirection of the cardiac output to working skeletal muscle, an organ with a large capability to recruit previously closed capillaries. On the other hand, decreases in $\dot{D}O_2$ are experienced by all organs, in particular those lacking the ability to increase capillarity, such as the kidney and the gut.

Whether the $\dot{D}O_2$–$\dot{V}O_2$ relationship in ARDS is a straight line or it is the manifestation of pathologic supply dependency has great clinical importance. If the latter is the case, then it makes sense to increase $\dot{D}O_2$ by fluid infusions, blood transfusions, or vasoactive substances until a $\dot{V}O_2$ plateau is reached. On the other hand, if the $\dot{D}O_2$–$\dot{V}O_2$ relationship in patients with ARDS is a straight line, lacking a $\dot{V}O_2$ plateau, then efforts to increase $\dot{D}O_2$ to supranormal levels may not be warranted.

It appears that survival of patients with ARDS is inversely related to their initial levels of $\dot{D}O_2$ and $\dot{V}O_2$. This was shown by Russell et al. (1990), who measured these parameters in 29 patients within 24 h from the onset of ARDS. However, in a randomized, prospective, double-blind study on the effect of prostaglandin E_1 in patients with ARDS, Bone et al. (1989) showed no improvement in survival, although patients given prostaglandin E_1 had significantly greater $\dot{D}O_2$ values than the control group.

Metabolic Markers of Tissue Hypoxia

Measures of $\dot{D}O_2$ and $\dot{V}O_2$ determine how much O_2 is offered and how much O_2 is taken by the tissues, but provide little information regarding the tissular O_2 requirements. In other words, $\dot{D}O_2$ and $\dot{V}O_2$ values that might be adequate for a patient at rest may be woefully lacking if the patient becomes agitated, septic, or enters a hypermetabolic state. Therefore, we need sensitive metabolic markers to help us determine the level of $\dot{D}O_2$ where anaerobic metabolism begins. Among possible markers of anaerobiosis are the concentration of lactate in blood, the products of adenine nucleotide metabolism, magnetic resonance spectroscopy, and tonometered gut mucosal pH.

Blood Lactate Concentration

Lactate is the end-product of anaerobic glycolysis and blood concentrations rise in response to hypoxia. The possibility that patients with O_2 supply dependency can be identified on the basis of their arterial lactate levels has been proposed by several authors (Kruse et al., 1990; Bakker & Vincent, 1991). In a study by Gilbert et al. (1986), patients with sepsis and elevated blood lactate concentration showed increases in $\dot{V}O_2$ when given infusions of fluids or blood transfusions. In that study, patients given dopamine or dobutamine also experienced increases in $\dot{V}O_2$, although this occurred regardless of their levels of serum lactate, suggesting that catecholamines may exert a direct positive effect on oxidative metabolism, a conclusion supported by the findings of increased resting energy expenditure in normal men given dopamine intravenously (Ruttiman *et al.*, 1991). Subsequent studies have confirmed that patients with sepsis or ARDS with elevated serum lactate levels respond to increases in $\dot{D}O_2$ produced by fluid or catecholamines with increases in $\dot{D}O_2$ (Vincent *et al.*, 1990a,b).

One of the drawbacks of using lactate as a marker of anaerobic metabolism is that it reflects the pooling from different tissue beds. Therefore, increased lactate production by a hypoxic organ may not be sufficient to alter the overall blood lactate concentration. Also, as shown by several investigators, the kinetics of lactate production and consumption are exceedingly difficult to predict, with some tissues producing and others consuming lactate (Gladden, 1991). Therefore, a high lactate value in the absence of hepatic dysfunction appears to be a reliable sign of tissue hypoxia, but a normal value cannot be taken as evidence of an adequate $\dot{D}O_2$.

The Products of Adenine Nucleotide Degradation

The products of adenine monophosphate (AMP) degradation, namely inosine, hypoxanthine, xanthine and uric acid have been proposed as metabolic markers of tissue hypoxia. Grum *et al.* (1985) noted an increase of these metabolites in the blood of critically ill patients with ARDS. However, this technique also suffers from the same drawbacks as blood lactate, since it is a global measurement with low sensitivity.

Magnetic Resonance Spectroscopy

A promising technique to help determine the onsent of anaerobiosis non-invasively, is phosphorus-31 nuclear magnetic resonance (^{31}P-NMR) spectroscopy. A magnetic resonance spectrometer consists of a radiotransmitter capable of directing high-frequency radio waves into a tissue sample placed inside a strong, homogeneous, magnetic field. This technique offers a non-invasive window into the adequacy of tissue oxygenation by measuring the levels of phosphocreatine, inorganic phosphate and ATP, as well as intracellular pH, in skeletal muscle, the brain and the heart (Gutierrez & Andry, 1989). Magnetic resonance spectroscopy has several technical limitations regarding the spatial localization of the signal. However, the major drawbacks of ^{31}P-NMR spectroscopy as a monitoring technique are the size of the magnet and the interference resulting from the proximity of metallic objects.

Individual Organ Perfusion and Metabolism

Systemic measures of $\dot{D}O_2$ and $\dot{V}O_2$ offer little information regarding the adequacy of O_2 supply to individual organs. This is an important consideration, since disturbances in tissue perfusion occur commonly in patients with

ARDS. Hypoperfusion and the accompanying decreases in tissue oxygenation set in motion a cascade of local regulatory responses that result in the redistribution of the cardiac output to different organs according to their metabolic need, with those organs with the highest metabolic rate receiving the greatest fraction of the cardiac output. Also, some organs are better prepared to regulate tissue perfusion than others. An example is skeletal muscle, whose capillary density can increase 20–30-fold during exercise and it is capable to withstand protracted periods of systemic hypoxia. This type of blood flow regulation is not available to other organs, such as the intestines, that depend heavily on autonomic reflex regulation.

Tonometric Determination of Gut Mucosal pH

A new technique capable of monitoring metabolic events in critically ill patients is the tonometric measurement of intestinal or gastric mucosal pH (pH_i). This parameter provides non-invasive metabolic information from the gut mucosa, a tissue that is at great risk during periods of hypoxia. Tonometry consists of a silastic balloon filled with saline that is inserted inside the intestines or the stomach. Since CO_2 is a freely diffusible gas, the PCO_2 in the outer layers of the gastric or intestinal mucosa comes into equilibrium with the PCO_2 in the saline contained in the silastic balloon. An approximation to the mucosal pH is obtained by applying the Henderson–Hasselbalch equation to concurrently measured mucosal PCO_2 and arterial HCO_3. The sensitivity of the intestinal and gastric mucosa to decreases in O_2 transport and sepsis has been demonstrated by several experimental studies (Grum et al., 1984; Fiddian-Green & Baker, 1987).

Unlike $\dot{D}O_2$ and $\dot{V}O_2$, whose interpretation requires knowledge of cellular energy demands, pH_i is an absolute measurement, since it represents an indirect measurement of the gastric mucosa anaerobic activity. During hypoxia or sepsis, blood flow is diverted from the splanchnic circulation and pH_i decreases as tissue hypoxia ensues and anaerobic sources of energy are recruited. Measurements of gastric pH_i are highly predictive of morbidity (Fiddian-Green et al., 1983; Gys et al., 1988) and of mortality (Fiddian-Green & Baker, 1987). In a recent study, Doglio et al. (1991) prospectively followed 80 consecutive patients and measured gastric pH_i upon admission to the ICU and again 12 h later. They stratified patients according to their pH_i values as normal pH_i (≥ 7.35) and low pH_i (< 7.35). As shown in Fig. 15.8, they found the lowest mortality in those patients with normal pH_i at both measuring periods (29%). Conversely, the highest mortality was noted in patients with low pH_i at admission and during the first 12 h in the ICU (87%).

In a multicentre, prospective, randomized study, Gutierrez et al. (1992) measured gastric pH_i in 260 patients admitted to the ICU with APACHE II scores between 15 and 25. Decreases in pH_i below 7.35 were treated with

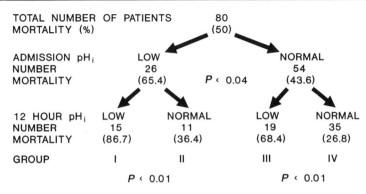

Figure 15.8 Patient mortality according to pH_i. Patient mortality according to gastric intramucosal pH measured in a group of 80 patients upon admission to the ICU and again 12 h later. Patients with low pH_i during the first 12 h had the highest mortality, whereas those able to maintain normal pH_i during that period had the lowest mortality. The APACHE II scores were similar for all four groups. (From Doglio *et al.*, 1991, with permission.)

therapy aimed at increasing $\dot{D}O_2$, including fluids, blood transfusions, and the infusions of dobutamine. They found that patients admitted with pH_i < 7.35 did not benefit from this resuscitation protocol. On the other hand, patients admitted that $pH_i \geq 7.35$, in whom pH_i-guided resuscitation was actively pursued whenever pH_i decreased below 7.35, had a 58% survival rate, compared to 42% for the control group (Fig. 15.9).

The different responses to pH_i-guided therapy among the study groups may be related to the role played by the gut during conditions of inadequate O_2 supply. It has been hypothesized that gastrointestinal hypoxia results in the translocation of bacteria and toxins from the lumen into blood, promoting the development of sepsis and multiple systems organ failure syndrome. Prompt therapeutic action, directed at increasing systemic $\dot{D}O_2$ in response to decreases in pH_i, could prevent these conditions, resulting in greater survival. On the other hand, increases in $\dot{D}O_2$ may be an ineffective therapy in patients admitted to the ICU after a period of protracted mucosal acidosis. In those patients a 'leaky' gut may have developed, allowing for the translocation phenomenon to occur. These findings emphasize the importance of prompt, and timely, therapy by increases in $\dot{D}O_2$ guided by changes in gastric mucosal pH.

Treatment of Impaired Oxygenation in ARDS

General Principles

There is no specific therapy for ARDS. In general, the treatment is directed toward maintaining adequate tissue oxygenation in vital organs, by supporting

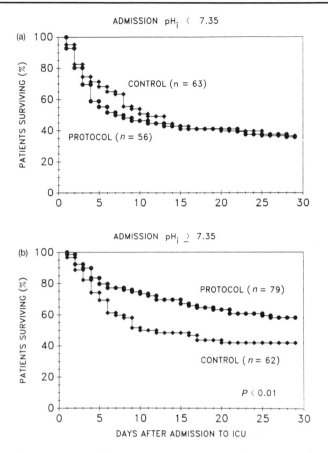

Figure 15.9 Survival curves for patients treated according to changes in gastric intramucosal pH. (a) Survival curves for patients admitted to the ICU with gastric mucosal pH < 7.35. There was no difference in survival between the study and the control group. (b) Survival curves for patients admitted with a gastric intramucosal pH ≥ 7.35. The study group, treated with therapy aimed at increases in DO_2 whenever the gastric mucosal pH decreased < 7.35, showed improved survival. (From Gutierrez *et al.*, 1992, with permission.)

the cardio-respiratory system, while allowing the alveoli-capillary membrane to recover its integrity. Given the nature of this chapter, we will focus on those aspects involved in the maintenance of arterial oxygenation, adequate oxygen delivery, and aerobic metabolism by the peripheral tissues.

Among the most important therapeutic principles in treating patients with ARDS are: (a) a vigorous search and treatment of associated conditions that may have precipitated, or complicated ARDS, i.e. sepsis, shock, anaemia, etc; (b) prompt recognition and treatment of complications, often of an iatrogenic nature, i.e. line sepsis, barotrauma (pneumothorax), improper ventilatory settings, the development of bowel ischaemia or acute renal failure, malnutrition, etc. Proper management of these patients requires the careful monitoring of haemodynamic, oxygen transport and metabolic variables. Therefore, we recommend the use of an arterial line for drawing of blood gases and continuous measurement of arterial blood pressure, a pulse oximeter to measure arterial O_2 saturation, a pulmonary artery catheter for measurement of the occlusion pressure and of cardiac output by the thermodilution method, a gastric tonometer for measurement of intramucosal pH as an index of tissue perfusion, and frequent measurements of blood lactate concentration.

Intubation and Mechanical Ventilation

Maintenance of adequate arterial oxygenation, defined as a haemoglobin O_2 saturation ≥ 0.90, is of paramount importance in the treatment of ARDS. Although this should be done while minimizing O_2 toxicity by keeping the $FIO_2 \leq 0.40$, the risk of oxygen toxicity should not be a major concern during the initial management of ARDS, and high levels of FIO_2 should be used as long as the patient is hypoxaemic. It should be remembered that the hypoxaemia of ARDS is mainly the result of shunting, and it is resistant to oxygen therapy. Therefore, patients with ARDS usually require high FIO_2 levels. Given the usually poor response to supplemental oxygen, patients with intractable hypoxaemia should be treated with mechanical ventilation. Among the main advantages of mechanical ventilation are: stabilization of the airway, better control of the tidal volume and functional residual capacity, the ability to apply PEEP and minimize shunt. Also, mechanical ventilation will decrease the O_2 cost of breathing, minimizing systemic O_2 consumption. Several comprehensive reviews on the use and pitfalls of mechanical ventilation in ARDS have been published recently (Bolin & Pierson, 1986; Marini, 1990; Stoller & Kacmareck, 1990).

Following intubation, the patient with ARDS should be ventilated with a tidal volume consisting of 8–10 ml kg^{-1} body weight with an FIO_2 of 1.0. This inspired O_2 fraction, in addition to eliminating $\dot{V}/\dot{Q}$ abnormalities, allows one to compute the degree of right-to-left shunt. Blood gases should be obtained 15 min after intubation for measurement of arterial PO_2, PCO_2, pH and O_2 saturation. This information will permit further adjustments of the ventilator. A pulse oximeter should be used thereafter to monitor arterial saturation continuously. Once the goal of adequate arterial oxygenation is achieved (≥ 0.90), the lowest possible FIO_2 capable of maintaining this level of O_2 saturation should be sought, and decreases in FIO_2 should be attempted as the clinical situation allows.

The lowest FIO_2 that can be administered for prolonged periods of time without the development of oxygen toxicity is unknown, although it appears that this can be done safely at FIO_2 levels ≤ 0.5. Pulmonary O_2

toxicity is a complex function of the alveolar O_2 concentration and the time of exposure. The damage that oxygen inflicts on the lung resembles ARDS in itself (Katzestein & Askin, 1990). Another complication of high FIO_2 levels is the washout of alveolar nitrogen, promoting atelectasis (denitrogenation) and further increases in shunt (Bolin & Pierson, 1986).

The Use of Positive End-Expiratory Pressure (PEEP)

As previously discussed, PEEP should be used to decrease the shunt fraction. To determine the optimal level of PEEP in a given patient, one should aim for that level of PEEP that maximizes $\dot{D}O_2$ while minimizing FIO_2, hopefully permitting adequate tissue oxygenation with an $FIO_2 < 0.50$. This should be done by applying stepwise increases of PEEP, usually at 5 cm H_2O intervals, as long as arterial PO_2 increases without declines in cardiac output.

Patient Monitoring

The most difficult aspect in the management of patients with ARDS is the ability to anticipate changes in clinical condition to allow the prompt institution of preventive measures. This may be possible by periodically monitoring haemodynamic parameters, $\dot{D}O_2$, $\dot{V}O_2$, OER, blood lactate concentration, and gastric mucosal pH (Fiddian-Green, 1991). A reasonable compromise between cost and optimal patient management is to measure these parameters every 6–8 h in patients with stable haemodynamics. A rapidly changing clinical condition may require more frequent measurements. As shown in other chapters, $\dot{D}O_2$ is calculated as the product of cardiac output and the arterial O_2 content, whereas $\dot{V}O_2$ can be measured directly from the expired gases, as long as $FIO_2 < 0.40$. Higher levels of FIO_2 may result in unacceptable errors in $\dot{V}O_2$. Perhaps the most practical method is to calculate $\dot{V}O_2$ using the Fick equation as cardiac output $\times (CaO_2 - C\bar{v}O_2)$.

The information provided by the above measurements should be used to determine the adequacy of $\dot{D}O_2$. As shown by Shoemaker $et\ al.$ (1988) survival in post-operative patients is a function of the oxygen debt. It is difficult to establish an absolute $\dot{D}O_2$ level to be used in every patient, although a level ≥ 600 ml min^{-1} m^{-2} has been proposed by some (Edwards, 1989). Alternatively, one could estimate the degree of oxygen debt from the levels of blood lactate and the gastric mucosal pH. Lactate levels > 2.2 (Gilbert $et\ al.$, 1986; Kruse $et\ al.$, 1990) and/or gastric mucosal pH < 7.32 should be taken as indicators of inadequate $\dot{D}O_2$ (Gutierrez $et\ al.$, 1992). Should that be the case, efforts should be made to increase cardiac output with fluid infusions and vasoactive substances, such as dopamine and dobutamine (Shoemaker $et\ al.$, 1986; Edwards $et\ al.$, 1989; Vincent $et\ al.$,

1990a,b). Arterial O_2 content should be increased with blood transfusions. It appears that a haemoglobin concentration of $12\,g\,dl^{-1}$ is adequate for O_2 delivery and optimal microvascular vasomotion (Messmer, 1991).

Conclusions

Although ARDS is associated with a high mortality rate, each patient that survives offers proof of the efficacy of intensive care principles in the treatment of this condition. In the final analysis, the most important aspect in the treatment of a patient with ARDS is the care and dedication given to that patient by the health care team, including physicians, nurses, respiratory therapists, dietitians, etc. Attention to detail and prompt response to pathological alterations are paramount. This includes the maintenance of aerobic metabolism by promoting adequate levels of $\dot{D}O_2$.

References

Annat G, Viale J, Pereival L *et al.* (1986) Oxygen delivery and uptake in the adult respiratory distress syndrome. *Am. Rev. Respiratory Dis.* **133:** 999–1001.

Ashbaugh DG, Bigelow DB, Petty TL & Levine EB (1967) Acute respiratory distress in adults. *Lancet* **2:** 319–23.

Bachofen M & Weibel ER (1977) Alteration of the gas exchange apparatus in adult respiratory insufficiency associated with septicemia. *Am. Rev. Respiratory Dis.* **116:** 589–615.

Bakker J & Vincent JL (1991) The oxygen supply dependancy phenomenon is associated with increased blood lactate levels. *J. Crit. Care* **6:** 152–9.

Bihari D, Smithies M, Gimson A & Tinker J (1987) The effects of vasodilation with prostacyclin on oxygen delivery and uptake in critically ill patients. *New Engl. J. Med.* **317:** 397–403.

Bolin R & Pierson D (1986) Ventilatory management in acute lung injury. *Crit. Care Clin.* **2:** 585–99.

Bone RC, Slotman G, Maunder R *et al.* (1989) Randomized double-blind, multicenter study of prostaglandin E_1 in patients with the adult respiratory distress syndrome. *Chest* **96:** 114–9.

Brigham KL & Meyrick BO (1986) State of the art: Endotoxin and lung injury. *Am. Rev. Respiratory Dis.* **133:** 913–27.

Brigham KL, Meyrick BO, Berry LC & Repine JE (1987) Antioxidants protect cultured bovine lung endothelial cells from injury by endotoxin. *J. Appl. Physiol.* **63:** 840–50.

Cain SM (1986) Assessment of tissue oxygenation. *Crit. Care Clin.* **2:** 537–50.

Carvalho AC, Bellman SM, Saullo VJ *et al.* (1982) Altered factors VIII in acute respiratory failure. *New Engl. J. Med.* **307:** 1113–19.

Clarke C, Edwards JD, Nightingale P *et al.* (1991) Persistence of supply dependency of oxygen uptake at high levels of delivery in adult respiratory distress syndrome. *Crit. Care Med.* **19:** 497–502.

Craddock PR, Fehr J, Brigham KL *et al.* (1977) Complement and leukocyte-mediated pulmonary dysfunction in hemodialysis. *New Engl. J. Med.* **296:** 769–74.

Danek SJ, Lynch JP, Weg JG & Dantzker DR (1980) The dependance of oxygen uptake on oxygen delivery in the adult respiratory distress. *Am. Rev. Respiratory Dis.* 387–95.

Dantzker DR (1986) Gas exchange in adult lung injury. *Crit. Care Clin.* **2:** 527–36.

Dantzker DR, Lynch JP & Weg JG (1980) Depression of cardiac output is a mechanism of shunt reduction in the therapy of acute respiratory failure. *Chest* **77:** 636–42.

Dantzker DR, Foresman & Gutierrez G (1991) Oxygen supply and utilization relationships. *Am. Rev. Respiratory Dis.* **143:** 675–9.

Doglio GR, Pusajo JF, Egurrola MA *et al.* (1991) Gastric mucosa pH as a prognostic index of mortality in critically ill patients. *Crit. Care Med.* **19:** 1037–40.

Dorinsky PM & Gadek JE (1989) Mechanisms of multiple nonpulmonary organ failure in ARDS. *Chest* **96:** 885–92.

Dorinsky PM, Costello JL & Gadek JE (1988) Relationship of oxygen uptake and oxygen delivery in respiratory failure not due to adult respiratory distress syndrome. *Chest* **93:** 1013–19.

Edwards DJ (1989) Optimal level oxygen transport in critically ill patients. In Vincent JL (ed.), *Update in Intensive Care and Emergency Medicine*, pp. 2–11. Berlin: Springer-Verlag.

Edwards DJ, Brown GC, Nightingale P *et al.* (1989) Use of survivors' cardiorespiratory values as therapeutic goals in septic shock. *Crit. Care Med.* **17:** 1098–103.

Ferrari-Baliviera E, Mealy K, Smith RL & Wilmore DW (1989) Tumor necrosis factor induces adult respiratory distress syndrome in rats. *Arch. Surg.* **124:** 1400–5.

Fiddian-Green RG (1991) Should measurements of tissue pH and PO_2 be included in the routine monitoring of intensive care unit patients? *Crit. Care Med.* **19:** 141–3.

Fiddian-Green RG & Baker S (1987) The predictive value of the stomach wall pH for complications after cardiac operations: a comparison with other forms of monitoring. *Crit. Care Med.* **15:** 153–6.

Fiddian-Green RG, McGough E, Pittenger G & Rothman ED (1983) Predictive value of intramural pH and other risk factors for massive bleeding from stress ulceration. *Gastroenterology* **85:** 613–20.

Fink MP, Fiallo V, Stein KL & Gardiner MW (1987) Systemic and regional hemodynamic changes after intraperitoneal endotoxin in rabbits. *Circ. Shock* **22:** 73–81.

Fowler AA, Hamman RF, Good JT *et al.* (1983) Adult respiratory distress syndrome: Risk with common predispositions. *Ann. Intern. Med.* **98:** 593–7.

Fowler AA, Hamman RF, Zerbe GO *et al.* (1985) Adult respiratory distress syndrome: Prognosis after onset. *Am. Rev. Respiratory Dis.* **132:** 472–8.

Gilbert EM, Haupt MT, Mandanas RH *et al.* (1986) The effect of fluid loading, blood transfusion and catecholamine infusion on oxygen delivery and consumption in patients with sepsis. *Am. Rev. Respiratory Dis.* **134:** 873–8.

Gladden BL (1991) Net lactate during progressive steady-level contractions in canine skeletal muscle. *J. Appl. Physiol.* **71:** 514–20.

Gregory GA, Kitterman JA, Phibbs RH *et al.* (1971) Treatment of the idiopathic respiratory-distress syndrome with continuous positive airway pressure. *New Engl. J. Med.* **284:** 1333–40.

Grum CM, Fiddian-Green RG, Pittenger GL *et al.* (1984) Adequacy of tissue oxygenation in intact dog intestine. *J. Appl. Physiol.* **56:** 1065–9.

Grum CM, Simon RH, Dantzker DR & Fox IH (1985) Evidence for adenosine tri-phosphate degradation in critically ill patients. *Chest* **88:** 763–7.

Gutierrez G (1991) Cellular energy metabolism during hypoxia. *Crit. Care Med.* **19:** 619–20.

Gutierrez G & Andry J (1989) Nuclear magnetic resonance measurements – clinical applications. *Crit. Care Med.* **17:** 73–82.

Gutierrez G & Pohil R (1986) Oxygen consumption is linearly related to O_2 supply in critically ill patients. *J. Crit. Care* **1:** 45–53.

Gutierrez G, Warley A & Dantzker DR (1986) Oxygen delivery and utilization in hypothermic dogs. *J. Appl. Physiol.* **60:** 751–7.

Gutierrez G, Pohil JP & Narayana P (1989) Skeletal muscle O_2 consumption and energy metabolism during hypoxemia. *J. Appl. Physiol.* **66:** 2117–23.

Gutierrez G, Palizas F, Doglio G *et al.* (1992) Gastric intra-mucosal pH as a therapeutic index of tissue oxygenation in critically ill patients. *Lancet* **339:** 195–99.

Gys T, Hubens A, Neels H *et al.* (1988) Prognostic values of gastric intramural pH in surgical intensive care patients. *Crit. Care Med.* **16:** 1222–4.

Hochachka PW (1986) Defense strategies against hypoxia and hypothermia. *Science* **231:** 234–41.

Inoue A, Yanagisawa M, Kimura S *et al.* (1989) The human endothelin family: Three structurally and pharmacologically distinct isopeptides predicted by three separate genes. *Proc. Natl. Acad. Sci. USA* **86:** 2863–7.

Johnson AR, Coalson JJ, Ashton J *et al.* (1985) Neutral endopeptidase in serum samples from patients with adult respiratory distress syndrome: Comparison with angiotensin converting enzyme. *Am. Rev. Respiratory Dis.* **132:** 1262–7.

Katzenstein A & Askin FB (1990) Acute lung injury patterns: Diffuse alveolar damage, acute interstitial pneumonia, bronchiolitis obliterans-organizing pneumonia. In Bennington JL (ed.), *Surgical Pathology of Non-neoplastic Lung Disease*, pp. 9–57. Philadelphia: W.B. Saunders.

Kreuzer F & Cain S (1985) Regulation of peripheral vasculature and tissue oxygenation in health and disease. *Crit. Care Clin.* **1:** 453–70.

Kruse JA, Haupt MT, Puri VK & Carlson RW (1990) Lactate levels as predictors of the relationship between oxygen delivery and consumption in ARDS. *Chest* **98:** 959–62.

Lee CT, Fein AM, Lippmann M *et al.* (1981) Elastolytic activity in pulmonary lavage fluid from patients with adult respiratory-distress syndrome. *New Engl. J. Med.* **304:** 192–6.

Lorente JA, Renes E, Gomez-Aguinaga M *et al.* (1991) Oxygen delivery-dependent oxygen consumption in acute respiratory failure. *Crit. Care Med.* **19:** 770–5.

Marcy TW & Marini JJ (1991) Inverse ratio ventilation in ARDS. Rationale and implementation. *Chest* **100:** 494–504.

Marini CE, Lodato RF & Gutierrez G (1989) Cardiopulmonary interactions in the cardiac patient in the intensive care unit. *Crit. Care Clin.* **5:** 533–49.

Marini JJ (1990) Lung mechanics in the adult respiratory distress syndrome: Recent conceptual advances and implications for management. *Clin. Chest Med.* **11:** 673–90.

Mathison JC, Wolfson D & Ulevith RJ (1988) Participation of tumor necrosis factor in the mediation of gram negative bacterial lipopolysaccharide-induced injury in rabbits. *J. Clin. Invest.* **81:** 1925–37.

Matthay MA (1990) The adult respiratory distress syndrome: Definition and prognosis. *Clin. Chest Med.* **11:** 575–80.

Messmer K (1991) Blood rheology factors and capillary blood flow. In Gutierrez G & Vincent JL (eds), *Update in Intensive Care and Emergency Medicine. Tissue Oxygen Utilization*, pp. 103–113. Berlin, New York: Springer-Verlag.

Meyrick B & Brigham K (1983) Acute effects of *E. coli* endotoxin on the pulmonary microcirculation of anesthetized sheep. Structure: function relationship. *Lab. Invest.* **48:** 458–70.

Mohsenifar A, Goldbach P, Tashkin DP & Campisi DJ (1983) Relationship between O_2 delivery and O_2 consumption in the adult respiratory distress syndrome. *Chest* **84:** 267–71.

Murray JF, Matthay MA, Luce J & Flick MR (1988) An expanded definition of the adult respiratory distress syndrome. *Am. Rev. Respiratory Dis.* **138:** 720–3.

Nelson DP, Beyer C, Samsel RW *et al.* (1987) Pathological supply dependence of O_2 uptake during bacteremia in dogs. *J. Appl. Physiol.* **63:** 1437–92.

Pepe PE (1986) The clinical entity of adult respiratory distress syndrome. Definition, prediction and prognosis. *Crit. Care Clin.* **2:** 377–403.

Pepe PE & Culver BH (1985) Independently measured oxygen consumption during reduction of oxygen delivery by positive end-expiratory pressure. *Am. Rev. Respiratory Dis.* **132:** 788–92.

Pepe PE, Potkin RT, Rous DH *et al.* (1982) Clinical predictors of acute respiratory distress syndrome. *Am. J. Surg.* **144:** 124–30.

Petty TL (1981) Adult respiratory distress syndrome: Historical prospective and definition. *Respiratory Med.* **2:** 99–103.

Rinaldo JE, Dauber JH, Christman JW & Rogers RM (1984) Neutrophil alveolitis following endotoxemia. *Am. Rev. Respiratory Dis.* **130:** 1065–71.

Ronco JJ, Phang T, Walley KR *et al.* (1991) Oxygen consumption is independent of changes in oxygen delivery in severe adult respiratory distress syndrome. *Am. Rev. Respiratory Dis.* **143:** 1267–73.

Russell JA, Ronco JJ, Lockhat D *et al.* (1990) Oxygen delivery and consumption and ventricular preload are greater in survivors than in non-survivors of the adult respiratory distress syndrome. *Am. Rev. Respiratory Dis.* **141:** 659–65.

Ruttiman Y, Shutz Y, Jequier E *et al.* (1991) Thermogenic and metabolic effects of dopamine in healthy men. *Crit. Care Med.* **19:** 1030–6.

Schumacker PT & Samsel RW (1990) Oxygen supply and consumption in the adult respiratory distress syndrome. *Clin. Chest Med.* **11:** 715–22.

Shibutani K, Komatsu T, Kubal K *et al.* (1983) Critical level of oxygen delivery in anesthetized man. *Crit. Care Med.* **11:** 640–3.

Shoemaker WC, Appel PL & Kram HB (1986) Hemodynamic and oxygen transport effects of dobutamine in critically ill general surgical patients. *Crit. Care Med.* **14:** 1032–7.

Shoemaker WC, Appel PL, Kram HB *et al.* (1988) Prospective trial of supranormal values of survivors as therapeutic goals in high-risk surgical patients. *Chest* **94:** 1176–86.

Stainsby WN & Otis AB (1964) Blood flow, oxygen tension, oxygen uptake, and oxygen transport in skeletal muscle. *Am. J. Physiol.* **206:** 858–66.

Stoller JK & Kacmarek RM (1990) Ventilatory strategies in the management of the adult respiratory distress syndrome. *Clin. Chest Med.* **11:** 755–72.

Tate RM & Repine JE (1983) Neutrophils and the adult respiratory distress syndrome. *Am. Rev. Respiratory Dis.* **128:** 552–9.

Tracey KJ, Lowry SF & Cerami A (1988) Chachetin/TNF-alpha in septic shock and septic adult respiratory distress syndrome. *Am. Rev. Respiratory Dis.* **138:** 1377–9.

Villar J, Manzano JJ, Blazquez MA *et al.* (1991) Multiple system organ failure in acute respiratory failure. *J. Crit. Care* **6:** 75–8.

Vincent JL, Roman A & Kahn RJ (1990a) Dobutamine administration in septic shock: Addition to a standard protocol. *Crit. Care Med.* **18:** 689–93.

Vincent JL, Roman A, Backer D & Kahn R (1990b) Oxygen uptake/supply dependency. Effects of short term dobutamine infusion. *Am. Rev. Respiratory Dis.* **42:** 2–7.

Wagner PD, Laravuso RB, Uhl RR & West JB (1974) Continuous distributions of ventilation–perfusion ratios in normal subjects breathing air and 100% oxygen. *J. Clin. Invest.* **54:** 54–68.

Warley A & Gutierrez G (1988) Chronic administration of sodium cyanate decreases O_2 extraction ratio in dogs. *J. Appl. Physiol.* **64:** 1584–90.

Weinberg PF, Matthay MA, Webster PR *et al.* (1984) Biological active products of complement and acute lung injury in patients with sepsis syndrome. *Am. Rev. Respiratory Dis.* **130:** 791–6.

West JB (1985) Ventilation–perfusion relationships. In Tracy TM (ed.), *Respiratory Physiology – The Essentials*, pp. 49–66. Baltimore: Williams & Wilkins.

Wiedemann HP, Matthay MA & Gillis CN (1990) Pulmonary endothelial cell injury and altered lung metabolic function. Early detection of the adult respiratory distress syndrome and possible functional significance. *Clin. Chest Med.* **11:** 723–36.

Zimmerman G, Renzetti A & Hill HR (1983) Functional and metabolic activity in granulocytes from patients with adult respiratory distress syndrome. *Am. Rev. Respiratory Dis.* **127:** 290–300.

16 Techniques for the Monitoring of Oxygen Transport and Oxygen Consumption

K.B. Hankeln

'Unfortunately for the understanding of circulatory function in the past, it was difficult to determine circulatory volume and flow, but easy to measure blood pressures. Therefore, blood pressure manometers have had a fatal influence on clinical practical mentality, even though most organs do not need pressure, but volume and flow.'

Jarisch A. Kreislauffragen
Dtsch Med. Wochenschrift 1928 54: 1211

Since the early research of Pflüger in 1872, the importance of flow-related variables in meeting the requirements of body metabolism has been recognized (Pflüger, 1872). However, the invention of the sphygmomanometer by the Italian paediatrician Riva Rocci in 1895 has had an overwhelming influence on patient management in every major speciality for over a century. Pressure-related measurements have dominated the field of treatment for routine, non-urgent patients and patients with severe life-threatening illnesses alike.

Shock from haemorrhage, sepsis, accidental injury and surgical trauma is largely due to tissue hypoxia from maldistributed flow and uneven vaso-constriction (Shoemaker *et al.*, 1973, 1983). This basic underlying physio-logic mechanism of shock may be precipitated or worsened by pre-existing associated illnesses, myocardial depression from anaesthetic agents, hypo-xaemia, failure to compensate for blood loss or fluid losses. Shock states are accompanied by increased body temperature and inflammatory responses. Diminished or inadequate oxygen consumption ($\dot{V}O_2$) results from poor tissue perfusion that inadequately supplies the body's increased metabolic needs. Circulatory responses to these metabolic needs include increased cardiac index (CI) and increased oxygen delivery ($\dot{D}O_2$).

Early in 1973 Shoemaker and co-workers were able to demonstrate that flow-related parameters were more valuable in predicting outcome than pressure-related measurements (Shoemaker *et al.*, 1973, 1983, 1988a,b; Shoemaker, 1978, 1987; Hankeln *et al.*, 1988; Singbartl, 1989). Therapy based on improving $\dot{V}O_2$ and $\dot{D}O_2$ was shown to reduce morbidity and mortality in critically ill post-operative patients (Shoemaker *et al.*, 1988a).

Changes in oxygen consumption were first described by Cuthbertson in 1936 in trauma patients suffering from fractures of the long bones. Guyton and colleagues then showed that the degree of reduction in oxygen consumption was related to survival or death (Guyton, 1959; Guyton & Crowell, 1961). This fact was confirmed by Shoemaker and co-workers in a large series of patients undergoing major surgery. Although confirmatory results were found by other investigators (Turner et al., 1982; Kuckelt, 1986; Shoemaker & Cain, 1987; Skootsky & Abraham, 1988; Tuchschmidt et al., 1989; Rieke et al., 1990), treatment based on flow-related variables, especially oxygen consumption and oxygen delivery, is not frequently practised.

The introduction of the Swan–Ganz catheter into therapy in 1971 (Ganz et al., 1971) made measurements of oxygen supply and delivery in critically ill patients possible. Oxygen delivery is defined as flow times the amount of oxygen contained in the arterial blood. The amount of oxygen transported and the amount of haemoglobin is determined mainly by the saturation of haemoglobin with oxygen, and cardiac output. While there have been several non-invasive techniques for measuring cardiac output (Bioimpedance Doppler; Nccom 3, Biomed Ltd., Irvine, CA; ACCUCOM, Datascope Corp, Paramus, NJ), oxygen delivery is presently measured invasively in the clinical environment.

Non-invasive measurements of oxygen consumption have been possible in the clinical environment since Neuhof and Wolf (1978) improved this technology for use at the bedside. There are several systems in clinical evaluation, some of which are integrated into ventilators and some of which are 'stand-alone' units: ELVIRA (Engstrom Co., 16120 Bromma, Sweden), MGM Metabolic Monitor (Medicor, Salt Lake City, Utah), Oxygen Consummeter (Draeger, Lübeck, Germany), MMC Beckman Metabolic Measurement Cart (Beckman Instruments, Orange, CA). However, only a few systems are commercially marketed for clinical use at the present time. One of these is the Datex Deltatrac (Hoyer Medizintechnik, Bremen, Germany/Datex Instrumentation Corp., PO Box, Helsinki, Finland). This is very compact and facilitates measurements of oxygen consumption in both spontaneously breathing and intubated patients.

There have been several commercial systems in clinical evaluation: MGM metabolic monitor (Medicor, Salt Lake City, Utah), Oxygen consummeter (Draeger Lübeck, FRG), MMC Beckman metabolic measurement cart (Beckman Instruments, Orange, Ca). However currently only two systems are commercially marketed for clinical use. Deltatrac (Hoyer Medizintechnik Bremen Germany/Datex Instrumentation Corp., P.O. Box Helsinki, Finland). This instrument is very compact and facilitates measurements of oxygen consumption in both spontaneously breathing and intubated patients. Another system is integrated into a ventilator system ELSA (Engström Company Bromma, Sweden).

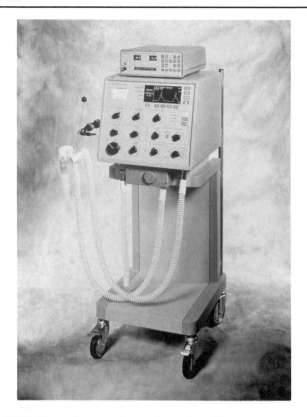

Figure 16.1   ELSA (Reproduced with permission from Engström, Bromma, Sweden).

Measurement of Oxygen Consumption

Oxygen consumption ($\dot{V}O_2$) in critically ill patients can be measured at the bedside by two different methods:

(1) *Invasive measurement*. Using the Fick principle, oxygen consumption is calculated using the oxygen transported in the patient's blood as indicator. Oxygen consumption is then calculated as the difference between the arterial and mixed venous oxygen contents multiplied by the patient's cardiac output.

(2) *Non-invasive technique*. Oxygen consumption is measured as the amount of O_2 taken from the respiratory gases. There are three possible techniques:

    (a) Measurement of O_2 consumption in an open system, using the Douglas bag. This method is widely used in cardiology but is inappropriate for the intensive or intra-operative setting because the patients have to be ventilated at elevated FiO_2 and the collection of the expired air via bag is relatively complicated.

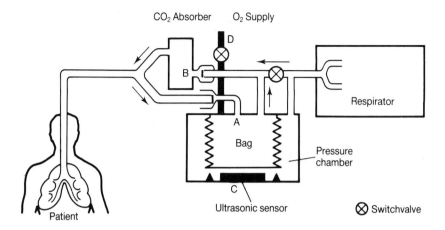

Figure 16.2   Closed system (S&W Kaloximet). The patient is ventilated with a bag (A). The carbon dioxide produced is removed by an absorber (B). The oxygen consumed is measured by an ultrasonic sensor that senses the bag excursion (C) and is replaced by an external supply (D).

(b) Measurement of O_2 in a closed system, taking spirometrical measurements (Fig. 16.2). Because the volumes measured are small, this technique is relatively complicated and rarely used (Lübbe et al., 1989).

(c) Measurement of inspiratory and expiratory O_2 concentrations and multiplying the difference by the minute ventilation (flow) (Fig. 16.3). This is the most widely used technique. It requires precise analysis of the oxygen content of the patient's inspired and expired air by appropriate sensors.

Instead of measuring flow (minute ventilation), a dilution technique was suggested by Meriläinen (1987) and Takala et al. (1989) which avoids potential problems with flow sensors. The Datex Deltatrac is based on their investigatory efforts.

Sensors for Measuring Oxygen Concentrations and Pressures

Electrochemical O_2 Sensor

The most popular sensor in routine measurements is the polarographic sensor using a liquid electrolyte. This 'Clark sensor' is also widely used in

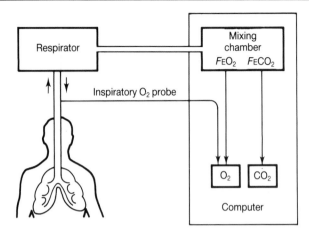

Figure 16.3 Open system measurement configuration in mechanically ventilated patients. Inspiratory probes are taken periodically and expiratory probes are taken from a mixing chamber. By additionally measured flow, oxygen consumption is calculated.

automated blood–gas analysers. Oxygen diffuses through a Teflon membrane into the electrolyte, which is usually potassium chloride. An electric current generated between a platinum cathode and a silver anode is proportional to the oxygen partial pressure. The response time, which depends on the thickness of the membrane, is around 100–200 ms in modern sensors.

One disadvantage of the Clark sensor is that the accuracy of measurement is dependent on ambient pressure. This also changes with the lung compliance, thus making $\dot{V}O_2$ measurements complex, especially in the inspiratory part.

Another disadvantage of the polarographic sensor is its non-linearity at high $\dot{V}O_2$ values. Its linearity will also change when it comes to the end of its lifetime (Braun *et al.*, 1982), which is typically 6–12 months (Fig. 16.4).

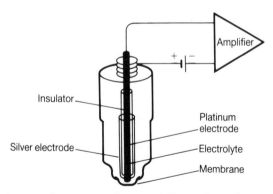

Figure 16.4 Polarographic sensor. Oxygen diffuses through a membrane into the measuring device, where a platinum cathode and silver chloride anode are separated by an electrolyte. The current is amplified and electronically displayed.

Fuel Cell

Another modification of the electrochemical principle is the fuel cell. In this sensor a gold cathode is separated from a lead anode by a potassium hydroxyde electrolyte. The oxygen diffuses through a membrane and creates a current, which is proportional to the amount of oxygen. Response time is mainly dependent on the thickness of the cell's membrane.

The lifetime of a cell working on this principle depends on the oxygen concentration to which it is exposed, so that frequent replacements are necessary. The typical lifetime is less than 6 months.

Zirconium Sensor

An alternative to electrochemical sensors is the zirconium dioxide sensor. This solid-state cell uses zirconium dioxide as electrode material. The cell has to be heated to 700–800°C which makes its use hazardous in the presence of anaesthetic agents. The typical response time is 100 ms and the lifetime of the cell around one year. The measuring characteristics are non-linear, making linearization of the measuring curve necessary.

Paramagnetic Sensor

Oxygen has a magnetic susceptibility which is 100 times higher than other common respiratory gases. This property has been used to construct analysers first by Pauling *et al.* (1946) and later by Hummel (1968). Since

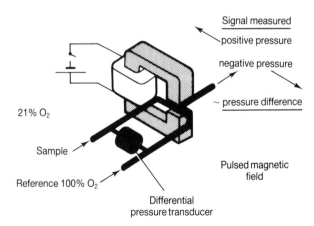

Figure 16.5 Datex paramagnetic differential pressure sensor. Sample and reference probes are transported through a magnetic field, which is switched on and off. The pressures inside and outside the field are measured by a differential pressure transducer. The pressure difference is proportional to the partial pressure of oxygen in the gas.

oxygen molecules in a non-homogeneous field tend to move to where the field strengths are higher, this principle can be used to measure oxygen concentrations. The response time is high (150 ms).

This sensor type was further improved by Meriläinen (1988). A rapid response sensor used in a modern instrument is shown in Fig. 16.5. According to the interaction between the pulsed magnetic field and the molecules, a pressure difference builds up which is proportional to the gas outside the field and inside the field. This pressure difference is proportional to the partial pressure of oxygen in the gas.

In early measuring devices an optical bench was used to measure the differences in oxygen pressures between two points. This principle was not successful because vibrations from ventilators and external noise caused frequent disturbances of the measurements.

Magnetoacoustic O_2 Sensor

The acoustic effect to measure gas fractions was first discovered by Alexander-Graham Bell a century ago. In this technique two microphones are used to measure the concentrations of a probe of unknown O_2 concentration and a reference gas with known oxygen content. This differential technique also makes use of the magnetic property of oxygen. The gas is exposed to an alternating magnetic field. Since the amplitude of the acoustic signal is directly proportional to the oxygen concentration, this technique can be used to measure oxygen fractions. (HP M 1025 A, Hewlett Packard Company, Waltham, Mass.)

Mass Spectrometers

Mass spectrometers have been used to measure respiratory gases, and their measurements are fast and accurate. However, their disadvantage is the sensitivity to moisture and mucus and also the elevated cost.

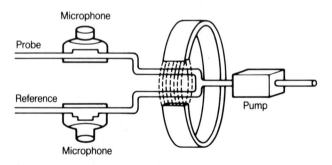

Figure 16.6   Schematic diagram of magnetoacoustic technique.

Factors Affecting Quality of Measurements

Since most of the gas analysers described measure gas partial pressures rather than percentage or concentration, experimentally verified algorithms are necessary to ensure accuracy at all relevant altitudes. Water vapour also has a direct effect on partial pressure measurements, so to correct this effect, measurements and calibration procedures have to be made under identical conditions. For example, 'water traps' based on a Peltier element, or special tubing material, e.g. Nafion®, PermaPure Inc., NJ, USA) which has selective permeability for water vapour, are needed to compensate for the effects of water vapour.

Sample Gas Pressure Effects from the Inspiratory Part

Sample gas pressure also has effects on the accuracy of the measurements. This pressure may change as the pressures needed to ventilate a patient are changing. While the oxygen partial pressure in the mixing chamber is always measured at ambient atmospheric pressure, the sample gas pressure may vary under ventilation with high positive end-expiratory pressure (PEEP) and high positive pressures. To compensate for these effects, pressure measurements must be taken to ensure the accuracy of the measurements.

In addition, in conditions of high inspiratory oxygen concentrations, this pressure-related effect may lead to incorrect $\dot{V}O_2$ readings. In some set-ups, complicated algorithms have been developed to compensate for these effects (Braun et al., 1982). Some researchers have suggested mechanical solutions such as pumps to constantly draw samples from the inspiratory part of the set-up, facilitating decompression to ambient conditions (Kreymann et al., 1989). We obtained good results in our set-up by taking a probe electronically trigged by the computer for the relevant respiratory cycle. This probe is collected in a bag and decompressed to ambient conditions before measurement of FiO_2.

Another problem in O_2 measurements is the potential error in stability of O_2 blenders. This problem was described by Noe et al. (1980) and in Hankeln et al. (1985) and Rau (1989). In our system set-up small changes in blender accuracy are corrected by taking a small probe from the inspiratory part of the set-up and subsequent decompression to ambient pressure.

Another source of errors may be small leakages in the patient's respiratory set-up. Errors may also occur because of mechanical dead space. Stokke and Burchardi (1982) have investigated the influence of dead space on end-tidal CO_2 and mixed expired O_2. Using the conventional set-up, they found measured mixed expired O_2 elevated in the presence of too low end-tidal CO_2. Exact separation of the inspired and expired air can be obtained by separating inspired and expired air by valves, thus increasing the accuracy of measurement of both $\dot{V}O_2$ and CO_2 production and additional lung function tests.

Another problem in the presence of a high FIO_2 is the relative errors in the readings of inspiratory and expiratory oxygen concentrations. The difference between inspiratory and expiratory oxygen concentrations is increasingly smaller as FIO_2 increases (Nelson, 1978; Rau, 1989). At FIO_2 higher than 80%, this error increases from 10% to ∞ thus making $\dot{V}O_2$ measurements impossible. (Westenskow et al., 1984).

In addition to precise measurements of the concentrations of all respiratory gases, the measurement of the ventilatory volumes is necessary. Several techniques for flow measurements are currently used.

Flow Sensors

The most commonly used sensors are pneumotachographs, hot wire anemometers, ultrasonic turbines, vortex flowmeters and differential pressure flowmeters. Under clinical conditions these measuring principles do not always work satisfactorily, because of the effects of humidity, production of mucus and salivation. In addition, the mixture of gases may vary and influence the dynamic properties of the sensor. Complex algorithms are needed to compensate for these effects. There are several factors affecting flow measurements.

Effects of Temperature, Pressure and Humidity on Respiratory Measurements

The volume of a gas (V) is influenced by ambient pressure and temperature. When gas volume is measured it is thus important to define at which temperature and pressure the measurement has been taken. The presence of other gases also affects the volume measurements. This complicates volume measurements in the operating theatre, where several agents for inhalation anaesthesia are used.

In the intensive care unit the situation is easier since only nitrogen is present besides oxygen and carbon dioxide. Also water vapour is always present in the respiratory gas and this also has to be taken into consideration. To compensate for temperature effects, the respiratory gas volumes are usually measured under STPD, ATPD or BTPS conditions.

STPD: standard temperature ($0°C = 273K$) and pressure $760\,mm\,Hg = 1013\,mbar$), dry gas.

ATPD: ambient temperature and pressure, dry gas.

BTPS: body temperature ($37°C$) and pressure ($P - 47\,mm\,Hg$), gas saturated with water vapour ($PH_2O = 47\,mm\,Hg$).

Conversion between each pair of volumes can be obtained by the following formulae:

$$V_{STPD} = \frac{P}{760} \times \frac{273}{273 + T} \times V_{ATPD}$$

$$V_{BTPS} = \frac{273 + 37}{273} \times \frac{760}{P - 47} \times V_{STPD}$$

Techniques to Measure Oxygen Consumption in the Clinical Setting

Closed Circuit Technique

In the closed circuit technique a subject breathes from a closed circuit. The carbon dioxide and water are subsequently removed and the missing oxygen is added via a calibrated flowmeter. Commercially this principle has been used in the S&W Kaloximet R system (Fig. 16.1). This system is based on the principle of a closed circuit rebreathing system with a CO_2 absorber. The decrease in the circulating gas volume is measured by an ultrasonic sensor and the oxygen is automatically replaced from an external oxygen supply. The flow of this oxygen represents the oxygen consumption.

In clinical tests Lübbe *et al.* (1989) found a correlation of 0.97 in comparison to invasively measured $\dot{V}O_2$ in post-operative cardiovascular patients.

Open Circuit Technique

Because of relative ease of adapting this system to ventilator circuits, the open circuit technique has gained more acceptance than the closed circuit technique.

In the open circuit method, the expired gases are collected in a bag or mixing chamber. The flow and the inspiratory as well as the expiratory concentrations of oxygen are measured. In addition the mixed expired carbon dioxide concentration is measured to calculate $\dot{V}CO_2$. Though the expiratory flow is also needed to calculate $\dot{V}O_2$, usually the expired flow is estimated using the Haldane equation.

Several systems based on this technique have been manufactured. (Siemens Elema OCC 980, Engström Metabolic Computer, Beckman Metabolic Measurement Cart MMC, MGM Metabolic Gas Monitor).

The underlying techniques were first applied clinically in 1978 by Neuhof and Wolf, thus allowing non-invasive measurements of $\dot{V}O_2$ at the bedside. The instrument for measuring $\dot{V}O_2$ consisted of an oxygen analyser, a pneumatic unit and an electronic calculator. The oxygen analyser was a paramagnetic analyser as described earlier and $\dot{V}O_2$ was calculated as the product of airflow and the differences in the oxygen concentrations in the inspired and expired air.

In spontaneously breathing patients, a constant flow was evacuated from a plastic hood, to allow $\dot{V}O_2$ measurements after some technical improvements. A typical example of recent 'state of the art' technology is the Datex Deltatrac metabolic monitor.

Invasive Measurement of $\dot{V}O_2$

An alternative for measuring $\dot{V}O_2$ is the use of the Fick principle. This technology is available at the bedside, since thermodilution methods are available to measure cardiac output (Fick, 1870; Ulmer, 1970; Ganz et al., 1971). The Fick method calculates the uptake or production of any substance as the arterio-venous difference multiplied by flow.

Since the introduction of the balloon floated Swan–Ganz catheter into clinical routine (Ganz et al., 1971), invasive measurements of $\dot{V}O_2$ are relatively easy in the operating room and the intensive care unit. Taking the oxygen bound to haemoglobin as the indicator, $\dot{V}O_2$ can be calculated as cardiac output times the difference between the oxygen content of the arterial blood (CaO_2) and the mixed venous blood ($C\bar{v}O_2$), respectively. Some rules must be observed to ensure the quality of the results (Nightingale, 1990). The blood probes have to be taken anaerobically and cardiac outputs should be taken at the end of expiration and averaged over at least three measurements.

$$\dot{V}O_2 = \text{blood flow} \times (CaO_2 - C\bar{v}O_2)$$

$$\dot{V}O_2 = \text{cardiac output} \times (CaO_2 - C\bar{v}O_2)$$

Since one gramme of haemoglobin can bind 1.36–1.39 ml of oxygen, and only a small amount of oxygen is dissolved in the plasma, depending on arterial partial pressure of oxygen, CaO_2 and $C\bar{v}O_2$ can be calculated as:

$$CaO_2 = 1.36 \times SaO_2 \times Hb + 0.031 \times PaO_2$$

and

$$C\bar{v}O_2 = 1.36 \times S\bar{v}O_2 \times Hb + 0.031 \times P\bar{v}O_2$$

Oxygen delivery ($\dot{D}O_2$) in turn is given by:

$$\dot{D}O_2 = CaO_2 \times \text{cardiac output}$$

The disadvantages of the method are that it requires pulmonary artery catheterization, it gives only a 'snapshot' of the $\dot{V}O_2$ and the results are not immediately available because, prior to the complex calculations, the blood probes have to be analysed for O_2 content.

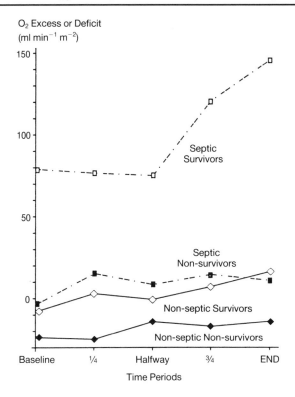

Figure 16.7   Oxygen balance in septic patients (dashed line) and non-septic patients (solid line) at five different time periods. Septic surviving patients have a significantly positive oxygen balance starting from midpoint until end of treatment. Septic patients have higher oxygen balances than non-septic patients and survivors of each group have higher oxygen balances than did the corresponding non-survivors.

In a study of a series of 55 critically ill patients who were monitored with a PA catheter for 317 monitoring days, DO_2 was determined by measuring blood probes for CaO_2 and $C\bar{v}O_2$ simultaneously to thermodilution cardiac output. All patients were intubated and artificially ventilated. In 25 patients, $C\bar{v}O_2$ was monitored by a fibre-optic catheter (Angiocard, Friedburg, Germany) to control the reliability of measurement and assessment of $\dot{V}O_2$ and $\dot{D}O_2$.

Data acquisition and processing were performed by a commercially available software (MEDAS Stephan Gmbh, Gackenbach, Germany) that rapidly processed the variables at the bedside. $\dot{V}O_2$ measurements were monitored by a precise system (MEMO, Mitronic Corp, Stuhr, Germany), which included a fast-response O_2 analyser (OM 11, Beckman, Fullerton, CA, USA). The system was programmed to measure and collect data automatically on a standard PC in 7 min intervals (Highscreen AT 386 SX microcomputer, VOBIS Gmbh, Aachen, Germany). $\dot{V}O_2$ values obtained by this non-invasive system were compared simultaneously with $\dot{V}O_2$ values calculated from the Fick equation. More than 16 000 $\dot{V}O_2$ values measured non-invasively were compared with 1354 $\dot{V}O_2$ values and a total of 764 $\dot{D}O_2$ values calculated from thermodilution cardiac index. All values were indexed to body surface area and body weight. Estimation of the rate of oxygen deficit or excess ($\dot{V}O_2$ measured $\pm$ $\dot{V}O_2$ need) was calculated according to previously described methods (Shoemaker *et al.*, 1988b) and displayed graphically throughout the monitoring period for surviving and non-surviving patients (Fig. 16.7, Tables 16.1 and 16.2).

Table 16.1   Non-invasively measured oxygen consumption (body temperature pressure saturated), estimated $\dot{V}O_2$ need and oxygen balance.

		Time point									
		Baseline		1/4		Halfway		3/4		End	
Non-invasive measurement of $\dot{V}O_2$ BTPS (ml min^{-1}m^{-2}), non-septic	S	112	(5.4)	123	(8.9)*	119	(6)	127	(7.1)*	136	(8.2)*
	NS	99	(6.8)	95	(7.3)*	104	(7)	101	(6.5)*	104	(7.8)*
$\dot{V}O_2$ BTPS (ml min^{-1}m^{-2}), septic	S	181	(11)*	183	(49)	182	(48)	220	(44)*	238	(20)*
	NS	120	(10)*	136	(13)	132	(7.3)	136	(8)*	132	(10)*
$\dot{V}O_2$ need (ml min^{-1}m^{-2}), non-septic	S	120	(1)	121	(1.3)	120	(1.3)	120	(1.3)	120	(1.3)
	NS	119	(3.2)	118	(3.2)	118	(2.9)	118	(2.9)	118	(2.9)
$\dot{V}O_2$ need indexed (ml min^{-1}m^{-2}), septic	S	127	(6)	127	(6)	127	(6)	127	(6)	127	(6)
	NS	124	(3.6)	125	(3.8)	125	(3.9)	126	(3.9)	124	(4.2)
$\dot{D}O_2$ (ml min^{-1}m^{-2}), non-septic	S	648	(45)	591	(37)	681	(35)	675	(35)	713	(31)*
	NS	600	(48)*	585	(45)	653	(52)	654	(52)	532	(43)*
$\dot{D}O_2$ (ml min^{-1}m^{-2})	S	691	(44)	755	(143)*	907	(148)*	933	(208)	925	(86)
	NS	567	(79)	510	(49)*	617	(53)*	656	(71)	611	(69)
Calculated oxygen debt (ml min^{-1}m^{-2})	S	−7.8	(5.8)	2.9	(9.5)	−0.9	(6.3)	6.6	(7.1)	15.6	(8.2)*
	NS	−23	(6.5)	−24	(8.4)	−14	(7.6)	−17	(7)*	14	(8.9)*
Calculated oxygen balance (ml min^{-1}m^{-2}), septic	S	77	(13)*	74	(44)	73	(43)*	117	(37)*	145	(9)*
	NS	−3.2	(10)*	14	(13)	7	(8)*	13	(8)*	8	(9)*

*Statistically different $P<0.05$.
S, survivor; NS, non-survivor.
All data mean ($\pm$SD) indexed for body surface.

Since the patients were sedated the $\dot{V}O_2$ demand was assumed to be 120 ml min^{-1}m^{-2}. The data were compared at (a) first available measurement, (b) the time that one-quarter of the monitored time elapsed, (c) halfway through the monitoring course, (d) at point three-quarters of total monitoring time, and (e) at the end of the monitoring period. This was necessary to ensure that the data were analysed at comparable periods, when the lengths of the critical illness varied.

Table 16.2 Measured oxgyen consumption $\dot{V}O_2\,kg^{-1}$ and oxygen delivery ($\dot{D}O_2\,kg^{-1}$) at five different timepoints in surviving (S) and non-surviving (NS) non-septic and septic patients.

		Time point				
		Baseline	1/4	Halfway	3/4	End
Non-invasive measurement of $\dot{V}O_2$ (ml min^{-1} kg^{-1}), non-septic	S	2.4 (0.1)	2.6 (0.9)*	2.5 (0.4)	2.7 (0.4)*	2.9 (0.5)*
	NS	2.1 (0.1)	2 (0.2)*	2.2 (0.2)	2.2 (0.1)*	2.2 (0.2)*
$\dot{V}O_2$ (ml min^{-1} kg^{-1}), septic	S	4.2 (0.3)*	4.2 (0.9)	4.2 (0.8)*	5.1 (0.7)*	5.6 (0.2)*
	NS	2.5 (0.2)*	2.8 (0.3)	2.7 (0.1)*	2.8 (0.2)*	2.6 (0.2)*
$\dot{D}O_2$ (ml min^{-1} kg^{-1}), non-septic	S	16.4 (3.3)	14.9 (4.6)	17.3 (2.6)	17.1 (2.5)	18 (2.2)
	NS	15.6 (1.44)	15 (1.2)	17 (1.3)	17 (1.2)	14 (1.3)
$\dot{D}O_2$ (ml min^{-1} kg^{-1}), septic	S	17 (1.2)	19 (3.8)	23 (3.5)	23 (4.9)	23 (2)
	NS	14 (1.8)	13 (1.3)	15 (1.4)	16 (1.9)	15 (1.8)

Means ($\pm$SD).
*Difference between survivors (S) and non-survivors (NS) statistically significant by analysis of variance.

Tables 16.3 and 16.4 summarise the data of the surviving and non-surviving patients for $\dot{V}O_2$ measured non-invasively, by direct Fick, comparison of $\dot{V}O_2$ and $\dot{D}O_2$ calculated from thermodilution measurements, and the estimated oxygen balance (deficits or excess) obtained at these five points. The patterns of surviving and non-surviving patients with and without sepsis were also obtained. Survivors in both the septic and non-septic groups had higher $\dot{D}O_2$ values compared with the values at the beginning of the observation period. The $\dot{D}O_2$ values when averaged throughout the observation period were significantly higher in the surviving patients (Fig. 16.8). The non-invasively measured $\dot{V}O_2$ values of survivors were similar to those of non-survivors at the beginning of monitoring, but significantly increased throughout monitoring and were significantly higher and statistically different at the end of the monitoring.

Table 16.3 Oxygen delivery and oxygen consumption measured invasively and non-invasively for survivors and non-survivors.

	Survivors		Non-survivors	
	Mean ($\pm$SEM)	Number	Mean ($\pm$SEM)	Number
$\dot{D}O_2$	732 (10)	439	620 (7.6)	364
$\dot{V}O_2$ invasive	130 (1.4)	404	113 (1.2)	360
$\dot{V}O_2$ non-invasive	134 (2.5)	328	124 (3.3)	281

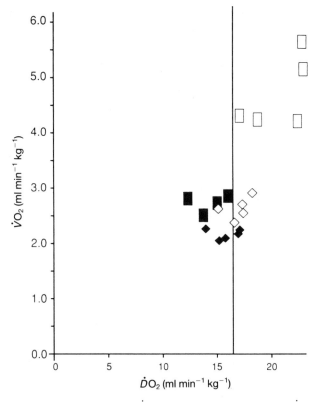

Figure 16.8   Oxygen consumption ($\dot{V}O_2$) versus oxygen delivery ($\dot{D}O_2$) in patients. □ Septic survivors; ■ septic non-survivors; ◇ non-septic survivors; ◆ non-septic non-survivor. There is a critical $\dot{V}O_2$ level in non-septic patients at $2.4\,\mathrm{ml\,min^{-1}\,kg^{-1}}$ and at $4\,\mathrm{ml\,min^{-1}\,kg^{-1}}$ in septic patients. There is also a critical level of $\dot{D}O_2$ at $16\,\mathrm{ml\,min^{-1}\,kg^{-1}}$ in septic patients.

Table 16.4   Comparative variables for 25 patients with continuous fibre-optic $S\bar{v}O_2$ measurements and non-invasive $\dot{V}O_2$ measurements.

	Mean (±SEM)	Number
$\dot{V}O_2$ direct Fick ($\mathrm{ml\,min^{-1}\,m^{-2}}$)	135 (5)	950
$\dot{V}O_2$ direct measurement ($\mathrm{ml\,min^{-1}\,m^{-2}}$)	132 (2)	1020

There was no statistically significant difference in $\dot{V}O_2$ values measured by direct Fick or non-invasive techniques (Tables 16.3 and 16.4). The calculated oxygen debt became positive during monitoring non-septic surviving patients, but continued to be negative in the non-survivors.

Sixteen (70%) of the surviving non-septic patients but only one (10%) non-survivor developed a calculated oxygen excess during the monitoring period.

When the patterns of patients who survived and those who died were looked at, it was found that there was a trend toward greater increases of $\dot{V}O_2$ and $\dot{D}O_2$ in the surviving patients, but $\dot{D}O_2$–$\dot{V}O_2$ patterns of non-survivors did not increase as much. This observation suggests that in the non-survivors, the circulatory defect did not respond to therapy or was not reversible. We found a critical level for $\dot{D}O_2$ that was similar to previously reported studies (Tuchschmidt et al., 1989), where $\dot{V}O_2$ had been measured with the Fick equation alone. Although a critical level for $\dot{V}O_2$ of $2.4\,\mathrm{ml\,min^{-1}\,kg^{-1}}$ was found in patients without sepsis and a critical level of $3.5\,\mathrm{ml\,min^{-1}\,kg^{-1}}$ in patients with septic complications, $\dot{V}O_2$ in septic patients was significantly higher at the beginning of treatment (Fig. 16.6).

Conclusions

Routine conventional monitoring focuses on readily superficial manifestations of shock such as haematocrit, blood pressure, heart rate and urine output. The variables may be adequate for the routine elective patients, but for patients who are critically ill or in shock, criteria must be provided to monitor haemodynamic and oxygen transport variables that may lead to improved outcome (Shoemaker, 1973; 1985).

In earlier studies (Guyton, 1959; Guyton & Crowell, 1961; Shoemaker et al., 1973; Kuckelt, 1986; Hankeln, 1988; Singbartl, 1989) evidence of reduced cardiac output and $\dot{D}O_2$ was found associated with reduced $\dot{V}O_2$. Furthermore, clinical as well as circulatory improvement occurred when these variables increased. A recent study (Shoemaker et al., 1988b) demonstrated that survivors of high-risk surgery had significantly less oxygen debt than did patients with organ failure or patients that subsequently died. Our findings are in agreement with these results. Techniques to measure $\dot{V}O_2$ independent of cardiac output are now available. Since reduced $\dot{V}O_2$ may be an important pathophysiological mechanism in shock states, continuous non-invasive monitoring of $\dot{V}O_2$ is a valuable measure of the circulatory status of inadequate or maldistributed peripheral blood flow.

The measurements should be supplemented with data from $\dot{D}O_2$ measurements. At present non-invasive techniques to measure these data are not available. Although there were little differences in the onset of monitoring, the oxygen balance became positive during treatment in both patients with and without septic complications.

Acknowledgements

This paper is dedicated to my first academic teacher Professor Dr h.c. Wolfgang Schmitz. I want to thank him with this paper for all his support of my training in the UK and USA, which contributed greatly to my scientific work.

References

Albrecht H (1988) Meßprinzipien des Oxyconsumeters. *Klinische Ernährung*. G. Klein Berger, Eckart HRSG; **30:** 52.

Braun U, Turner E & Freiboth K (1982) Ein Verfahren zur Bestimmung von O_2 Aufnahme und CO_2 Abgabe am beatmeten Patienten. *Anästhesie* **31:** 307.

Browning JA, Lindberg SE, Turney SZ & Chodoff P (1982) The effects of fluctuating FIO_2 on metabolic measurements in mechanically ventilated patients. *Crit. Care Med.* **10:** 82.

Cuthbertson, DP (1936) Further observations on disturbance of metabolism caused by injury with particular reference to the dietary requirements of fracture cases. *Br. J. Surg.* **23:** 505.

Crowell JW & Smith EE (1964) Oxygen deficiency and irreversible hemorrhagic shock. *Am. J. Physiol.* **206:** 313.

Dow, Ph (1956) Estimation of cardiac output and central blood volume by dye dilution. *Physiol. Rev.* **6:** 77.

Fick A (1870) Über die Messung des Blutquantums in den Herzventrikeln. *Sitzung der Phys. Med. Ges. Würzburg* Bd II: XVI.

Ganz W, Donoso R, Marcus HS et al. (1971). A new technique for measurement of cardiac output by thermodilution in man. *Am. J. Cardiol.* **27:** 392.

Guyton AC & Crowell JW (1961) Dynamics of the heart in shock. *Fed. Proc.* **20 (Suppl. 9):** 51.

Guyton AC (1959) A continuous cardiac output recorder employing the Fick principle. *Circ. Res.* **7:** 661.

Hankeln KB, Senker R, Schwarten J et al. (1988) Evaluation of prognostic indices based on hemodynamic and oxygen transport variables in shock patients with adult respiratory distress syndrome. *Crit. Care Med.* **15:** 1.

Hankeln KB, Michelsen H, Schipulle M et al. (1985) Microcomputer-assisted monitoring system for the measuring and processing of cardiorespiratory variables: Preliminary results of clinical trials. *Crit. Care Med.* **13:** 426.

Hankeln KB, Gronemeyer R, Held A & Böhmert F (1985) Use of continuous noninvasive measurement of oxygen consumption in patients with adult respiratory distress syndrome following shock of various etiologies. *Crit. Care Med.* **19(5):** 642.

Hummel H (1968) Ein neuer magnetischer Sauerstoffmesser mit sehr kurzer Einstellzeit und hoher Selektivität. *Chem. Ing. Techn.* **40:** 947.

Kreymann G, Gottschall S & Großer S (1989) Nichtinvasives Monitoring des Gasaustauschs. Methodische Voraussetzungen und klinische Anwendung. *Anästh. Intensivmedizin* **24:** 43.

Kuckelt W (1986) *Interdisziplinäre Intensivtherapie.* Berlin: **108:** 166–78.

Lübbe N, Seitz W, Bornscheuer A & Verner L (1989) Erste klinische Erfahrungen mit dem S&W Kaloximet R, einem Gerät zur O_2 Verbrauchsmessung in Anästhesie und Intensivmedizin. *Anästhesie* **38:** 157.

Meriläinen PT (1988) A fast differential paramagnetic O_2 sensor. *Int. J. Clin. Monit. Comp.* **5:** 195.

Meriläinen PT (1987) Metabolic monitor. *Int. J. Clin. Monit. Comp.* **4:** 167.

Nelson LD, Anderson HB & Hernando Garcia H (1978) Clinical validation of a new metabolic monitor suitable for use in critically ill patients. *Crit. Care Med.* **15:** 951.

Neuhof H & Wolf H (1978) Method for continuously measured oxygen consumption and cardiac output for use in critically ill patients. *Crit. Care Med.* **6:** 155.

Nightingale P (1990) Practical points of oxygen transport principles. *Intensive Care Med.* **16 (Suppl. 2):** 173.

Noe FE, Whitty AJ, Davies KH *et al.* (1980) Noninvasive measurement of pulmonary gas exchange during anesthesia. *Anaesthesia Analgesia* **59:** 263.

Pflüger E (1872) Über die Diffusion des Sauerstoffs, den Ort und die Gesetze der Oxydationsprozesse im tierischen Organismus. *Pflüger's Arch.* **6:** 43.

Pauling L, Wood RE & Studevant JH (1946) Oxygen meter. *J. Am. Chem. Soc.* **68:** 795.

Rau M (1989) Zur Anwendbarkeit des Fickschen Prinzips für die Herzzeitvolumenmessung beim beatmeten Patienten auf der Intensivstation Diss. Hamburg.

Rieke H, Weyland A, Hoeft A *et al.* (1990) Kontinuierliche HZV Messung nach dem Fickschen Prinzip in der Kardioanästhesie. *Anästhesie* **39:** 13.

Schumacker PT & Cain SM (1987) The concept of a critical oxygen delivery. *Intensive Care Med.* **13:** 223.

Shoemaker WC, Montgomery ES, Kaplan E *et al.* (1973) Physiologic patterns in surviving and nonsurviving shock patients. *Arch. Surg.* **106:** 630.

Shoemaker WC, Appel P & Bland R (1983) Use of physiologic monitoring to predict outcome and to assist clinical decisions in the critically ill postoperative patients. *Am. J. Surg.* **146:** 43.

Shoemaker WC, Appel P & Kram HB (1988a) Prospective trial of supranormal values of survivors as therapeutic goals in high risk surgical patients. *Chest* **94:** 1176.

Shoemaker WC (1978) Pathophysiology of Shock and Shock syndromes. Textbook of Critical Care. In Shoemaker, Thompson & Holbrook (eds). Saunders 1984 and Cardiac output for use in critically ill patients. *Crit. Care Med.* **6:** 155.

Shoemaker WC, Appel P & Kram HB (1988b) Tissue oxygen debt as a determinant of lethal and nonlethal postoperative organ failure. *Crit. Care Med.* **16:** 1117.

Shoemaker WC (1987) Evaluation of oxygen transport patterns to the pathophysiology and therapy of shock states. *Intensive Care Med.* **13:** 230.

Singbartl G (1989) Kardiozirkulatorische und pulmonale Veränderungen bei Patienten mit isolierter cerebraler Läsion. I Hämodynamik *Anästhesie* **38:** 116.

Skootsky S & Abraham E (1988) Continuous oxygen consumption measurement during initial emergency department resuscitation of critically ill patients. *Crit. Care Med.* **16:** 706.

Stokke T & Burchardi H (1982) Einfache Trennung von In und Exspirationsgas während maschineller Beatmung. *Anästhesie* **31:** 293.

Takala J, Kenäinen O, Väisänen P & Kari A (1989) Measurement of gas exchange in intensive care: Laboratory and clinical validation of a new device. *Crit. Care Med.* **17:** 1041.

Tuchschmidt J, Fried J & Suzunney R (1989) Early hemodynamic correlates of survival in patients with septic shock. *Crit. Care Med.* **719:** 17.

Turner E, Braun U, Leitz KH *et al.* (1982) Überwachung der Gesamtsauerstoff aufnahme bei koronarchirurgischen Eingriffen. *Anästhesie* **31:** 280.

Ulmer HE (1970) Grundlagen der Thermodilutionsmethode zur Fluß und Volumenbestimmung. *Prakt. Anästhesie Wiederbel.* **2:** 78.

Westenskow DR, Cutler CA & Wallace WD (1984) Instrumentation for monitoring gas exchange and metabolic rate in critically ill patients. *Crit. Care Med.* **12:** 183.

17 Controversies in Oxygen Supply Dependency

Paul T. Schumacker and Richard W. Samsel

Cellular Basis for Oxygen Demand

The cells that comprise the tissues of the body are obligated to perform a variety of functions necessary for cell survival, including growth, membrane transport, biosynthesis, cellular repair, and other maintenance processes. Cells also perform facultative services as part of their contribution to the specific function of the tissue, including contractile, biosynthetic, motile, ion or protein transport, or other metabolic activities. Since most of these processes involve a decrease in the entropy of the cell or its environment, they require energy expenditure on the part of the cell. The cells obtain this energy by oxidizing hydrocarbons and capturing a portion of the free energy released in the form of high-energy phosphate compounds, such as ATP. Cellular enzymes mediate specific biochemical reactions, using the energy released by hydrolysis of ATP. By maintaining the concentration of ATP in the cell, specific enzyme systems are provided with a ready source of the energy required for obligatory and facultative chores. The effective concentration of ATP (the energy charge) is maintained in most cell types by electron transport system of the mitochondria.

Under normal circumstances, oxygen is present within the mitochondria at concentrations far in excess of that required to maintain oxidative phosphorylation. However, when oxygen supply to the tissue becomes limited, local oxygen consumption may fall if the local mitochondrial oxygen concentration becomes inadequate to deal with the flux of reducing equivalents generated by intermediary metabolism. In this state of hypoxia, cellular oxygen consumption ($\dot{V}O_2$) becomes oxygen supply-limited, and cell energetic processes can become limited by lack of energy supply. When facultative functions fail, organ system function deteriorates. When cellular obligatory functions fail, cell homeostasis is threatened. If energy supply is limited for a sufficient time, irreversible changes in tissue and cellular function arise.

Systemic and Tissue Regulation of O_2 Supply

Given that the cell metabolic rate normally determines tissue $\dot{V}O_2$, a major role of the lungs and cardiovascular system is to maintain the delivery of oxygen to each cell in accord with its metabolic demand. Since the oxygen demand of tissues such as skeletal muscle may vary widely, the cardio-vascular system must be capable of effecting dramatic changes in the magnitude and distribution of oxygen transport. This control mechanism involves an interplay between systemic autonomic reflex systems and local tissue microvascular responses (Cain, 1987). One example of this dual-control mechanism is seen in strenuous muscular exercise, where ratio of whole body oxygen supply to demand is reduced. In this state, increases in sympathetic nervous system activity cause a generalized increase in α-adrenergic vasoconstrictor tone. This increases vascular resistance in many vascular beds susceptible to autonomic regulation, preserving oxygen supply for the working muscle groups. Within the working muscles, local metabolic vasodilation competes with the increase in autonomic-mediated tone, thereby reducing local vascular resistance and augmenting the local O_2 delivery in accord with the increased O_2 demand (Granger et al., 1975).

Under normal resting conditions, a reduction in the ratio of oxygen supply to demand caused by reduced cardiac output or a fall in arterial blood oxygen content appears to elicit a similar response. For example, during severe arterial hypoxaemia the peripheral chemoreceptors mediate a reflex increase in sympathetic nervous system tone while local metabolic vaso-dilation maintains local tissue flow in accord with tissue oxygen demands (Bredle et al., 1988b). The effectiveness of metabolic vasodilation becomes apparent when the arterial hypoxaemia is especially severe. In this situation, the metabolic vasodilatory competition with autonomic vaso-constriction (termed autoregulatory escape) (Granger et al., 1976) can reduce systemic arterial blood pressure to the point where myocardial perfusion is compromised, and acute cardiac failure soon follows.

In healthy tissues, microvascular responses to reduced oxygen delivery may in some circumstances complement the local metabolic control of blood flow by augmenting the extent of tissue oxygen extraction. This increase in tissue oxygen extraction that occurs when O_2 delivery is reduced is thought to involve multiple levels of the microcirculation. At the precapillary level, metabolic feedback from parenchymal cells dilates terminal arterioles (or precapillary sphincters, where they exist) thereby increasing the density of perfused capillaries (Granger et al., 1975, 1976; Granger & Shepherd, 1979). This decreases intercapillary distance and increases capillary transit time, thereby facilitating greater O_2 extraction along capillaries without limiting unloading by diffusion. In normal tissues, these mechanisms defend tissue normoxia (i.e. maintain supply-independent O_2 uptake) until O_2 extraction reaches 65–75% (Schumacker & Cain, 1987; Cain, 1978; Pepe & Culver, 1985; Gutierrez et al., 1986; Nelson et al., 1987b).

Experimental evidence for the above mechanisms is extensive. For example, studies using intravital microscopy in thin muscle preparations have shown that decreasing the PO_2 elicits an increased diameter of arterioles, an increase in capillary flow velocity, and a decrease in the mean intercapillary distance (Prewitt & Johnson, 1976; Lindbom et al., 1980). Conversely, a high tissue PO_2 decreased the number of capillaries receiving blood flow (Lindbom et al., 1980). Granger and co-workers found increases in capillary filtration coefficient during hypoxia in skeletal muscle hypoxia, which was evidence in support of capillary recruitment (Granger et al., 1976). In pump-perfused small intestine, Granger et al. (1982) found that capillary filtration coefficient increased when blood flow was reduced, and that $\dot{V}O_2$ was maintained until a critically low blood flow was reached. Collectively, these studies suggest that local metabolic control of perfused capillary density and red cell flow acts to maintain cellular O_2 availability as the O_2 supply changes.

Effective coupling of local O_2 delivery to local perivascular O_2 demand protects tissue metabolism from hypoxic damage by preventing the appearance of anoxic regions when O_2 delivery is reduced (Granger et al., 1976, 1982; Granger & Nyhof, 1982). However, even healthy tissues exhibit a critical O_2 delivery, below which further reductions in delivery cause a fall in tissue $\dot{V}O_2$ (Schumacker & Cain, 1987). Although O_2 extraction can increase further below the critical point, supply-dependent O_2 uptake occurs because this increase is not sufficient to maintain $\dot{V}O_2$.

Laboratory studies of whole animals (Cain, 1977; Long et al., 1988) or isolated tissues (Bredle et al., 1989; Gutierrez et al., 1990; Schlichtig et al., 1991) consistently demonstrate a biphasic relationship between O_2 delivery and uptake. At normal or high levels of O_2 transport a region of supply-independent O_2 uptake is found, whereas a region of O_2 supply dependency is seen below a critical O_2 delivery threshold. Surprisingly, many tissues appear to reach O_2 supply dependency at the same critical O_2 extraction in the range of 60–65%. In this regard, isolated liver (Samsel et al., 1991), skeletal muscle (Bredle et al., 1988a), kidney (Schlichtig et al., 1991), intestine (Nelson et al., 1988), and heart (Walley et al., 1988) demonstrate similar critical O_2 extraction ratios among differing species and laboratories.

Clinical Observations of Apparent 'Pathological O_2 Supply Dependency'

Beginning with the report of Powers et al. (1973) a large number of clinical studies have focused attention on the relationship between O_2 delivery and uptake in patients with different forms of cardiovascular disease. Although major differences exist among these studies, a common element is the observation that changes in systemic oxygen delivery appear to cause parallel changes in systemic $\dot{V}O_2$. Because this occurs when systemic O_2 delivery is normal or even high, it suggests that the normal vascular mechanisms controlling tissue oxygen extraction may be impaired in a state of pathological O_2 supply dependency (Cain, 1984). Diseases in which this unexpected O_2 supply dependency has been reported include the adult respiratory distress syndrome (ARDS) (Powers et al., 1973; Danek et al., 1980; Mohsenifar et al., 1983; Bihari et al., 1987), chronic obstructive lung disease (Brent et al., 1984; Albert et al., 1986), sepsis syndrome (Kaufman et al., 1984; Abraham et al., 1984; Haupt et al., 1985; Astiz et al., 1986; Wolf et al., 1987; Pittet et al., 1990), pulmonary vascular disease (Mohsenifar et al., 1988), pulmonary hypertension (Mohsenifar et al., 1988). Pneumocystis pneumonia (Ronco et al., 1990), silicosis (Albert et al., 1986), congestive heart failure (Mohsenifar et al., 1987) and obstructive sleep apnoea (Williams & Mohsenifar, 1989). A criticism of some (but not all) of these studies focuses on the statistical problem arising from the use of the thermodilution cardiac output measurement in the calculation of both O_2 uptake and O_2 delivery (Archie, 1981). Since clinical studies are usually limited to only 2 or 3 data points per patient, the analysis has typically focused on whether a line drawn through these points on a plot of delivery versus $\dot{V}O_2$ has a significant slope or not. Since both the supply-independent and supply-dependent regions are not generated in such studies, the finding of a positive slope suggests that the region studied was below the critical point, whereas the finding that the slope is zero implies that the points were within the region of O_2 supply-independent uptake. Since the use of shared variables in the analysis tends to augment the slope of such a regression, the question of whether the effect is real or artifactual arises.

The group of investigators led by Powers (Powers et al., 1973) agreed that independent measurement of dependent and independent variables was most desirable (Moreno et al., 1986). However, they also argued that (a) if the error in cardiac output determinations and blood gas analyses were known, and (b) if the changes in O_2 delivery were large in relation to the cardiac output measurement error, then a procedure could be applied to correct the slope of the regression line through grouped data for the amount introduced by the coupled variables (Stratton et al., 1987). In that report, they presented a statistical analysis to correct the regression lines accordingly. Moreover, a retrospective analysis of two previous studies (Powers et al., 1973; Danek et al., 1980) suggested that a significant correlation was still present after the shared variable component of the slope was removed. Unfortunately, the outcome of that statistical correction is highly sensitive to the error estimate for the cardiac output determination. Since the accuracy of thermodilution measurements is difficult to quantify precisely, conclusions reached based on data corrected by this method must still be made with caution.

More recent studies of the relationship between O_2 delivery and uptake in critically ill patients have circumvented this methodological weakness by measuring O_2 uptake independently from analysis of inspired–expired gas analysis. To date, several independent studies have failed to detect an abnormal relationship between O_2 supply and uptake in patients with sepsis or ARDS (Annat *et al.*, 1986; Carlile & Grays 1989; Ronco *et al.*, 1991b). Collectively, this work fuels the suspicion that so-called pathological O_2 supply dependency may not, in fact, represent a failure in tissue oxygen extraction mechanism.

Animal Studies of Oxygen Supply Dependency in Models of Disease

To date, a large number of animal studies have been carried out in an effort to learn more about the physiology and pathophysiology of oxygen extraction by tissues. Collectively, these studies have added to our understanding of factors that influence the relationship between oxygen delivery and uptake, although clear similarities and differences exist between these models and the clinical diseases they resemble. Experimental animal studies have generally avoided the methodological shortcomings of many of the clinical studies, in the sense that a single experimental intervention can be studied in comparison with strict experimental controls. Laboratory studies can also avoid the statistical problems arising from analysis of data with shared variables, since independent measurements of delivery and O_2 consumption are feasible with invasive measurements made under controlled laboratory conditions. Finally, laboratory studies permit a more complete assessment of the relationship between delivery and uptake than is generally possible in clinical studies. For example, the assessment of a critical O_2 delivery requires measurements at deliveries above and below the critical point. Since an extended period of O_2 supply-dependent $\dot{V}O_2$ is injurious to tissues, interventions that reduce O_2 delivery significantly in clinical studies are not feasible.

A number of investigators have explored the relationship between O_2 delivery and uptake in acute models of tissue injury in anaesthetized animals. In one study, Pepe and Culver (1985) measured critical oxygen deliveries in an oleic acid-induced model of lung oedema. When O_2 delivery was reduced by positive end-expiratory pressure (PEEP) or by limiting venous return, whole body $\dot{V}O_2$ remained constant until delivery fell below 13 ml min^{-1} kg^{-1}. Since this critical delivery was not different from non-injured controls, they concluded that acute direct lung injury was not associated with systemic consequences for oxygen extraction. Using a similar model of acute lung injury, Long and colleagues (Long *et al.*, 1988) found that systemic critical oxygen deliveries were not impaired by lung injury alone, or its treatment with PEEP or high inspired oxygen fractions. By contrast with the above studies, Dorinsky and co-workers (1988) reported finding an apparent increase in the critical oxygen delivery in anaesthetized dogs given phorbol myristate acetate to induce a vascular injury. Although limited by the lack of a direct comparison to controls, these findings suggested that neutrophil activation and/or direct vascular injury may hinder the ability of tissues to adjust O_2 extraction in response to changes in blood flow and oxygen transport.

The observation that many of the patients demonstrating abnormal supply dependence of oxygen uptake in clinical studies of ARDS were also septic led Nelson and colleagues (Nelson et al., 1987a) to examine the effects of bacterial sepsis on oxygen extraction in anaesthetized dogs. They found a significantly increased critical O_2 delivery in animals infused with washed P. aeruginosa organisms, compared with sham-infused controls. While the mechanism underlying this disruption was not apparent, numerous studies dating back to the mid-1950s (Zweifach et al., 1956; Zweifach & Thomas, 1956) had suggested that bacterial endotoxins are capable of initiating profound changes in vascular smooth muscle reactivity to contracting agonists. When oxygen supply to a tissue is reduced, increases in tissue O_2 extraction appear to depend on effective reductions in micovascular blood flow to tissue regions with low metabolic demands, coupled with metabolic vasodilation in resistance vessels supplying regions with relatively high metabolic activity. Vascular injury that disrupts either the intrinsic constrictor or relaxing properties of blood vessels may undermine tissue O_2 extraction by impairing the efficient microvascular distribution of blood flow with respect to O_2 demand. Indeed, when Nelson et al. studied the effects of E. coli endotoxin on whole body and intestinal oxygen extraction in response to progressive hypovolaemia, an impaired critical extraction ability was found (Nelson et al., 1988). Endotoxin appeared to disrupt adjustments of extraction both in whole body and simultaneously in an isolated segment of small intestine. Moreover, the autoperfused intestine segment reached its critical point at a significantly higher *systemic* O_2 delivery, suggesting that the regulation of oxygen delivery among organs as a functions of systemic O_2 supply was also impaired.

If the oxygen extraction impairment found in the isolated intestine by Nelson et al. was extrapolated to the entire gut, it was apparent that this, by itself, was inadequate to explain the overall impairment seen at the whole body level in the same study. This suggestion that additional tissues were involved led Samsel and colleagues (1988) to explore O_2 extractions in isolated canine hindlimb (mostly skeletal muscle) during endotoxaemia. Surprisingly, hindlimb was not impaired in its ability to increase O_2 extraction in respone to reduced O_2 delivery, while whole body was impaired. Moreover, this model showed no evidence of a redistribution of systemic blood flow toward skeletal muscle, as has been suggested in prior studies of experimental sepsis (Wright et al., 1971; Finley et al., 1975). In a subsequent study of pump-perfused hindlimb, Bredle and colleagues (Bredle *et al.*, 1989) found a small but significant impairment in local hindlimb critical oxygen delivery.

One mechanism thought to contribute to the increases in oxygen extraction in tissues such as intestine is an increase in perfused capillary density (Shepherd, 1978, 1982). In a recent study, Drazenovic and colleagues (1992) compared morphologic measurements of perfused capillary density in intestinal mucosa in normal controls and a group of endotoxin-challenged animals. Interestingly, the normal controls showed a correlation between tissue oxygen extraction ratio and perfused capillary density, measured by infusion of colloidal carbon. This suggested that regulation of perfused capillary density may contribute to physiological changes in local O_2 delivery, thereby contributing to the maintenance of tissue $\dot{V}O_2$. Unlike controls, endotoxin-challenged animals showed no relationship between gut O_2 delivery or extraction and mucosal capillary recruitment. Although perfused capillary density was slightly lower in endotoxin-challenged animals, these results suggested that loss of regulatory control, rather than massive microembolization of capillaries, was the case. A failure to recruit capillaries in response to encroaching tissue hypoxia may render the tissue more susceptible to anoxic damage by limiting the ability to maintain supply-independent $\dot{V}O_2$ in the face of limited tissue O_2 supply.

The intrinsic vascular mechanisms underlying the defect in oxygen extraction ability in endotoxaemia could conveivably reflect an impaired contractile function, an impaired relaxation response, or a combination of both. To address this, Wylam and co-workers (1990) studied the *in vitro* responses of 3-mm rings of conduit arteries harvested from anaesthetized dogs administered endotoxin 4–5 h previously. In this model, contractile responses to increasing log doses of phenylephrine were not significantly different from sham-infused controls. When vessels pre-contracted with phenylephrine (EC_{50}) were relaxed with nitroprusside, a similar, complete relaxation was found in both control and experimental groups. However, when pre-contracted vessels were relaxed with acetylcholine a significantly impaired relaxation was found in the rings harvested from endotoxin-treated animals. These findings suggested that impaired endothelial-mediated relaxation via endothelial-derived relaxing factor (functionally equivalent to nitric oxide radical) release may have contributed to an impaired microvascular regulation of oxygen delivery. In a study of endotoxin effects in rat aorta, Joulu-Schaeffer *et al.* (1990) found impaired contractile responses to noradrenaline. Moreover, normal contractile function was restored acutely by addition of N^G-monomethyl-L-arginine, an inhibitor of nitric oxide synthase. This suggested that the impaired intrinsic contractility was mediated by excessive release of nitric oxide. Since similar results were obtained in rings functionally denuded of their endothelium, this excess nitric oxide appears to have originated within the smooth muscle cells, which are incapable of synthesizing nitric oxide in normal tissues. By implication, endotoxin administration appears to initiate the expression of this enzyme within vascular myocytes. Collectively, these findings suggest that both the endothelium and smooth muscle components of the vascular wall may contribute to an impaired vascular regulation in endotoxaemia, through mechanisms that involve alterations in the L-arginine-dependent production of nitric oxide.

Conceivably, other factors that interfere with normal regulation of vascular tone might also interfere with the efficient extraction of oxygen by tissues. In a study of anaesthetic agents, Van der Linden and colleagues (1991) compared the effects of various anaesthetics on critical oxygen extraction during progressive haemorrhage in dogs. Interestingly, halothane, enflurane, isoflurane and alfentanil all reduced the critical oxygen extraction ratio, compared to that seen during pentobarbital-anaesthetized controls. In that study, a correlation was also found between the reduction in systemic vascular resistance caused by the anaesthetic agent and the extent of impairment in the critical oxygen extraction ratio. These findings suggest that direct pharmacological vasodilation may undermine adjustments in whole body oxygen extraction ratio by allowing some tissues to 'steal' O_2 delivery in excess of tissue need under conditions where supply is limited. Similar results with halothane were reported by Hershenson and colleagues (1988).

Similarities and Contrasts Between Animal and Human Studies

Although some similarities can be seen between experimental and clinical studies, marked differences also exist. Perhaps the most notable difference between laboratory and clinical studies relates to the magnitude of the apparent tissue oxygen extraction impairment seen. Many of the clinical studies of pathological O_2 supply dependency show an abnormal relationship between O_2 supply and uptake at very high deliveries where the extraction ratio is 30% or less. Even the patients undergoing coronary artery bypass surgery reported by Shibutani et al. (1983) appear to demonstrate onset of supply dependency when O_2 extraction is in the range of 30–35%, and these patients were not acutely ill. By comparison, even the most severe experimental models do not produce defects of this magnitude. For example, even after challenge with high doses of intravenous endotoxin the critical O_2 extraction ratio still reached levels of 45–50% (Nelson et al., 1988). Why should such a difference exist between humans and animal models?

The clear determination of a critical O_2 delivery requires measurement of points above and below the critical threshold. Because O_2 supply limitation below the critical threshold is almost certainly injurious to tissues, measurements of a biphasic relationship between O_2 delivery and uptake in normal humans have not been reported previously. The lack of such data has led to the speculation by Dantzker and colleagues that humans would not exhibit such a relationship (Dantzker et al., 1991). They argue that humans normally maintain an O_2 delivery at or near the critical threshold. If this were the case, then any reduction in delivery from the normal level would necessarily cause the onset of O_2 supply dependency. According to their theory, increases in delivery above the normal level can only occur as a physiological response to increasing O_2 demand, analogous to the way that exercise elicits increases in O_2 transport. If this hypothesis were correct, it would imply that humans are incapable of manifesting large increases in systemic O_2 extraction in response to reduced O_2 delivery, yet data to the contrary exist (Schlichtig et al., 1986). It would also imply that humans can only achieve O_2 extractions in the range of 30–40% at the critical point, compared to other species that achieve critical extractions of 55% or more. While the Shibutani et al. (1983) clinical study did appear to show an onset of O_2 supply dependency at extractions of less than 40%, they analysed a collection of single data points from many patients, as opposed to a range of values from a single patient. Such a collective analysis could obscure the response that would have been seen in a single patient. Moreover, one animal study has suggested that the intravenous opiate anaesthetic alfentanil may depress normal tissue O_2 extraction ability (Van der Linden et al., 1991). The possibility that the fentanyl anaesthesia used in the Shibutani et al. (1983) study could have contributed to the low extractions is thus a possibility.

An alternative to the Dantzker et al. explanation (Dantzker et al., 1991) is that the magnitude of human O_2 supply dependency results have been overestimated by the noise introduced when shared variable analysis was used. When this 'noise' is combined with the limitation that only 2 or 3 data points per patient can easily be obtained, the potential for overestimating the degree or presence of O_2 supply dependency is magnified. Preliminary reports suggest that humans do, indeed, demonstrate the same biphasic relationship between O_2 supply and uptake (Ronco et al., 1991a) seen experimentally, with critical O_2 extraction ratios in accord with the values reported from animal studies. However, clinical studies utilizing independent measurements of O_2 delivery and uptake also suggest strongly that prior estimates of pathological O_2 supply dependency overestimated its magnitude. Even if pathological O_2 supply dependency does not exist to the degree originally thought, animal studies have clearly demonstrated that conditions that disrupt control of peripheral O_2 transport can limit tissue O_2 extraction responses in states where O_2 delivery is limited. The question of whether these factors contribute to localized tissue hypoxia when O_2 delivery is still within the normal range is still unanswered. An important lesson learned from the experimental studies is that disrupted oxygen extraction in tissues is difficult to measure, even under controlled laboratory conditions. Consequently, a disrupted oxygen extraction ability could still contribute to local tissue hypoxia and consequent organ dysfunction in critical illness, without necessarily causing the large changes in $\dot{V}O_2$ previously reported in response to moderate changes in O_2 delivery.

References

Abraham E, Shoemaker WC & Cheng PH (1984) Cardiorespiratory responses to fluid administration in peritonitis. *Crit. Care Med.* **12:** 664–7.

Albert RK, Schrijen F & Poincelot F (1986) Oxygen consumption and transport in stable patients with chronic obstructive pulmonary disease. *Am. Rev. Respiratory Dis.* **134:** 678–82.

Annat G, Viale JP, Percival C et al. (1986) Oxygen delivery and uptake in the adult respiratory distress syndrome. Lack of relationship when measured independently in patients with normal blood lactate concentrations. *Am. Rev. Respiratory Dis.* **133:** 999–1001.

Archie JP, Jr (1981) Mathematic coupling of data: a common source of error. *Ann. Surg.* **193:** 296–303.

Astiz M, Rackow EC & Weil MH (1986) Oxygen delivery and utilization during rapidly fatal septic shock in rats. *Circ. Shock* **20:** 281–90.

Bihari D, Smithes M, Gimson A & Tinker J (1987) The effects of vasodilation with prostacyclin on oxygen delivery and uptake in critically ill patients. *New Engl. J. Med.* **317:** 397–402.

Bredle DL, Bradley WE, Chapler CK & Cain SM (1988a) Muscle perfusion and oxygenation during local hyperoxia. *J. Appl. Physiol.* **65:** 2057–62.

Bredle DL, Chapler CK & Cain SM (1988b) Metabolic and circulatory responses of normoxic skeletal muscle to whole-body hypoxia. *J. Appl. Physiol.* **65:** 2063–8.

Bredle DL, Samsel RW, Schumacker PT & Cain SM (1989) Critical O_2 delivery to skeletal muscle at high and low PO_2 in endotoxemic dogs. *J. Appl. Physiol.* **66:** 2553–8.

Brent BN, Matthay RA, Mahler DA et al. (1984) Relationship between oxygen uptake and oxygen transport in stable patients with chronic obstructive pulmonary disease. *Am. Rev. Respiratory Dis.* **129:** 682–6.

Cain SM (1977) Oxygen delivery and uptake in dogs during anemic and hypoxic hypoxia. *J. Appl. Physiol.* **42:** 228–34.

Cain SM (1978) Effects of time and vasoconstrictor tone on O_2 extraction during hypoxic hypoxia. *J. Appl. Physiol.* **45:** 219–24.

Cain SM (1984) Supply dependency of oxygen uptake in ARDS: Myth or reality. *Am. J. Med. Sci.* **288:** 119–24.

Cain SM (1987) Gas exchange in hypoxia, apnea, and hyperoxia. In *Handbook of Physiology: The Respiratory System IV*, pp. 403–20. Bethesda: American Physiological Society.

Carlile PV & Gray BA (1989) Effect of opposite changes in cardiac output and arterial PO_2 on the relationship between mixed venous PO_2 and oxygen transport. *Am. Rev. Respiratory Dis.* **140:** 891–8.

Danek SJ, Lynch JP, Weg JG & Dantzer DR (1980) The dependence of oxygen uptake on oxygen delivery in the Adult Respiratory Distress Syndrome. *Am. Rev. Respiratory Dis.* **122:** 387–95.

Dantzker DR, Foresman B & Gutierrez G (1991) Oxygen supply and utilization relationships. A reevaluation. *Am. Rev. Respiratory Dis.* **143:** 675–9.

Dorinsky PM, Costello JL & Gadek JE (1988) Oxygen distribution and utilization after phorbol myristate acetate-induced lung injury. *Am. J. Med. Sci.* **138:** 1454–63.

Drazenovic R, Samsel RW, Wylam ME *et al.* (1992) Regulation of perfused capillary density in canine intestinal mucosa during endotoxemia. *J. Appl. Physiol.* **72:** 259–65.

Finley RJ, Duff JH, Holliday RL *et al.* (1975) Capillary muscle blood flow in human sepsis. *Surgery* **78:** 87–94.

Granger DN, Kvietys PR & Perry MA (1982) Role of exchange vessels in the regulation of intestinal oxygenation. *Am. J. Physiol.* **242:** G570–4.

Granger HJ & Nyhof RA (1982) Dynamics of intestinal oxygenation: interactions between oxygen supply and uptake. *Am. J. Physiol.* **243:** G91–6.

Granger HJ & Shepherd AP (1979) Dynamics and control of the microcirculation. *Adv. Biomed. Engng* **7:** 1–63.

Granger HJ, Goodman AH & Cook BK (1975) Metabolic models of microcirculatory regulation. *Fed. Proc.* **34:** 2025–30.

Granger HJ, Goodman AH & Granger DN (1976) Role of resistance and exchange vessels in local microvascular control of skeletal muscle oxygenation in the dog. *Circ. Res.* **38:** 379–85.

Gutierrez G, Warley AR & Dantzker DR (1986) Oxygen delivery and utilization in hypothermic dogs. *J. Appl. Physiol.* **60:** 751–7.

Gutierrez G, Marini C, Acero AL & Lund N (1990) Skeletal muscle PO_2 during hypoxemia and isovolemic anemia. *J. Appl. Physiol.* **68:** 2047–53.

Haupt MT, Gilbert EM & Carlson RW (1985) Fluid loading increases oxygen consumption in septic patients with lactic acidosis. *Am. Rev. Respiratory Dis.* **131:** 912–16.

Hershenson MB, O'Rourke PP, Schena JA & Crone RK (1988) Effect of halothane on critical levels of oxygen transport in the anesthetized newborn lamb. *Anesthesiology* **64:** 174–9.

Joulou-Schaeffer G, Gray GA, Fleming I, *et al.* (1990) Loss of vascular responsiveness induced by endotoxin involves L-arginine pathway. *Am. J. Physiol.* **259:** H1038–43.

Kaufman B, Rackow EC & Falk JL (1984) The relationship between oxygen delivery and consumption during fluid resuscitation of hypovolemic and septic shock. *Chest* **85:** 336–40.

Lindbom L, Tuma RF & Arfors KE (1980) Influence of oxygen on perfused capillary density and capillary red cell velocity in rabbit skeletal muscle. *Microvasc. Res.* **19:** 197–208.

Long GR, Nelson DP, Sznajder JI *et al.* (1988) Systemic oxygen delivery and consumption during acute lung injury in dogs. *J. Crit. Care* **3:** 249–55.

Mohsenifar Z, Goldbach P, Tashkin DP & Campisi DJ (1983) Relationship between O_2 delivery and O_2 consumption in the adult respiratory distress syndrome. *Chest* **84:** 267–71.

Mohsenifar Z, Amin D, Jasper AC *et al.* (1987) Dependence of oxygen consumption on oxygen delivery in patients with chronic congestive heart failure. *Chest* **92:** 447–50.

Mohsenifar Z, Jasper AC & Koerner SK (1988) Relationship between oxygen uptake and oxygen delivery in patients with pulmonary hypertension. *Am. Rev. Respiratory Dis.* **138:** 69–73.

Moreno LF, Stratton HH, Newell JC & Feustel PJ (1986) Mathematical coupling of data: correction of a common error for linear calculations. *J. App. Physiol.* **60:** 335–43.

Nelson DP, Beyer C, Samsel RW *et al.* (1987a) Pathological supply dependence of O_2 uptake during bacteremia in dogs. *J. Appl. Physiol.* **63:** 1487–92.

Nelson DP, King CE, Dodd SL *et al.* (1987b) Systemic and intestinal limits of O_2 extraction in the dog. *J. Appl. Physiol.* **63:** 387–94.

Nelson DP, Samsel RW, Wood LDH & Schumacker PT (1988) Pathological supply dependence of systemic and intestinal O_2 uptake during endotoxemia. *J. Appl. Physiol.* **64:** 2410–19.

Pepe PE & Culver BH (1985) Independently measured oxygen consumption during reduction of oxygen delivery by positive end-expiratory pressure. *Am. Rev. Respiratory Dis.* **132:** 788–92.

Pittet JF, Lacroix JS, Gunning K *et al.* (1990) Prostacyclin but not phentolamine increases oxygen consumption and skin microvascular blood flow in patients with sepsis and respiratory failure. *Chest* **98:** 1467–72.

Powers SR, Mannal R, Neclerio M *et al.* (1973) Physiologic consequences of positive end-expiratory pressure. *Ann. Surg.* **3:** 265–71.

Prewitt RL & Johnson PC (1976) The effect of oxygen on arteriolar red cell velocity and capillary density in rat cremaster muscle. *Microvasc. Res.* **12:** 59–70.

Ronco JJ, Montaner JSG, Fenwick JC *et al.* (1990) Pathologic dependence of oxygen consumption on oxygen delivery in acute respiratory failure secondary to AIDS-related *Pneumocystis carinii* pneumonia. *Chest* **98:** 1463–6.

Ronco JJ, Fenwick JC, Phang PT *et al.* (1991a) O_2 delivery, O_2 consumption and the critical O_2 delivery threshold for anaerobic metabolism in septic and nonseptic dying patients. *Am. Rev. Respiratory Dis.* **143:** A82 (abstract).

Ronco JJ, Phang PT, Walley KR *et al.* (1991b) Oxygen consumption is independent of changes in oxygen delivery in severe Adult Respiratory Distress Syndrome. *Am. Rev. Respiratory Dis.* **143:** 1267–73.

Samsel RW, Nelson DP, Sanders WM *et al.* (1988) Effect of endotoxin on systemic and skeletal muscle O_2 extraction. *J. Appl. Physiol.* **65:** 1377–82.

Samsel RW, Cherqui, D, Pietrabissa A *et al.* (1991) Hepatic oxygen and lactate extraction during stagnant hypoxia. *J. Appl. Physiol.* **17:** 186–93.

Schlichtig R, Cowden WL & Chaitman BR (1986) Tolerance of unusually low mixed venous oxygen saturation. *Am. J. Med.* **80:** 813–18.

Schlichtig R, Kramer DJ, Boston R & Pinsky MR (1991) Renal O_2 consumption during progressive hemorrhage. *J. Appl. Physiol.* **70:** 1957–62.

Schumacker PT & Cain SM (1987) The concept of a critical oxygen delivery. *Intensive Care Med.* **13:** 223–9.

Shepherd AP (1978) Intestinal O_2 consumption and Rb extraction during arterial hypoxia. *Am. J. Physiol.* **234:** E248–51.

Shepherd AP (1982) Metabolic control of intestinal oxygenation and blood flow. *Fedn Proc.* **41:** 2084–9.

Shibutani K, Komatsu, T. Kubal K *et al.* (1983) Critical level of oxygen delivery in anesthetized man. *Crit. Care Med.* **11:** 640–3.

Stratton HH, Feustel PJ & Newell JC (1987) Regression of calculated variables in the presence of shared measurement error. *J. Appl. Physiol.* **62:** 2083–93.

Van der Linden P, Gilbart E *et al.* (1991) Effects of anesthetic agents on systemic critical O_2 delivery. *J. Appl. Physiol.* **71:** 83–93.

Walley KR, Becker CJ, Hogan RA *et al* (1988) Progressive hypoxemia limits left ventricular oxygen consumption and contractility. *Circ. Res.* **63:** 849–59.

Williams AJ & Mohsenifar Z (1989) Oxygen supply dependency in patients with obstructive sleep apnea and its reversal after therapy with nasal continuous positive airway pressure. *Am. Rev. Respiratory Dis.* **140:** 1308–11.

Wolf YG, Cotev S, Perel A & Manny J (1987) Dependence of oxygen consumption on cardiac output in sepsis. *Crit. Care Med.* **15:** 198–203.

Wright CJ, Duff JH, McLean APH & MacLean LD (1971) Regional capillary blood flow and oxygen uptake in severe sepsis. *Surg. Gynecol. Obstet.* **132:** 637–44.

Wylam ME, Samsel RW, Umans JG *et al.* (1990) Endotoxin impairs endothelium-dependent relaxation of canine arteries in vitro. *Am. Rev. Respiratory Dis.* **142:** 1263–7.

Zweifach BW & Thomas L (1956) The role of epinephrine in the reactions produced by the endotoxins of gram negative bacteria. The changes produced by endotoxin in the vascular reactivity of epinephrine in the rat mesoappendix and the isolated perfused rabbit ear. *J. Exp. Med.* **104:** 881–96.

Zweifach BW, Nagler AL & Thomas L (1956) The role of epinephrine in the reactions produced by the endotoxins of gram negative bacteria. *J. Exp. Med.* **103:** 865–80.

Appendix I: Glossary of Terms

AaPO$_2$ Alveolar–arterial PO_2 difference (Equivalent to $P[A - a] O_2$ or $PaO_2 - PaO_2$ or A − a PO_2)

ARDS   Adult respiratory distress syndrome

BSA   Body surface area

C   Specific heat
CaO$_2$ Arterial blood oxygen content
CcO$_2$ End-capillary oxygen content
CHF   Congestive heart failure
CI   Cardiac index
COP   Colloid osmotic pressure
CPAP   Continuous positive airway pressure
C$\bar{v}$O$_2$ Mixed venous blood oxygen content
CVP   Central venous pressure

$\dot{D}O_2$ Oxygen delivery
2,3-DPG   2,3-Diphosphoglycerate
DRG   Diagnostic related group

FiO$_2$ Fractional concentration of inspired oxygen

GITS   Gut-derived infectious toxic shock

Hct   Haematocrit
Hb   Haemoglobin content
HR   Heart rate

IABP   Intra-aortic balloon pump
ICU   Intensive care unit
ISS   Injury severity score

JVP   Jugular vein pressure

LAP	Left atrial pressure
LCWI	Left cardiac work index
LV	Left ventricular
LVSWI	Left ventricular stroke work index
$M\bar{A}P$	Mean arterial pressure
MR	Metabolic rate
MSOF	Multiple systemic organ failure
NMR	Nuclear magnetic resonance
NIR	Near-infrared
OER	Oxygen extraction ratio
OUC	Oxygen utilization coefficient
PADP	Pulmonary artery diastolic pressure
PAFC	Pulmonary artery flotation catheter
PAOP	Pulmonary artery occlusion pressure
P_AO_2	Alveolar oxygen tension
PaO_2	Arterial oxygen tension
PAP	Pulmonary artery pressure
PAWP	Pulmonary artery wedge pressure
Pb	Barometric pressure
PCO_2	Carbon dioxide tension
PCWP	Pulmonary capillary wedge pressure
PEEP	Positive end-expiratory pressure
P_IO_2	Inspired oxygen tension
PMNL	Polymorphonuclear leukocyte
Pmv	Hydrostatic pressure of microvascular space
$Ppmv$	Hydrostatic pressure of perimicrovascular space
$P\bar{v}O_2$	Mixed venous oxygen tension
PVR	Pulmonary vascular resistance
P_{50}	PO_2 at 50% oxygen saturation
$\dot{Q}$	Cardiac output
$\dot{Q}s/\dot{Q}T$	Shunt fraction or venous admixture
RAP	Right atrial pressure
RCWI	Right cardiac work index
RER	Respiratory exchange rate
RQ	Respiratory quotient
RV	Right ventricular
RVSWI	Right ventricular stroke work index

S	Specific gravity
SaO_2	Percentage saturation of haemoglobin with oxygen in arterial blood
$S\bar{v}O_2$	Percentage saturation of haemoglobin with oxygen in mixed venous blood
SVI	Stroke volume index
SVR	Systemic vascular resistance
SWI	Stroke work index
T	Temperature
t	Time
V	Volume
$\dot{V}A$	Alveolar ventilation
$\dot{V}CO_2$	Carbon dioxide production rate
$\dot{V}E$	Expired ventilation
$\dot{V}O_2$	Oxygen consumption rate
VO_2	Volume of oxygen
$\dot{V}/\dot{Q}$	Ventilation/perfusion ratio
WP	Wedge pressure

Appendix II: Standard Equations

Haemodynamic Equations

SV $\quad$ = Stroke volume = $\dfrac{\text{Cardiac output}}{\text{Heart rate}}$ (ml)

CI $\quad$ = Cardiac index = $\dfrac{\text{Cardiac output}}{\text{BSA}}$ (litres min^{-1} m^{-2})

SVI $\quad$ = Stroke volume index = $\dfrac{\text{CI}}{\text{Heart rate}}$ (ml m^{-2})

or SVI $\quad$ = $\dfrac{\text{SV}}{\text{BSA}}$ (ml m^{-2})

SVR $\quad$ = Systemic vascular resistance = $\dfrac{\text{M\={A}P} - \text{RAP}}{\text{Cardiac output}} \times 80$ (dyne s cm^{-5})

SVRI $\quad$ = Systemic vascular resistance index = $\dfrac{\text{M\={A}P} - \text{RAP}}{\text{CI}} \times 80$ (dyne s cm^{-5} m^{-2})

PVR $\quad$ = Pulmonary vascular resistance = $\dfrac{\text{P\={A}P} - \text{PAWP}}{\text{Cardiac output}} \times 80$ (dyne s cm^{-5})

PVRI $\quad$ = Pulmonary vascular resistance index = $\dfrac{\text{P\={A}P} - \text{PAWP}}{\text{CI}} \times 80$ (dyne s cm^{-5} m^{-2})

RVSWI $\quad$ = Right ventricular stroke work index = SVI $\times \dfrac{(\text{P\={A}P} - \text{RAP})}{\text{CI}} \times 0.0136$ (g min^{-1} m^{-2})

LVSWI $\quad$ = Left ventricular stroke work index = RVI $\times \dfrac{(\text{M\={A}P} - \text{PAWP})}{\text{CI}} \times 0.0136$ (g min^{-1} m^{-2})

Oxygen Transport Equations

CaO_2 = Arterial oxygen content = Hb × SaO_2 × K + dissolved oxygen (ml dl^{-1})

$C\bar{v}O_2$ = Mixed venous oxygen content = Hb × $S\bar{v}O_2$ × K + dissolved oxygen (ml dl^{-1})

K is taken to be 1.34, 1.36, 1.38 or 1.39 depending on results from in-vivo or in-vitro studies. In actual practice the influence on CaO_2 and $C\bar{v}O_2$ calculation is small.

$$\text{Dissolved arterial oxygen content} = \begin{array}{l} PaO_2 \text{ (in mm Hg)} \times 0.003) \text{ (ml dl}^{-1}) \\ \text{or } PaO_2 \text{ (in kPa)} \times 0.0225 \text{ (ml dl}^{-1}) \end{array}$$

$$\text{Dissolved mixed venous oxygen} = \begin{array}{l} P\bar{v}O_2 \text{ (in mm Hg)} \times 0.003) \text{ (ml dl}^{-1}) \\ \text{or } P\bar{v}O_2 \text{ (in kPa)} \times 0.0225 \text{ (ml dl}^{-1}) \end{array}$$

Arterial – mixed venous oxygen content difference
$$= CaO_2 - C\bar{v}O_2 \text{ (ml dl}^{-1})$$

$\dot{D}O_2$ = Oxygen delivery = cardiac output × CaO_2 × 10 (ml min^{-1})
$\dot{V}O_2$ = Oxygen consumption = cardiac output × $CaO_2 - C\bar{v}O_2$) × 10 (ml min^{-1})

$$\text{Fick equation: cardiac output} = \frac{\dot{V}O_2}{CaO_2 - C\bar{v}O_2}$$

In clinical practice the terms $\dot{D}O_2$ and $\dot{V}O_2$ are used to denote indexed values of oxygen delivery and consumption.

$$\text{OER} = \text{Oxygen extraction ratio} = \frac{CaO_2 - C\bar{v}O_2}{CaO_2} \text{ (\%)}$$

$$\text{or OER} = \frac{SaO_2 - S\bar{v}O_2}{SaO_2} \text{ (\%)}$$

$$Qs/Q\text{T} = \text{Pulmonary venous admixture} = \frac{CcO_2 - CaO_2}{CcO_2 - C\bar{v}O_2} \text{(\%)}$$

where CcO_2 is ideal pulmonary capillary oxygen content calculated from the alveolar gas equation solved for oxygen.

(Pulmonary venous admixture is sometimes referred to as shunt fraction or degree of intrapulmonary shunting.)

Other indices of oxygen exchange in popular use are:

$P(\text{A–a})O_2$ = alveolar to arterial oxygen tension gradient = $PAO_2 - P_aO_2$ mm Hg or kPa

Although the actual physiological term is $P(\text{A} - \text{a})O_2$, clinicians use $\text{A} - \text{aD}O_2$; the two terms are synonymous.

$P\text{A}O_2$ is ideal alveolar oxygen tension calculated from the alveolar gas equation.

$PaO_2/F\text{I}O_2$ is the ratio of arterial oxygen tension to fractional inspired oxygen concentration (%).

Fractional inspired oxygen concentration (%)

$$[\text{FI}O_2] = \frac{\text{inspired oxygen concentration}}{100}$$

e.g. 60% oxygen = $\text{FI}O_2$ of 0.6.

$P\text{A}O_2/F\text{I}O_2$ is alveolar PO_2 to inspired oxygen concentration (%).

In the last two equations oxygen tensions are in mm Hg.

Index